D0537021

Jerry Baker's

Vital Vinegar

COOKBOOK "CURES"

500+ Healing Recipes for a Happier, Healthier You!

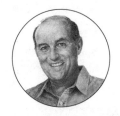

www.jerrybaker.com

Other Jerry Baker Books:

Vinegar Solutions for Savvy Seniors
Goof Proof Your Life!
Jerry Baker's Live Rich, Spend Smart, and Enjoy Your Retirement
Jerry Baker's Vinegar: The King of All Cures!
Jerry Baker's Fix It Fast and Make It Last
Jerry Baker's Solve It with Vinegar!
America's Favorite Practical Problem Solvers
Jerry Baker's Can the Clutter
Jerry Baker's Speed Cleaning Secrets
Grandma Putt's Old-Time Vinegar, Garlic, and 101 More Problem Solvers
Jerry Baker's Supermarket Super Products

Jerry Baker's Supermarket Super Gardens
Jerry Baker's Bug Off!
Jerry Baker's Terrific Garden Tonics!
Jerry Baker's Backyard Problem Solver
Jerry Baker's Green Grass Magic
Jerry Baker's Great Green Book of Garden Secrets
Jerry Baker's Old-Time Gardening Wisdom

Jerry Baker's Backyard Birdscaping Bonanza
Jerry Baker's Backyard Bird Feeding Bonanza
Jerry Baker's Year-Round Bloomers
Jerry Baker's Flower Garden Problem Solver
Jerry Baker's Perfect Perennials!

Jerry Baker's Grow Younger, Live Longer
Healing Remedies Hiding in Your Kitchen
Jerry Baker's Cure Your Lethal Lifestyle
Jerry Baker's Top 25 Homemade Healers
Healing Fixers Mixers & Elixirs
Jerry Baker's Supermarket Super Remedies
Jerry Baker's The New Healing Foods
Jerry Baker's Anti-Pain Plan
Jerry Baker's Oddball Ointments and Powerful Potions
Jerry Baker's Giant Book of Kitchen Counter Cures

To order any of the above, or for more information on Jerry Baker's amazing home, health, and garden tips, tricks, and tonics, please write to:

Jerry Baker, P.O. Box 1001, Wixom, MI 48393

Or, visit Jerry Baker online at:

jerrybaker.com

Vital Vinegar

COOKBOOK "CURES"

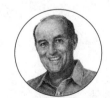

www.jerrybaker.com

Published by American Master Products, Inc.

Executive Editor: Kim Adam Gasior
Writer: Vicki Webster
Design and Layout: Alison McKenna
Copy Editor: Nanette Bendyna
Production Editor: Sydney Francois
Indexer: Nan Badgett

Publisher's Cataloging-in-Publication Data
provided by Five Rainbows Cataloging Services

Names: Baker, Jerry, author.
Title: Vital vinegar cookbook "cures" : 500+ healing recipes for a happier, healthier you! / Jerry Baker.
Description: Wixom, MI : American Master Products, 2018.
Identifiers: ISBN 978-0-922433-19-3 (hardcover)
Subjects: LCSH: Vinegar. | Cooking (Vinegar) | Functional foods. | Formulas, recipes, etc. | Cookbooks. | BISAC: COOKING / Specific Ingredients / General. | HEALTH & FITNESS / Diet & Nutrition / General.
Classification: LCC TX819.V5 B35 2018 (print) | DDC 641.6/2--dc23.

Printed in the United States of America
2 4 6 8 7 5 3 hardcover

TABLE OF CONTENTS

INTRODUCTION

Judging from the hoopla vinegar is getting in culinary and health-care circles these days, you'd think it was a brand-new product. But this versatile megastar has been pleasing people's palates and curing their ills since before the dawn of recorded history. This book combines both of those talents into a collection of recipes that will delight even the most finicky foodies—while delivering dynamic nutrition that can help alleviate or prevent a whole lot of common ailments.

We'll start in Chapter One with fabulous, foolproof formulas for making your very own vinegar, beginning with apple cider vinegar—or ACV, as it's known to natural health care gurus from coast to coast. From there, your health-giving hit parade continues with how to craft ultra-simple versions of wine, malt, and rice vinegars that stand head and shoulders above anything you'll find in your local supermarket.

But that's not all! You'll also learn easier-than-pie techniques for infusing vinegar with herbs, spices, fruits, and vegetables. These vivacious blends can turn a run-of-the-mill recipe into a dynamite dish worthy of a five-star restaurant. The additives also give the vinegar some health-giving "muscle power." Depending on the "infusables" you use, these potent potions can fend off cold and flu viruses (see page 27), help keep your ticker in tip-top shape (page 17), and do much, much more.

You'll find even more homemade health in the form of fortified vinegars (page 25), which are thickened, ready-in-a-flash blends of vinegar mixed with herbs, spices, fruits, and/or vegetables. You whip 'em up in a blender or food processor and use them as nutritious (and delicious) dips, salad dressings, or toppings for anything from meat, pasta, and baked potatoes to your favorite desserts. Tip: If, like most folks these days, you and your family aren't getting all the fruits and vegetables you need to maintain your daily quota, these yummy concoctions are just what the doctor ordered to up your intake the fast, fun, and easy Jerry Baker way!

Beginning in Chapter Two and continuing through Chapter Ten, you'll discover how to put the astounding healing power of vinegar to work in simple-to-make, scrumptious recipes that literally run the culinary gamut from soup to nuts. Just to whet your appetite, here's a sampling of the body- and mind-boosting treats we have in store for you:

A sensational salad dressing that can help support your immune system, maintain healthy blood pressure, and relieve respiratory disorders (*Maple-Balsamic Vinaigrette*, page 36).

A sweet and simple salad that delivers a load of benefits for your lungs, liver, blood, and digestive system—and can help protect your skin from sun damage (*French Carrot Salad*, page 72).

Dandy DIY pickles that'll cool you down fast when the weather turns steamy—plus help boost brain function and enhance your body's ability to lose weight (*Pickled Chard Coolers*, page 114).

A champ of a chili that supports eye health, weight-loss efforts, and a healthy nervous system (*Mango Chicken Chili*, page 177).

A bracing vegetable blend that can ease joint pain by fighting inflammation and help maintain a healthy gastrointestinal system (*Veggie Bake Casserole*, page 203).

A cheery chicken sandwich that shores up your defenses against colds and seasonal allergies; boosts heart health; and encourages deep, restful sleep (*Open-Face Gruyère Chicken Melt*, page 233).

A dilly of a dip that can help your heart health, keep you hydrated, and lower anxiety (*Avocado-Cucumber Salsa*, page 268).

A delicious drink that tastes just like apple pie—and can boost your digestion and battle dangerous free radicals throughout your body (*Apple Pie Power Drink*, page 327).

A peach of a peach cake that supports healthy skin, provides a potent load of antioxidants, and can give a big boost to your immune system (*Balsamic Peach Bundt Cake*, page 350).

But wait—there's more! In each chapter, you'll also find **Culinary Q & As,** which provide answers to **CULINARY Q & A** nutritional questions and food-prep dilemmas of all kinds. For example, you'll learn a guaranteed way to ease muscle cramps using mustard (page 133), and you'll discover the secret for getting the most from dried herbs and spices (page 13).

Kitchen Capers give you nifty nuggets of wisdom that (for instance) will stop onion tears in their tracks (page 84) and keep cottage cheese fresh longer (page 274). You'll also learn a simple trick for adding instant elegance, delicious flavor—and health-giving goodness— to everything from meat to desserts (page 233).

Instant Gratification offers ready-in-a-flash recipes for dishes that are as good for you as they are easy. To whet your appetite, *Super Food—Super Fast* (page 71) puts the nutritional firepower of kale to work in minutes. And *A Honey of a Honey Mustard* (page 132) creates a condiment better than anything you can get at your local deli!

Cure It Quick recipes taste great and deliver targeted health benefits for your body and your mind. The delicious *Joint-Soothing Nectar* on page 4 promotes blessed relief from arthritis aches. The *Fast-Acting Headache Relief* recipe lives up to its promise (see page 38), and *Dandy Dandelion Detox Salad* (page 74) works its magic by supporting your liver.

A+ Ingredients list select benefits you can gain from each recipe. For instance, see the box at right for the health-giving ingredients in *Salt & Vinegar Potatoes with Yogurt-Scallion Dip* on page 293.

Bear in mind that the recipes in this book can't do anything on their own. The key to good health is to eat a varied, well-balanced diet with all the nutrients the human body needs. It's also crucial to couple healthy eating habits with sound sleep and regular exercise.

With all this terrific food ahead of you, time's a wastin'. So let's hit the kitchen and discover how these vinegar-enhanced recipes can lead to good health and a long life!

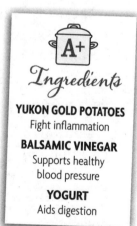

A+

Ingredients

YUKON GOLD POTATOES
Fight inflammation

BALSAMIC VINEGAR
Supports healthy blood pressure

YOGURT
Aids digestion

COMING TO TERMS WITH VINEGAR

Vinegar can be made from any substance that's sweet enough to ferment (when the sugar content changes to alcohol). Once that happens, a second fermentation turns the alcohol to acetic acid (a.k.a. vinegar). Here's a rundown of some of the most popular types of vinegar:

Apple cider vinegar is mild with just a slight flavor of (surprise!) apple. It's the vinegar of choice for most health- and beauty-care purposes. But it's also highly versatile in the kitchen and makes a fine recipe stand-in for just about any other kind of vinegar. You can make your own ACV by following the simple instructions on page 4.

Distilled white vinegar (a.k.a. white vinegar) is made from grain alcohol. It's the vinegar of choice for pickles, and, in small amounts, for many of the food-related tips and tricks throughout this book. However, beware of using white vinegar in large quantities in recipes because its sour, harsh taste can overpower more delicate flavors.

Wine vinegars come in red, white, sherry, and champagne varieties. They're the most versatile vinegars for recipes. While you can buy some excellent wine vinegars, home-made versions are generally far superior. The do-it-yourself process is simple—and fun (see *DIY Wine Vinegar* on page 5 for the ultra-easy directions).

Balsamic vinegar is made from the unfermented juice of Trebbiano and Lambrusco grapes, which grow only in the Modena and Reggio areas of Italy. The juice is boiled down to a sweet, fruity syrup and then aged in wooden barrels for many years. Fortunately, modern producers have found ways to speed up the process, making prices affordable.

Malt vinegar, which is made from barley and other grains, is mild and sweet. While it's best known as a condiment for fish and chips, you can substitute it for other types of vinegar in almost any dish. But because it's so mild, you may want to add a little more than the recipe calls for. To make your own, see *Merry Malt Vinegar* on page 7.

Rice vinegar is made from rice wine. Japanese varieties have a delicate, subtle flavor, while Chinese versions tend to be sweet and sour. While rice vinegar is an essential ingredient in Asian cuisine, it can also add zip to standard American fare. For one easy-does-it version, see *Nice Rice Vinegar* on page 6.

Infused vinegars are made by immersing herbs, fruits, vegetables (or combinations thereof) in vinegar and letting them steep for anywhere from a week to several months. You can buy excellent commercial versions, but it's a snap to make your own for a lot less money. You'll find a sampling of customizable formulas in Chapter One.

Chapter One

Heavenly Homemade Vinegar

You can find commercial versions of all the vinegars used throughout this book. So why bother to make your own? Here's why: Because the process can be a lot of fun, it's simpler than pie, and you know exactly what's gone into the final product. Plus, whether you use your DIY vinegars in your own cooking or gift them to friends, you'll have the delightful satisfaction of saying, "I made it myself!"

CLASSIC APPLE CIDER VINEGAR

This is the vinegar your grandma—and her grandma—used to make. Granted, it does take its good ol' time to reach full potency, but it's quick and easy to throw together.

YIELD: about 2 ½ cups	PREP: 5 minutes	WAIT: 6–8 months

6 ripe apples, unpeeled and diced (cores and all)*

2 cups of distilled or filtered water (or enough to cover the apples)

½ package of active dry yeast

* *Use organic apples if at all possible.*

1. Put the apples into a large glass jar, then add the water and yeast.

2. Securely cover the jar with cheesecloth and a rubber band, and set it in a place that's warm (about 80°F).

3. Let it sit until the natural sugars have created hard cider (about 3 months, but test it periodically—your taste buds will tell you when it's "ripe").

4. Strain out the apples, then pour the liquid back into the jar. Re-cover with a clean cloth and keep in a warm spot until the alcohol has turned to vinegar, which should take another 3 to 4 months.

5. When ready, pour the vinegar into a sterilized glass bottle or jar and store it at room temperature.

Note: *Homemade vinegar will last longer if you pasteurize it (see the Culinary Q & A at right).*

To sterilize bottles or jars, fill them with boiling water, let them sit for 10 minutes, then empty them. Wait until they've reached room temperature, or close to it, before pouring in the vinegar. Also soak the corks or bottoms of the stoppers for 10 minutes in boiling water.

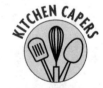

Cure It QUICK!

JOINT-SOOTHING NECTAR The combination of apple cider vinegar and tart cherry juice can work wonders for arthritis sufferers. To put this dynamic, delicious duo to work, simply mix 1 cup of each in a glass jar with a tight, non-metallic lid. Then once or twice a day, stir 2 teaspoons of the mixture into a tall glass of water, and drink it up. Store the blend in the refrigerator, where it'll keep for up to two weeks. It can help relieve your muscle and joint pain quick!

DIY WINE VINEGAR

Store-bought wine vinegars are generally rushed through the fermentation process, which makes them highly acidic and lacking in flavor. This homemade vinegar has a smooth, full-bodied taste that gives a delicious boost to everything from soups and sauces to (of course) vinaigrette dressings. And it's a snap to make your own.

YIELD: about 6 cups   **PREP:** 10 minutes   **WAIT:** 11–12 weeks

Good-quality red or white wine

1 cup of distilled or filtered water

8-oz. bottle of vinegar mother*

* Available in wine- and beer-making supply stores or buy it online.

1. Mix 2 cups of wine and the water in a ½-gallon wide-mouth glass jar, then add the mother. Cover the jar with a double layer of cheesecloth and secure with a rubber band.

2. Set the jar in a warm (70° to 90°F), dark spot. Over the next 1½ weeks, add 2½ more cups of wine three separate times. If a thin film has formed on the surface, add the wine through a plastic or stainless steel funnel. Do not stir or shake the liquid, as it needs to remain still.

3. Let the jar sit for 10 weeks, sniffing the contents often. If the liquid ever gives off a scent like that of furniture polish, dispose of it, wash the jar, and start over.

4. When the vinegar smells sharp and crisp, strain it into sterilized bottles through a funnel lined with a coffee filter.

5. Cap or seal the bottles tightly and store them in a dark place at room temperature.

CULINARY Q & A

? Can pasteurizing my homemade vinegar help it last longer?

! Yes. Homemade vinegar will stay in excellent condition if you pasteurize it. To do so, heat the vinegar to exactly 155°F in a stainless steel saucepan for 30 minutes. Store it in a bottle at room temperature away from direct sunlight. Once the bottle has been opened, the vinegar will retain its full flavor for three months, then will gradually begin to lose its zip.

NICE RICE VINEGAR

If you want a mild vinegar that has a hint of sweetness, give this perky potion a try. Rice vinegar is known for its health-boosting abilities—it helps your body soak in as much of the nutrients from the foods you eat as possible, and it aids in digestion.

YIELD: about 16 ounces	**PREP:** 5 minutes	**WAIT:** 3 weeks–6 months

2 cups of cooked rice, with cooking water

1–2 oz. of vinegar mother

1 qt. or so of distilled or filtered water

1. Put the rice, along with any cooking water, in a stone crock or large glass jar. Add the mother, and fill the container to the top with the water.

2. Cover the container with a double layer of cheesecloth, secure it with a rubber band, and set the mixture in a dark, warm place (60° to 80°F is ideal, but the warmer the temperature, the faster the blend will ferment).

3. Wait for 3 weeks, remove the cover, and sample. If the flavor is tart and acidic, your batch is done. If you taste even a hint of alcohol, replace the cheesecloth and check back periodically.*

4. When it's ready, strain the liquid through cheesecloth into a clean container. Re-cover, and set it in the fridge for 1 to 2 hours, or until the liquid is no longer cloudy. Store in sterilized bottles with tight seals.

* It can take from 3 weeks to 6 months to reach full flavor, depending on temperature, materials, and bacteria levels.

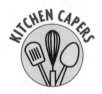

KITCHEN CAPERS

If you prefer, you can substitute rice wine for the vinegar mother. The fermentation process will take longer, but the final results will be the same. The Shaoxing brand of wine (available in most Asian markets) is an excellent choice.

CULINARY Q & A

? What exactly is "vinegar mother"?

! Vinegar mother (a.k.a. *Mycoderma aceti*) is a substance composed of cellulose and *Acetobacter* bacteria. When exposed to air, it turns alcohol into acetic acid. The mother develops naturally as alcoholic liquids ferment, but adding it to your vinegar-in-the-making speeds up the process.

MERRY MALT VINEGAR

Wine vinegar isn't the only kind that's far superior to commercial brands. Once you have sampled the richer, heartier flavor of homemade malt vinegar, the store-bought stuff will never cut the mustard at your house again!

YIELD: about 1 gallon	**PREP:** 5 minutes	**WAIT:** 7 days minimum

Your favorite beer or ale*

Distilled or filtered water

Vinegar mother

* *It must be free of preservatives and have an alcohol content between 5 and 7 percent. If it's higher than that, dilute it with another part or two of water after you pour it into the container.*

1. Mix 3 parts beer or ale with 1 part water in a container.** Cover it with cheesecloth, and set it in a dark area at room temperature for 24 hours.

2. Remove the cloth, and add the vinegar mother. Re-cover, put the container in a dark spot, and leave it to ferment for at least a week.

3. Taste the liquid. If it's ready, strain, pasteurize (if it suits you), and bottle it. Or, if needed, let it age longer, tasting it every week or so. (It can age as long as you'd like.)

** *The best, and most user-friendly, vessel for this purpose is a crock or a glass beverage container with a spigot at the bottom (like the ones sold for dispensing iced tea). Just make sure the spigot is made of wood, plastic, or stainless steel—not aluminum, which will react with the vinegar.*

KITCHEN CAPERS If you keep one or more batches of vinegar of any kind "cooking" continuously, empty and wash the container(s) about every six months. You can replace the mother with a fresh version, or retain a piece of the old one.

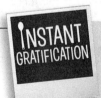

INSTANT GRATIFICATION

Ultra-Easy Wine Vinegar

This recipe is no-muss, no-fuss! Simply put 1 pound of raisins in a bowl and add 2 quarts of distilled or filtered water. Cover the bowl with cheesecloth, secure with a rubber band, and leave in a warm place for four months, until it tastes of vinegar. Strain out the raisins, pour the vinegar into sterilized glass jars or bottles, and store at room temperature.

FESTIVE FRUIT SCRAP VINEGAR

Here's a fun, easy—and thrifty—way to make use of leftover fruit peelings and cores that you would otherwise toss in the garbage can or the compost bin.

YIELD: about 1 gallon	**PREP:** 5 minutes	**WAIT:** about 6-8 weeks

Fruit peelings, cores, or overripe fruit, scrubbed and chopped (seeds removed)

Raw sugar

Distilled or filtered water

1 cup of unfiltered apple cider vinegar or vinegar mother (optional)

1. Put your fruit scraps in a wide-mouth glass jar or ceramic crock that holds at least a gallon of liquid.

2. Mix 1 cup of sugar per gallon of water until you have enough to cover the fruit (multiply as needed). Add a little extra because the scraps will swell up.*

3. Cover the container with cheesecloth, secured with a rubber band, and set it in a warm, dark place. Let it sit for at least 2 weeks, or until bubbles stop forming.

4. Strain the liquid into a clean jar and re-cover. Leave for a month, and start tasting it every few days.

5. When it's to your liking, strain through several layers of damp cheesecloth into sterilized bottles or jars, and seal each one with a cork or plastic lid. Then discard or compost the solids, and enjoy your fruity creation!

Add apple cider vinegar or vinegar mother, if desired, to speed up the fermentation process.

KITCHEN CAPERS

The smaller your chunks of fruit are, the faster they'll ferment. Just make sure the pieces are big enough to strain out easily when the vinegar has reached its peak—don't use pureed fruit!

INSTANT GRATIFICATION

Malt Vinegar Salt

This is perfect sprinkled on popcorn, corn on the cob, or French fries. Mix 6 tablespoons coarse or kosher salt, 1 tablespoon cornstarch, and ¼ cup malt vinegar to make a paste. Spread into a thick layer on a rimmed baking sheet. Leave uncovered, at room temperature for 24 hours, or until hardened. Break up pieces in a food processor, or with a fork, until you have a coarse salt. Seal in a container, and store in a cool, dry place for up to three months.

TURN-OF-THE-CENTURY RASPBERRY VINEGAR

This recipe dates back to around 1900, but it's still popular today, and for good reason: It's more complex and full-bodied than fruit-infused vinegars, with a flavor that's tart, tangy, fruity, and sweet all at once. Give it a try—you and your family will love it!

YIELD: about 2 ½ quarts   **PREP:** 30 minutes   **WAIT:** about 2 months

5 qts. of fresh red or black raspberries

2 qts. of distilled or filtered water

1 lb. of sugar

1. Wash and slightly crush (don't mash!) 1 quart of the berries. Transfer to a bowl, and add the water. Cover the bowl loosely with cheesecloth, but don't secure it.

2. Set the bowl in a warm spot (80°F is ideal), and let it sit overnight. In the morning, strain out and dispose of the solids. Pour the remaining liquid back into the bowl.

3. Add another quart of berries to the liquid, and repeat steps 1 through 3 until all the fruit has been used.

4. After all the berries have been through the first three steps, add the sugar, and stir until it's dissolved. Put the bowl, loosely covered, in a warm place. Leave it still for about 2 months, or until the vinegar tastes ready. Then strain it into sterilized glass bottles, and store at room temperature.

KITCHEN CAPERS

No matter what kind of vinegar you're making from scratch, keep this timely tip in mind: The wider the mouth of your jar is, the more wild bacteria the contents will capture, and the faster the fermenting process will be.

CULINARY Q & A

? Why is it so important to use distilled or filtered water when you're making vinegar. What's wrong with plain old tap water?

! In a word, chemicals. The chlorine and other substances contained in most municipal water supplies can kill or at least contaminate the mother. If that happens, your vinegar will be ruined and all your effort will be for naught.

CUTTING-EDGE COCONUT VINEGAR

Coconut vinegar is a traditional favorite in the Philippines, but here in the USA it's recently achieved true superstar status in nutritional circles. Health gurus tell us that it delivers the same almost-magical benefits of apple cider vinegar, with a better taste and (according to some experts) a bigger supply of vitamins A, C, and D.

YIELD: about 1 quart	**PREP:** 5 minutes	**WAIT:** about 1–3 months

1 qt. of coconut water*

¼ cup of sugar

1 tbsp. of vinegar mother

Available in health-food stores and most supermarkets.

1. In a medium-size saucepan, heat the coconut water until it begins to steam.

2. Remove the pan from the heat, add the sugar, and stir until it's dissolved.

3. Pour the mixture into a glass jar, cover it with cheesecloth, and set it in a dark place at room temperature. Let it sit for about a week, or until the liquid has turned to alcohol.

4. When the taste is to your liking, add the vinegar mother.

5. Return the container to its dark place, and leave it for 1 to 3 months, or until it's turned to coconut vinegar. Use it in the recipes coming up, or as a substitute for apple cider vinegar in health tonics.

KITCHEN CAPERS If you see a scum forming on your vinegar-in-the-making, don't disturb it. It's the vinegar mother. Eventually, it'll sink to the bottom and continue its job. But if you see or smell any mold, toss the whole batch out and start over.

CULINARY Q & A

? Help, please! Most vinegar-making instructions say to set the jar in a cool, dark spot during the fermentation process, but I really don't have a space like that to spare. What can I do?

! Here's what: Simply swaddle the jar in thick fabric to protect it from the light. Clean, thick dish or hand towels will work fine.

NEW ENGLAND MAPLE VINEGAR

Combined with sunflower oil, this classic New England creation makes an easygoing summer salad dressing. But it is also just as delicious drizzled on its own over a bed of mixed greens or even dropped into a martini.

YIELD: about 10 cups	PREP: 5 minutes	WAIT: about 4 weeks

3 ⅓ cups of unfiltered apple cider vinegar

3 cups of pure maple syrup

1 ⅓ cups of dark rum

⅞ cup of water

1. Pour the apple cider vinegar into a large glass jar or ceramic crock. Add in the maple syrup, rum, and water, and stir thoroughly to combine.

2. Cover the container with cheesecloth, secure it with a rubber band, and store it in a cool, dark place for 4 weeks.

3. Keep tasting the vinegar until you notice a smooth, tart, and sweet flavor with no hint of alcohol burn.

4. When the flavor is just right and to your liking, strain the finished vinegar into smaller containers, and store them at room temperature.

KITCHEN CAPERS

Do not use DIY vinegar of any kind for making infused vinegars or for pickling or canning. For these purposes, you need an acidity level of at least 5 percent. Wine-making suppliers sell testing kits, but it's easier to use commercial vinegars, which reach or surpass the 5 percent threshold.

Cure It QUICK!

THE SAMURAIS' SECRET WEAPON These Japanese warriors claimed they owed their strength and power to an infused vinegar called *Tamago-su*, or egg vinegar. Folks in Japan still use it to maintain good health and slow down the aging process. It works its magic by helping to prevent both the formation of damaging free radicals and the buildup of LDL (bad) cholesterol in your body. To make your own supply, simply immerse a whole, raw egg in 1 cup of rice vinegar, and let it sit, covered, for seven days. When the week's up, you'll find that everything has dissolved into the vinegar except the transparent membrane that was just inside the shell. Discard the membrane, and stir the egg-infused vinegar thoroughly. Store the tonic in a glass jar with a tight-fitting lid. Then, three times a day, stir 1 or 2 teaspoons of the vinegar into a glass of hot water, and drink to a long, healthy life.

ELEGANT HERBAL VINEGAR

Homemade herbal vinegars pack a flavor punch you will never find in store-bought versions, and they're as easy to make as a pot of tea. What's more, the final product looks as grand as anything you'd buy at a fancy-food boutique—for just a fraction of the price. This recipe makes a single quart, but multiply the ingredients as desired.

YIELD: 1 quart	**PREP:** 10 minutes	**WAIT:** about 2–4 weeks

2 cups of fresh herb leaves,* gently washed and dried

1 qt. of good-quality vinegar

* *Use whatever herbs or herb combos you fancy.*

1. Pack the herbs loosely into a sterilized 1-quart canning jar.

2. Heat the vinegar until it's just warm (don't let it boil!), pour it over the herbs, and cover the jar with a non-metallic lid.

3. Put your filled jar in a dark place at room temperature (like a kitchen cabinet), and let it sit for a couple of weeks.

4. When the time's up, open the lid and sniff. If you detect a rich, herbal aroma, your "crop" is ready. Otherwise, close the jar, and check again every week.

5. When the scent is just right, strain out the solids, pour the flavored vinegar into pretty sterilized bottles, and tuck a fresh herb sprig or two into each one.

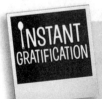
INSTANT GRATIFICATION

Pop Goes the Tomato!
When summertime gives you sweet, ripe tomatoes, pick 'em off the vine, and split them down the middle. Put them in a pan, cover them with maple vinegar, and cook until the tomatoes burst. During the breakdown process, the sugars in the vinegar are caramelizing and adding their flavor to the tomatoes. The result: an amazing addition to eggs, fish, pasta, pizza—or anything tomatoes adorn!

KITCHEN CAPERS

If you are short on dark indoor storage space, try this ancient trick: Start by filling your jar(s) with herbs as described above and add room-temperature vinegar. Then set the jars in a sunny location, indoors or out, until the flavor and aroma are just right (which could take anywhere from a week to two months).

FOUR THIEVES VINEGAR

One of the most famous—and curative—herbal vinegars of all time came to us courtesy of a quartet of convicted robbers who lived in 17th-century France. Numerous variations have evolved over the centuries, but this is one of the most popular and easiest to make.

YIELD: about 2 quarts	PREP: 5 minutes	WAIT: 6-8 weeks

2 tbsp. of dried food-grade lavender

2 tbsp. of dried mint

2 tbsp. of dried rosemary

2 tbsp. of dried sage

2 tbsp. of dried thyme

4–8 minced fresh garlic cloves

1 32-oz. bottle of unfiltered apple cider vinegar

1. Put the first six ingredients* in a large glass jar, and pour the vinegar over them.

2. Cover the jar tightly, and leave it in a cool, dark place for 6 to 8 weeks, shaking it daily if possible.

3. When the time's up, strain the tonic into smaller containers for easier use. Store them away from heat and light. Use the tonic as needed following the directions in "Good Things from Bad Guys" on page 27.

* *Many herbal-supply stores and online herbal retailers sell this 6-part blend all mixed up and ready to go.*

KITCHEN CAPERS When you're making vinegar of any kind (from scratch or infused) and the only jars you have are equipped with metal lids, cover the openings with plastic wrap before you screw on the caps. Otherwise, the vinegar will react with the metal, and your handiwork will be worthless.

CULINARY Q & A

? Will any type of dried herbs work for my Four Thieves Vinegar? Can I use what's already in my spice rack? Will it affect the quality of my vinegar?

! Actually, the herbs and spices in those little jars are processed to destroy any bacteria and other microorganisms, but that also destroys vitamins, minerals, proteins, and other nutrients. Instead, buy organic herbs from the grocery store, a health-food store, an herb shop, or a reputable website that specializes in organic herbs and spices.

MIGHTY SPICY VINEGAR

When you are looking for a hearty vinegar with a kick, this recipe will do the trick! It's robust and perfect for making marinades, mustards, or other full-bodied spreads and dips. Believe it or not, it's even delightful in many dessert recipes, such as in the Super Spice Cake on page 348. Not sure? Try it for yourself!

YIELD: about 2 cups	**PREP:** 10 minutes	**WAIT:** 1–4 weeks

2 tsp. of allspice berries

2 tsp. of coriander seeds

1 tsp. of mustard seeds

1 tsp. of whole cloves

1 3-inch cinnamon stick

1 bay leaf

1-inch piece of fresh ginger, peeled

2 cups of good-quality malt vinegar

1. Crush the spices slightly (don't grind them!), and bundle them up in a muslin or cheesecloth pouch for easy removal later.*

2. Combine the spices and vinegar in a stainless steel saucepan and heat to 110°F. Immediately remove the pan from the heat, and let the vinegar cool slightly.

3. Pour the contents into a sterilized glass jar, cover it tightly, and set it in a dark place at room temperature (like a kitchen cabinet). Shake the container every couple of days.

4. After 7 days, taste the vinegar. If the flavor is not to your liking, it needs more time to sit. Replace the lid and keep checking once a week for a month or so, or until you are satisfied with the finished vinegar.

5. Strain out the solid spices, and pour the liquid into one or more sterilized bottles. Seal them tightly, and store your vinegar in a cool, dry place for up to 3 months.

Or if you prefer, simply drop the spices into the vinegar and strain them out later.

KITCHEN CAPERS

Using the basic directions for Mighty Spicy Vinegar (above), you can produce rich, intense vinegars from a variety of different flavorings. Use 2 to 4 tablespoons of seeds or spices per 2 cups of vinegar. See "Spice Up Your Life..." (on page 19) for some excellent combo suggestions.

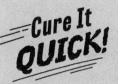

ST. HILDEGARD'S TICKER TUNE-UP TONIC

The medieval German nun St. Hildegard of Bingen was also a renowned herbalist. She routinely prescribed this herbal vinegar tonic to improve blood circulation, help relieve heart conditions, and generally keep her patients' tickers in tip-top shape. And you know what? It works every bit as well today as it did back in the 1100s. To make about 5 cups of elixir, proceed as follows: Mix 10 to 12 large sprigs of fresh parsley, 1 quart of red or white wine, and 2 tablespoons of white vinegar in a saucepan, and boil for 10 minutes. Add 9 ounces of raw honey, reduce the temperature to medium, and stir until the honey is thoroughly blended in. Remove the pan from the heat. When the mixture is cool enough to handle safely, strain it and pour it into bottles with tight caps. Store them in a cool, dark place, and take 1 tablespoon of the tonic three times a day.
Note: *Needless to say, this tonic is not a replacement for top-notch medical care!*

HERBAL VINEGAR ALL-STARS

There's virtually no limit to the herbal combinations (some with a jolt of citrus zest) that work beautifully for infused vinegars. These very versatile blends are some of the best.

All-Star Blend	Ingredients
Basil-orange	White wine vinegar, basil, and the peel from one orange
Dill-peppercorn	Apple cider vinegar, dill, and black peppercorns
Garlic-chive	Rice vinegar; 2 or 3 peeled, chopped garlic cloves; and chives
Lemon-thyme	White wine vinegar, the peel from one lemon, and thyme
Parsley-thyme	Sherry vinegar, parsley, thyme, rosemary, and bay
Pure garlic	Red or white wine vinegar, 12 crushed garlic cloves
Sage-rosemary	Red wine vinegar, sage, and rosemary
Shallot-pepper	Apple cider vinegar, chopped shallots, and hot red peppers
Tarragon-garlic	Malt vinegar, tarragon, garlic chives, whole cloves, and chopped garlic cloves
Ultra-lemony	Champagne vinegar, lemon balm, lemongrass, lemon thyme, and lemon zest

PEACHY KEEN VINEGAR

Peaches are full of antioxidants and essential nutrients that help to keep you healthy from head to toe. You couldn't ask for a better way to use them than in this delicious recipe.

YIELD: about 1 quart	**PREP:** 25 minutes	**WAIT:** about 8-48 hours

4 cups of overripe peaches (6-7 fruits), peeled, pitted, and roughly chopped

3 cups of white wine vinegar

½ cup of honey

1. Bring all of the ingredients to a simmer in a large saucepan. Cook, stirring occasionally, for 15 minutes. Then remove the pan from the heat, cover, and let cool to room temperature.

2. Puree the mixture until smooth (about 10 seconds). Strain through a fine sieve into a large nonreactive bowl.

3. Line the sieve with cheesecloth, place it over another nonreactive bowl, and pour the peach mixture into the sieve. Don't press on the solids!

4. Cover the bowl—sieve and all—with plastic wrap, and let the mixture strain in the refrigerator for about 8 hours, or up to 2 days.

5. Remove the cover and the sieve. Discard the solids, and pour the vinegar into sterilized bottles or jars.

KITCHEN CAPERS

When a recipe calls for lemon juice, use lemon vinegar instead. Besides adding its own taste, it'll enhance the flavor, texture, and appearance of the other ingredients. To make it, see the Culinary Q & A box below.

CULINARY Q & A

? Do you have a recipe that'll use all of my leftover fruit—I hate to waste it!

! This quick and easy Fruity Vinegar is a great way to add extra vitamins and nutrients to your recipes. Cut your choice of fruit into pieces, pack into a sterilized jar, and cover completely with white wine vinegar. Cap the jar tightly, and set it aside to steep. In a week or so, the vinegar will be ready to use.

CHRISTMASSY CRANBERRY VINEGAR

This beautiful ruby-red blend is a delicious treat at any time of the year, but it makes an especially useful addition to your entertaining repertoire throughout the winter holiday season, from Thanksgiving through New Year's Day.

YIELD: about 1 gallon	PREP: 35 minutes	WAIT: about 1 week

6 cups of fresh cranberries, washed and drained

2 cups of sugar

1 gal. of red wine vinegar

6-inch cinnamon sticks

Extra cranberries (optional)

1. In a large pot, bring the berries, sugar, and vinegar to a simmer (not a boil!). Simmer gently, uncovered, for about 30 minutes.

2. Remove the pan from the heat, cover, and let it sit for 8 to 12 hours.

3. Line a colander with cheesecloth or a large coffee filter, set it into a bowl, and pour in the cranberry mixture. Discard or compost the berries.

4. Gather up some attractive bottles. Insert a cinnamon stick and, if desired, several fresh cranberries into each bottle, and pour in the infused vinegar. Seal each bottle with a cork or a decorative stopper, and let them all sit for a week or so to let the cinnamon flavor intensify.

KITCHEN CAPERS Fancy glass bottles that previously held sauces, oils, or fancy commercial vinegars make great containers for your homemade supply. Craft-supply stores and online retailers sell corks in all shapes and sizes, as well as artistic stoppers that can be used over and over again.

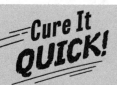

Cure It QUICK!

SAY "CHEERS!" TO YOUR HEALTH Christmassy Cranberry Vinegar (above) is loaded with heart-healthy compounds, as well as disease-fighting, anti-aging antioxidants. And recent studies have shown that sparkling wine may be even more helpful for our tickers than red wine. Put 'em together, and what have you got? This power-packed way to toast the new year—or any other festive occasion: Pour 1 tablespoon of cranberry vinegar into a champagne flute, and fill 'er up with bubbly. Give it a stir, and hoist your glass to good health, good times, and good friends!

BERRY LOVELY VINEGAR

Mix this vitamin-rich vinegar with olive oil, and drizzle it over a bed of mixed greens, chopped pecans, and some whole raspberries for a delicious, healthy treat.

YIELD: 2 quarts	PREP: 15 minutes	WAIT: 3 weeks

3 cups of fresh blackberries, red raspberries, or black rasp-berries, lightly crushed

5 tbsp. of honey

1 qt. of red wine vinegar

1. Combine all of the ingredients in a large bowl. Fill the bottom pot of your double boiler with water. Pour the mixture into the top pot, and bring it to a boil.

2. Turn down the heat and simmer for about 10 minutes.

3. Ladle the mixture into a sterilized, wide-mouthed jar, and seal it tightly.

4. Put the jar in a cool, dark place, and let it sit for about 3 weeks. Give it a taste to see if it's ready. If not, reseal the jar, and check back in a few days.

5. If it's ready, strain the mixture directly into sterilized bottles, using a funnel lined with a coffee filter. Press down firmly on the fruit to extract as much juice as possible. Discard or compost the solids.

6. Seal and label the bottles, and store them in a dark place at room temperature.

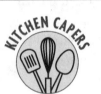

If yellow raspberries are the apples of your eye (and taste buds), substitute a light, mild vinegar for the red wine vinegar. Champagne, white wine, or sherry vinegars will all give you lovely, palate-pleasing results. You won't be able to get enough!

INSTANT GRATIFICATION

A Berry Fine Beverage

Drink a toast to your creative efforts with this simple libation: Mix 1 teaspoon of raspberry vinegar with about ¼ cup of sparkling water in an 8-ounce tumbler. Add ice to about the halfway mark, then fill 'er up with sparkling water. Add a couple of fresh berries and a mint leaf or two if you like. Then stir and enjoy! (See Chapter Nine for more delicious vinegar-spiked drinks, both with and without alcohol.)

SOUR CHERRY VINEGAR

Tart cherries are full of pain-soothing compounds and rich antioxidants, making this sweet-tart vinegar a health superstar! And it's easy to make any time of the year.

YIELD: about 16 ounces	PREP: 10 minutes	WAIT: 2 days

3 cups of red wine vinegar

1 ½ cups (about 7 ¾ oz.) of dried sour cherries

1. Combine the vinegar and cherries in a large glass jar with a tight-fitting lid, and let it stand at room temperature for 2 days.

2. Strain the mixture through a fine sieve into a saucepan, pressing down on the cherries with a spoon to extract as much of the juice as possible. Discard or compost the spent cherries.

3. Bring the vinegar to a boil over high heat, then immediately remove the pan from the stove.

4. Cool the garnet-toned, aromatic liquid to room temperature, and pour it into one 16-ounce or two 8-ounce sterilized jars.

 KITCHEN CAPERS

Bring rice to a whole new level by replacing one-third of the cooking water with the Sour Cherry Vinegar (above). Or, whisk it with any nut oil, such as walnut, almond, or hazelnut, for a vinaigrette that's out of this world.

SPICE UP YOUR LIFE...

With spiced vinegar. Here's just a sampling of marvelous matchups to try:

Type of Vinegar	Compatible Spices
Apple cider or white wine	6 whole, peeled garlic cloves; 1 teaspoon each of black peppercorns, caraway seeds, and whole cloves
Balsamic	1-inch piece of fresh ginger, peeled; 1 small hot red pepper; 1 teaspoon each of black peppercorns and whole cloves
Red wine	1 whole cracked nutmeg; a 3-inch cinnamon stick; and 1 teaspoon each of allspice berries, black peppercorns, juniper berries, and whole cloves
Sherry	1-inch piece of fresh ginger, peeled; a 3-inch cinnamon stick; 1 bay leaf; and 2 teaspoons each of allspice berries and celery seeds

MARVELOUS MANGO VINEGAR

This delightful—and healthy—concoction is just one example of a fortified vinegar. Try it poured over vanilla ice cream or stirred into a glass of sparkling water (see "The Thick of Things" on page 25 for more combos with flavorful fortitude).

YIELD: about 2 ½ cups	PREP: 10 minutes	WAIT: none

2 large ripe mangoes (about 2 ½ cups), peeled and diced

½ cup of vanilla-scented sugar syrup (see Vanilla-Scented Sugar Syrup, below)

Pinch of salt

½ cup of champagne vinegar

1. Puree the first three ingredients in a blender.

2. Add the vinegar and take a taste. If the mixture is too sweet to suit you, add more vinegar; if it's too tart, add more sugar.

3. Strain the mixture through a fine strainer into a bowl or pitcher.

4. Pour the blend into a sterilized bottle or jar that has a non-metallic lid, and store it in the refrigerator.

When you make a fruit vinegar, whether fortified or infused, that calls for sugar or honey, use the amount specified in the recipe, but taste the finished blend. If it's too sweet to suit you, gradually add more vinegar; if it's too tart, mix in more sweetener until the flavor is just right.

Vanilla-Scented Sugar Syrup

This sweet treat makes a tasty addition to fortified fruit vinegars of all kinds. It's also delicious stirred into iced tea and other cold beverages—including many of the vinegar-based drinks coming up in Chapter Nine. To make the syrup, put 4 cups of sugar and 1 cup of water in a pan and bring to a boil over high heat. Lower the heat to a simmer and cook for about four minutes, stirring occasionally. Let the syrup cool to room temperature, and stir in 2 tablespoons of pure vanilla extract. Pour the blend into a glass jar, cap it tightly, and store it at room temperature. (This recipe makes about 3 ¼ cups of syrup.)

RAVISHING ROSE HIP VINEGAR

Few folks think of rosebushes as fruit crops. But ounce for ounce, their fruits (a.k.a. hips) have 20 times more vitamin C than oranges. Unfortunately, heating or processing the hips destroys much of their vitamin content—but this tasty vinegar retains every bit of it.

YIELD: about 16 ounces	PREP: 5 minutes	WAIT: 4-6 weeks

1 cup of rose hips, washed

2 cups of unfiltered apple cider vinegar (more if needed)

1. Smash the rose hips carefully or pulse them a few times in a food processor.

2. Put them in a sterilized glass jar, and cover completely with the vinegar. Seal the jar tightly, and set it in a cool, dark place.

3. When the taste is right (usually 4 to 6 weeks), strain the vinegar thoroughly through clean muslin or a paper coffee filter. Make sure you get out all the seeds and (especially) the little hairs, which can deliver a powerful sting to your throat.

4. Transfer the vinegar to a sterilized bottle, cap or cork it, and store it in a cool, dark place. It should keep for up to 6 months.

Note: *This vinegar is delicious in sauces, marinades, and dressings.*

Harvest rose hips, from wild or backyard bushes, after the first frost, when the fruits are still firm and either bright red or orange (depending on the variety). Once the hips turn darker in color, they'll taste sweeter, but they will have lost much of their vitamin C content.

CULINARY Q & A

? Can I use rose petals in vinegar as well? Do you have a recipe?

! Yes! Rose petals have natural oils that help to moisturize dry skin, reduce stress, and soothe irritation. Here's how to make rose petal vinegar: Pack fresh, organic red rose petals (about 2 cups) into a sterilized glass jar, and cover with warm white wine or champagne vinegar. Let it cool to room temperature, then seal and place in a cool, dark spot for a week. Strain out the petals. Add it to baths or rub onto your skin directly to use.

ULTRA-EASY HOT-PEPPER VINEGAR

If you like spicy food, try this zesty recipe. It's simpler than most and never fails to produce fast, fiery results. Plus, it's full of potent antioxidants and vitamin C. See the Culinary Q & A box below for more of the health-boosting benefits.

YIELD: 8-10 ounces	PREP: 10 minutes	WAIT: 7 days

12-15 hot peppers of your choice, washed and pierced with a needle

2 sprigs of fresh parsley

White wine vinegar

1. Pack the peppers and parsley into an 8- to 10-ounce sterilized bottle or jar.

2. Fill the container with enough white wine vinegar to cover the peppers and parsley completely, and cover it with a tight-fitting lid.

3. Let the mixture steep for 7 days at room temperature. Then tuck it into the refrigerator, and use it to your heart's (and tummy's) content.

4. Whenever you use some of your spicy potion, replace it with enough fresh vinegar to completely cover the peppers and parsley. It should keep for at least 3 to 4 months.

 KITCHEN CAPERS For an extra-special visual treat, make your Hot-Pepper Vinegar using peppers in different shapes and colors. Fill fancy bottles or jars, add a hand-written label, and you'll have some of the best Christmas, birthday, or hostess gifts in town!

CULINARY Q & A

? How is Hot-Pepper Vinegar good for you, and how much should I take?

! Medical research has shown that vinegar and capsaicin (the chemical that gives hot peppers their heat) team up to help you lose or maintain weight by boosting your metabolism; fend off colds and infectious diseases; and stimulate sweat glands, which enable your body to keep its cool in steamy weather. There is no precise dose for Hot-Pepper Vinegar. Simply add it to your menu to jump-start your system and generally keep your body functioning on all its "cylinders."

GARDEN HARVEST VINEGAR

Vegetable vinegars offer up intense flavor and power-packed nutrition in a versatile liquid form. You can use any combination of veggies you like, or try this aromatic and tantalizing favorite—you'll be tempted to swig it straight from the bottle!

YIELD: about 16 ounces	PREP: 10 minutes	WAIT: 1–3 weeks

3 long, thin slices of carrot

2 long slices of
    red bell pepper

1 asparagus spear

1 long, thin slice of celery

2 green beans

2 pea pods

2 garlic cloves, peeled

1 sprig of parsley

2 black or green olives

2 tsp. of whole peppercorns

16 oz. (or more if needed)
    of white wine vinegar

1. Wash vegetables, and pat dry. Pack all of the ingredients into a large glass jar, starting with the long, thin items. Then fill in the gaps with the smaller ones.

2. Pour in the white wine vinegar to completely cover the vegetables. Seal the jar tightly, and set it in a dark place at room temperature.

3. Let the mixture steep for about 1 to 3 weeks, or until it reaches your desired flavor.

4. Strain the vinegar into a sterilized bottle, cap it tightly, and use it in your favorite recipes.

KITCHEN CAPERS The vegetables listed in Garden Harvest Vinegar (above) are just the beginning! Have fun creating your own variations on the theme. For example, use leeks instead of garlic, green peppers instead of red, or replace the parsley with basil. Your mix-and-match options are endless!

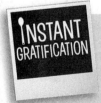

INSTANT GRATIFICATION

Versatile Vegetable Vinegar

If hot peppers aren't your cup of tea, any veggies can add a flavorful punch to vinegar. Here are some options: 1 pound of sweet onions, peeled and sliced; 1 pound of bell peppers (red, green, yellow, or purple), seeded and chopped; 6 garlic cloves, peeled and crushed; or 3 bunches of green onions, thinly sliced. Put whichever variation you choose in a sterilized glass jar with 1 quart of red or white wine vinegar. Close the lid tightly, and let it age for at least 30 days. Strain it through cheesecloth until the liquid runs clear, and pour it into sterilized bottles.

NIFTY NASTURTIUM VINEGAR

Edible flowers lend themselves perfectly to delicious, nutritious vinegars. Nasturtium vinegar is one of the most popular, and it adds a distinctive flavor to soups and stews. Grow your own edible flowers, or purchase from an organic online retailer.

YIELD: 1 quart	**PREP:** 10 minutes	**WAIT:** 6 weeks

1 qt. of freshly picked nasturtium flowers

1 large onion, finely chopped

6 whole peppercorns

2 whole cloves

1 garlic clove, minced

1 qt. of white wine or sherry vinegar

1. Look through the freshly picked flowers and remove any dead or damaged ones. Then rinse them gently in water, and pat dry.

2. Combine all of the ingredients in a sterilized glass jar, cover it, and set it in a cool, dark place for about 6 weeks.

3. Strain the liquid into one or more sterilized bottles, and enjoy!

KITCHEN CAPERS Always make sure that any flowers you use in your vinegars have been organically grown and haven't been treated with chemical pesticides or foliar fertilizers. Never use florist flowers of any kind—they're guaranteed to be chock-full of toxins!

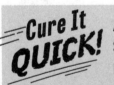

Cure It QUICK!

A SIMPLE SORE-THROAT SOOTHER Whether the pain is caused by the *Streptococcus* bacteria or a virus, this tasty beverage will make it vanish: Just mix 1 tablespoon each of rose hip vinegar and raw honey in 1 cup of warm water, and sip the potion slowly. Repeat as desired once or twice a day. Before you know it, you'll be ready to warble a tuneful melody!

CULINARY Q & A

? What other flowers can I use to create infused vinegars?

! The flowers of all culinary herbs make delicious infused vinegars. You can also try these flower-garden favorites: chamomile, cottage pinks, chrysanthemums, English daisies, johnny-jump-ups, marigolds, pansies, red clover, and violets.

THE THICK OF THINGS

When you want the flavor of an infused vinegar but you want it now, a fortified vinegar is the answer to your wish. It's a thickened blend of vinegar mixed with herbs, spices, fruits, and/or vegetables. You whip it up in a blender or food processor and use it as a dip, salad dressing, or topping for anything from meat, pasta, and baked potatoes to your favorite desserts. Another big advantage over infused vinegars is that because you use the fortified versions immediately (or close to it), the acidity level is a moot point—which means you can safely use your homemade vinegar as the base. As far as ingredients go, the sky's the limit, but these are some versatile—and terrifically tasty—mixtures:

Fortified Vinegar	Ingredients
Carrot	1 cup of sliced carrots, ½ cup of unfiltered apple cider vinegar, ½ cup of water, 3–4 tablespoons of honey (optional)
Cucumber, celery, & onion	1 large cucumber, 2 cups of chopped celery, 1 small chopped onion, 1 cup of champagne vinegar, 1 cup of water
Garlic	8 garlic bulbs, peeled, and 1 cup of unfiltered apple cider vinegar
Honeydew	2 cups of chopped honeydew melon, ¼ cup of champagne vinegar, ¼ cup of water
Kale-mustard	2 cups of kale, ¼ cup of unfiltered apple cider vinegar, ¼ cup of water, 2 tablespoons of dry mustard
Lemon	1 whole lemon (including peel), chopped, 2 tablespoons of champagne vinegar, ½ cup of water
Mint	2 cups of fresh mint leaves, 1 cup of malt or red wine vinegar, 2 tablespoons of honey
Parsley	2 cups of fresh parsley, ½ cup of red wine vinegar, ½ cup of water
Raspberry	1 cup of raspberries (fresh or frozen), 3 tablespoons of red wine vinegar, ½ cup of Vanilla-Scented Sugar Syrup (see page 20)
Strawberry	2 cups of fresh strawberries, 1 cup of sugar, ½ cup of champagne vinegar

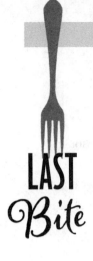

MORE VINEGAR-MAKING TIPS & TRICKS

THE START OF IT ALL

Historians speculate that vinegar was discovered by accident at least 10,000 years ago, when a wine vat was opened prematurely. The result was a not-so-tasty, but much more versatile, liquid. In the late 1300s, master vinegar makers in France developed what is still called the Orleans method, by which they could make continuous batches by adding fresh wine or cider to oak barrels that contained remnants of the previous batch (a.k.a. the "mother"). Infused vinegars soon followed, and by the late 1700s, Parisian street markets offered more than 50 varieties of flavored cooking vinegar. Among the most popular were pepper, clove, chicory, mustard, fennel, ginger, pistachio, and truffle. Fast forward to 1869, when the H.J. Heinz Company became the very first to mass produce and distribute vinegar. And the rest, as they say, is history!

DE-POLLUTE YOUR PRODUCE

Before you use fresh fruits, vegetables, herbs, or flowers in a vinegar recipe, clean them thoroughly. To do that, simply mix 2 tablespoons of vinegar (any kind), 1 tablespoon of lemon juice, and 1 cup of water in a small spray bottle. Keep the bottle by the sink, and spray all your fruits and veggies thoroughly. Then rinse 'em with clear water, and you're good to go!

Do yourself a favor and use this on all of your fresh produce, whether you intend to make vinegar from it or eat it. After all, even organically grown crops generally contain stuff that you'd rather not eat, like the residue from manure tea, garlic- or citrus-based pesticides—or plain old garden-variety dirt.

CULINARY Q & A

? I've heard that some fruits and vegetables retain more pesticide residue than others. Is this true? And if so, what are the most problematic ones?

! Yes, it is true. And unfortunately, some of the healthiest of the bunch—including apples—rank highest on the list. The list changes slightly from time to time, but the Environmental Working Group publishes annual rosters of the good and the bad. For the latest ratings, check www.ewg.org.

GOOD THINGS FROM BAD GUYS

Here's the full scoop on the Four Thieves Vinegar on page 13: In the 17th century, the bubonic plague (a.k.a. the Black Death) swept across Europe, killing at least half the population. French folklore tells us that in Marseilles, four men repeatedly looted the homes of deceased victims but, miraculously, never got sick. According to one version of the story, after the thieves were arrested, they were forced to bury the dead, with the promise that if they survived, they would go free. Well, survive they did—apparently thanks to an herbal vinegar tincture concocted by one of the bad guys, who happened to be an herbalist. As the gang's resistance to the disease became well known, other folks began using the potion. Today, natural health gurus still swear by the amazing healing power of Four Thieves Vinegar. And here's a trio of ways to use this wonder "drug."

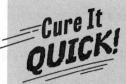

RASPBERRY SORE-THROAT SOLUTION
When it feels like there's a four-alarm fire raging in your throat, this cooling potion can douse the flames fast. Put 2 cups of ripe red raspberries in a bowl, and add 2½ cups of white wine vinegar. Pour the mixture into a saucepan, stir in 1 cup of sugar, and bring to a low boil. Simmer for 15 minutes, and remove from the heat. When the mixture has cooled almost to room temperature, strain it through a sieve or cheesecloth, pressing on the berries to extract as much juice as possible. Pour the potion into a glass bottle, store it in the refrigerator, and gargle with it as needed. You'll be feeling better in no time!

Fight colds, flu, and other illnesses. Adults should take 1 tablespoon of Four Thieves Vinegar three times a day. The dosage for children is 1 teaspoon three times a day. How you take it is your call. For example, you can sip it from a spoon, add it to salad dressing, or mix it with water, fruit juice, or herbal tea.

Prevent colds and flu. Use the same quantities (1 tablespoon for adults, 1 teaspoon for children), but for prevention purposes, taking the potion once a day should do the trick. For additional resistance, you can also add a tablespoon or so to your bathwater, and breathe in the healing vapors while you're soaking your worries away.

Kill germs. Fend off airborne viruses as well as surface bacteria by filling a spray bottle with equal parts of Four Thieves Vinegar and water, and spraying it into the air and onto surfaces in your home and office.

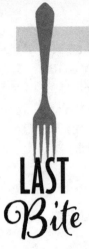

5 SIMPLE SECRETS TO VERY FINE VINEGAR

When you're making infused vinegars of any kind, make sure to keep this handful of helpers in mind to produce the very best batch possible:

1. Let your taste be your guide. There are no rules when it comes to making flavored vinegars. Use whatever kinds of vinegar and herbs, spices, fruits, vegetables, or flowers that appeal to you.

2. Don't scrimp on the "infusables." If you don't use enough, the flavor will be weak. As a general rule, you want to use about 2 cups of herbs or 4 cups of flowers per quart of vinegar—but let your eyes and nose be your guides.

3. Use high-quality vinegar. Don't try to economize by using the cheap stuff. If the vinegar you start with doesn't taste good, the finished product won't either—no matter how much flavoring you pack into it.

4. Use only the finest fresh herbs or flowers. Anything that's limp, yellowing, or (heaven forbid!) turning brown is too far gone to make high-quality vinegar.

5. Don't put 'em on display. Decorative bottles filled with infused vinegar can look beautiful on a windowsill with the light streaming through them. But that light will make the flavor fade fast. You can make a few just-for-show batches if you want to, but keep your cooking and gift-giving supply in a cool, dark place. A pantry works well; so does a kitchen cabinet that's far away from the stove, the refrigerator, or any other heat source.

Always remember that when it comes to infused vinegars, the right steeping time is strictly a matter of taste. The longer the flavorings remain in the vinegar (of course), the stronger the finished product will be. Your best course of action: Sample your "crop" after a week or so and every week thereafter until the intensity meets your approval. Generally, most of the flavor is extracted after a month. If you want an extra-intense vinegar, after 30 days or so, strain it, add fresh flavorings, and continue steeping and sampling until your taste buds say, "This is it!"

VINEGAR & HERBS—A POWER-PACKED HEALTH-CARE PAIR

When it comes to solving specific health problems—or simply maintaining your vim and vigor—herbal vinegars are genuine miracle workers. For the ultra-simple formula, see Elegant Herbal Vinegar on page 12. Of course, the herbs you want to use depend on the job(s) you have in mind for them. Here are some of the best choices:

Herbal Vinegar	How It Helps Your Health
Basil	Fights colds and flu, eases migraines, helps relieve stress, helps cure depression, and removes warts
Bay	Helps prevent tooth decay and eases the pain of head- and stomachaches
Chamomile	Helps reduce pain and inflammation in the digestive tract and relaxes both body and nerves
Dill	Calms upset stomachs, helps relieve muscle spasms, freshens breath, and stimulates the flow of breast milk in nursing mothers
Garlic	Kills bacteria, clears lung congestion, promotes good blood sugar and cholesterol levels, boosts circulation, and acts as an antihistamine
Marjoram & oregano	Act as effective antiseptics, soothe sore throats, and relieve aching joints and muscles
Parsley	Aids digestion, supports healthy blood pressure, keeps your immune system healthy, helps maintain strong bones, helps heal the nervous system, relaxes stiff muscles, and eases joint pain
Peppermint	Energizes mind and body and relieves nausea and upset stomachs
Rosemary	Stimulates memory, boosts energy, and helps chase the blues away
Sage	Restores vitality and strength, fights fevers, and soothes mucous membrane tissue—thereby curing mouth ulcers and sore gums and throats
Thyme	Helps detoxify the body (especially the liver), boosts the immune system, fights fatigue, and fends off parasites

Note: *If you're on medication of any kind (even aspirin); you suffer from high blood pressure, diabetes, or any other chronic condition; or you're pregnant or think that you might be pregnant, check with your doctor before you dose yourself with these or any other herbs.*

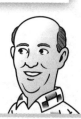

Chapter Two

Dynamite Dressings, Marinades, & Sauces

There is no easier way to enjoy all the delights of vinegar than to use it in dressings, marinades, and sauces. That (of course) is what this chapter is all about. You'll find scads of simple ways to perk up salads, meats, or just about any other edibles—and treat yourself and your family to better health while you're at it. So what are you waiting for?

BALSAMIC VINAIGRETTE

While this delicious dressing is terrific on any kind of tossed salad, it's also perfect for basting grilled vegetables or fish, or as a marinade for chicken.

YIELD: about 3 ¼ cups   **PREP:** 5 minutes

1 cup of balsamic vinegar

¼ cup of sweet vermouth

1 large shallot, minced

Salt and pepper to taste

2 cups of extra virgin olive oil

1. Mix the balsamic vinegar, vermouth, minced shallots, and salt and pepper together in a bowl.

2. Slowly whisk in the olive oil until it's well blended. Then add it to the salad or meat of your choice.

3. If you don't use this dressing immediately, refrigerate it in a tightly closed container for up to 30 days. Shake well before using.

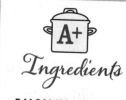

Ingredients

BALSAMIC VINEGAR
Helps fight free radicals

SHALLOTS
Help calm anxiety

EXTRA VIRGIN OLIVE OIL
Promotes cardiovascular health

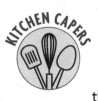

KITCHEN CAPERS The key to making a successful vinaigrette dressing is to create what chemists call an emulsion. To do that, first, whisk together all of the ingredients except the oil. Once they are thoroughly combined, slowly dribble in the oil as you whisk it into the vinegar mixture.

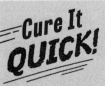

Cure It QUICK!

SPARE-TIRE DEFLATOR Repeated scientific tests have proven that balsamic vinegar helps eliminate belly fat, which can lead to conditions like heart disease, sleep apnea, and type 2 diabetes. It works by activating genes that cause your body to distribute fat more evenly, rather than storing it at your waist. The jury is still out on the exact amount, but a good quantity to aim for is 5 teaspoons a day, which is the amount researchers have found to increase insulin sensitivity in diabetics. How you take the Big B is your call: Sip it straight from a spoon; stir your ration into juice, tea, or water; drizzle it over vegetables or fruit; or use it in the recipes you'll find throughout this book (including the Balsamic Vinaigrette, above).

CREAMY RASPBERRY DRESSING

Serve this winner as a topping for juicy fresh fruit, or enjoy it on a salad made with baby spinach or Bibb lettuce, fresh raspberries, and toasted walnuts.

YIELD: about ⅔ cup	**PREP:** 5 minutes	**WAIT:** 3–4 hours

⅓ cup of plain yogurt

¼ cup of fresh raspberries

3 tbsp. of raspberry vinegar

2 tbsp. of mayonnaise

1 tbsp. of Dijon mustard

1 tsp. of sugar

1. Whisk all of the ingredients together in a large bowl until they are combined thoroughly.

2. Cover the mixture tightly, and chill it for several hours, so the flavors can blend. Add ground black pepper to taste, if desired.

3. Drizzle it over your salad, and dig in!

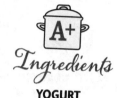

KITCHEN CAPERS

When you're making a vinaigrette dressing recipe, you don't have to use the quantities of vinegar and oil that are listed. Use whatever proportions you prefer. If you're not sure, start with 2 parts vinegar to 3 parts oil, and experiment until you find the balance you like.

A+

Ingredients

YOGURT
Helps reduce bloating

RASPBERRIES
Enhance brain function

MAYONNAISE
Promotes healthy skin

CULINARY Q & A

? I've been careful to use fat-free dairy products. But recently I heard that full-fat dairy products are not as bad for us as previously believed. Is that true?

! Yes! Recent studies show that the only types of fat that really hurt you are the man-made varieties like trans fats and the refined polyunsaturated fats found in canola and other vegetable oils. So full-fat dairy products are A-okay!

Here's another kicker: During the manufacturing process, low-fat and fat-free dairy products are stripped clean of a key health-giving ingredient found in whole milk: conjugated linoleic acid (CLA), a fat that's been proven to fight disease and help fend off abdominal fat deposits.

FRUITY VINAIGRETTE DRESSING

Heart-healthy extra virgin olive oil is paired with vitamin-rich orange juice, disease-fighting honey, and fresh ginger for an all-around full-body health boost!

YIELD: about ¾ cup   **PREP:** 10 minutes

¼ cup of extra virgin olive oil

3 tbsp. of orange juice

2 tbsp. of lemon juice

2 tbsp. of raspberry or red wine vinegar

1 tbsp. of raw honey

½ tbsp. of prepared mustard

1 tsp. of grated fresh ginger

1. Combine all of the ingredients in a tightly lidded jar.

2. Shake well to thoroughly mix the ingredients together. Refrigerate the mixture until you are ready to use it.

3. Just before serving, shake again to mix thoroughly. Add it to chopped fruit or pour it over a green salad and top with chicken or ham.

A+ Ingredients

ORANGE JUICE
Helps maintain healthy bones

RAW HONEY
Alleviates allergies

GINGER
Helps relieve inflammation

Always taste a dressing before you put it on your salad since it's all but impossible to adjust the ingredients once everything's mixed together. But don't use a spoon. Instead, grab a piece of lettuce or a carrot, dip it into the dressing, and take a bite. You will know exactly how the end result will taste.

KITCHEN CAPERS

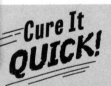
Cure It QUICK!

GIVE SAD A DRESSING DOWN If you suffer from seasonal affective disorder (SAD), the winter months can be miserable. But here's good news: This simple vinaigrette dressing just might help lift your spirits. To make it, whisk together ¼ cup each of flaxseed oil, lemon juice, and white balsamic vinegar; 1 tablespoon of Dijon mustard; and 1 minced garlic clove. Season with salt and pepper, and toss the dressing with your favorite salad greens.

The secret ingredient is the flaxseed oil. It can up your levels of essential fatty acids, which are often low in SAD sufferers.

HEARTY HERBAL DRESSING

This fragrant, egg-thickened mixture is perfect with a seafood salad, drizzled over sliced fresh-from-the-garden tomatoes, or used as a dressing for potato or chicken salad.

YIELD: about 1 cup	PREP: 10 minutes	WAIT: 30 minutes

3 tbsp. of red wine vinegar

1 tbsp. of Dijon mustard

1 large egg yolk

Salt and freshly ground black pepper to taste

⅔ cup of extra virgin olive oil

¼ cup of chopped fresh parsley

2 large shallots, minced

2 tbsp. of capers, drained

2 tbsp. of snipped fresh chives

1. Whisk the first three ingredients together in a medium-size bowl. Season with salt and pepper.

2. Whisk in the olive oil in a slow, steady stream until the mixture is thick.

3. Stir in the remaining ingredients.

4. Let the dressing sit for about 30 minutes, so the flavors can develop fully. Stir one time just before serving.

A+ Ingredients

EGG YOLK
Supports cardiovascular health

SHALLOTS
Help calm anxiety

CHIVES
Support digestion

KITCHEN CAPERS
To keep your refrigerator clean and odor-free, simply wipe the shelves and walls—inside and out—with a half-and-half solution of vinegar and water. For the top, use paper towels or a cloth dipped in full-strength vinegar.

CULINARY Q & A

? Do I need to use homemade salad dressings right away, or can I make them ahead of time and store them for future use?

! While it is true that most salad dressings are at their peak of flavor at the time you make them, you can store any of them in the refrigerator. Make sure you use a glass jar—not plastic, which absorbs the ingredients' aromas—and cover the jar with a tight-fitting lid. The contents should be fine for up to two weeks, but when it starts to change color, toss the dressing out.

MAPLE-BALSAMIC VINAIGRETTE

Balsamic vinegar is often used in heart-healthy diets because it is low in fat, cholesterol, and sodium while high in calcium, iron, and potassium.

YIELD: about 1¾ cups	PREP: 10 minutes

½ cup of balsamic vinegar

¼ cup of pure maple syrup

2 tsp. of Dijon mustard

Salt and pepper to taste

1 cup of extra virgin olive oil

1. Add the balsamic vinegar, maple syrup, mustard, and salt and pepper to your blender, and then pulse to combine.

2. With the motor still running, add the olive oil in a slow but steady stream, until the mixture is thoroughly blended together.

3. Serve this vinaigrette immediately atop your favorite salad, or pour it over the meat of your choice as a marinade. If you are saving it for later use, cover it and refrigerate.

Ingredients

BALSAMIC VINEGAR
Maintains healthy blood pressure

MAPLE SYRUP
Boosts the immune system

DIJON MUSTARD
Helps ease respiratory disorders

KITCHEN CAPERS

To remove built-up film and hard-water stains from a blender, pour 1 cup of vinegar and ¼ cup of baking soda into the jar. Once the bubbling subsides, add 2 cups of water and run the machine on high for three to four minutes. Rinse with clear water, and use a small brush to remove any lingering marks.

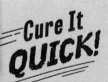

PARSLEY PAIN PULVERIZER This frilly herb has amazing power to help ease the pain of arthritis and other joint problems. This simple vinaigrette is one of the tastiest ways to take your healthy "medicine." To make it, mix 2 tablespoons of coarsely chopped fresh parsley with 2 tablespoons of red wine vinegar and salt and pepper to taste (if desired). Then slowly whisk in 2 tablespoons of extra virgin olive oil. Toss it with salad greens, or dribble it onto a baked potato or half an avocado.

BALSAMIC BLUE CHEESE DRESSING

If you're a blue cheese lover, you know that those bottled dressings can be bland to say the least. So do yourself a favor and give this handy, homemade version a try. You will never want to buy store-bought dressing again!

YIELD: 1 cup   **PREP:** 5 minutes

¼ cup of balsamic vinegar

¼ tsp. of salt

⅛ tsp. of hot-pepper sauce (optional)

Freshly ground black pepper to taste

½ cup of extra virgin olive oil

⅔ cup of crumbled blue cheese*

* *Roquefort and Gorgonzola work well also.*

1. Whisk the balsamic vinegar, salt, hot pepper sauce (if desired), and freshly ground black pepper together in a small bowl.

2. Slowly drizzle in the oil, whisking until well combined.

3. Stir in the blue cheese. Serve immediately, or cover and refrigerate until ready to use.

A+

Ingredients

HOT-PEPPER SAUCE
Supports digestion

BLACK PEPPER
Aids weight loss

BLUE CHEESE
Helps strengthen bones and teeth

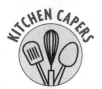

KITCHEN CAPERS
To give instant pizzazz to store-bought blue cheese or creamy ranch dressing, spike it with a tablespoon or so of vinegar. Use any herb-, vegetable-, or fruit-infused flavor you have on hand, or go with balsamic or wine vinegar.

CULINARY Q & A

? What's the best way to store blue cheese?

! Put it in an airtight container in your refrigerator's vegetable bin. The high humidity is perfect for all cheeses.

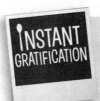

INSTANT GRATIFICATION

Fast Fruit Salad Dressing
Fabulous fruit toppings don't come any easier than this: Just mix a tablespoon of peach- or blueberry-spiced vinegar with 1 tablespoon of either sour cream, plain yogurt, or mayonnaise, and pour it over chunks of your favorite fruits.

CREAMY HORSERADISH VINAIGRETTE

To get the tang—and the anti-inflammatory, antioxidant, and disease-fighting health benefits—of horseradish without the four-alarm firepower of the fresh root, this is the recipe to reach for. Try it on a green salad or as a marinade.

YIELD: ⅓ cup   **PREP:** 5 minutes

2 tsp. of champagne vinegar

2 tsp. of horseradish cream

½ tsp. of kosher or sea salt

¼ tsp. of freshly ground black pepper

¼ cup of extra virgin olive oil

1. Whisk the first four ingredients together in a nonreactive bowl until thoroughly blended.

2. Continue to whisk as you slowly pour the oil in a thin stream down the side of the bowl, then stir until well combined.

3. Taste the mixture, and add more salt and pepper if needed. If the flavor is too salty for you, whisk in another spoonful of vinegar, until the taste is to your liking.

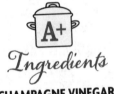

A+ Ingredients

CHAMPAGNE VINEGAR
Supports healthy weight loss

HORSERADISH CREAM
Boosts immunity

EXTRA VIRGIN OLIVE OIL
Promotes cardiovascular health

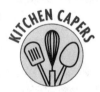

KITCHEN CAPERS

If you simmer any marinade or dressing to reduce it slightly, you'll have a slightly thicker sauce that you can serve on the side during a meal or use as the base for another sauce.

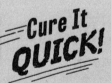

Cure It QUICK!

FAST-ACTING HEADACHE RELIEF A headache is your body's way of telling you that something has gotten out of whack. So the next time the throbbing starts, don't simply pop a painkiller. Instead, make yourself a green salad and top it with a vinaigrette made from equal parts of apple cider vinegar and extra virgin olive oil. You should feel relief almost immediately. The reason: Research has shown that regardless of what triggers the pain in your head, your body's system, which is normally slightly acidic, turns overly alkaline. The malic acid in apple cider vinegar will restore proper balance before you know it!

RED HOT HORSERADISH DRESSING

If you're a fiery-food fan, try this steamy, spicy winner! Drizzle it over your favorite mixed green salad to really ramp up the heat. Your taste buds will be begging for more!

YIELD: about 1 cup   **PREP:** 5 minutes

⅓ cup of red wine vinegar

¼ cup of soy sauce

¼ cup of sugar

1 tbsp. of grated fresh horseradish

Hot-pepper sauce to taste

½ cup of extra virgin olive oil

1. Thoroughly mix the red wine vinegar, soy sauce, sugar, horseradish, and hot-pepper sauce together in a small bowl.

2. Slowly and steadily whisk in the olive oil, until the mixture is fully combined.

3. Dress a salad of your choice with the mighty mix, and get ready to dig in! Or, cover and refrigerate for later use.

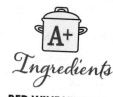

Ingredients

RED WINE VINEGAR
Promotes heart health

HORSERADISH
Boosts liver function

HOT-PEPPER SAUCE
Supports your metabolism

KITCHEN CAPERS

When you're fresh out of hot-pepper sauce, just mix 1 teaspoon of vinegar with ¾ teaspoon of cayenne pepper for each teaspoon of sauce you need.

CULINARY Q & A

? My family and I love fresh horseradish. But every time I grate the roots, my eyes burn like crazy, and the tears flow like Niagara Falls. Is there any way to avoid this agony?

! There sure is! Simply chop off a chunk or two of the root, put the pieces in a blender or food processor, and add a spoonful or so of vinegar. Then put the cover on and let 'er rip. If you use a hand grater, sprinkle the cut end of the root with vinegar, then pull a plastic bag over the whole shebang, and grate inside that fume-containing cover. Either way, your eyes will stay dry, with no burning sensation.

MIGHTY MUSTARD DRESSING

Mustard is extremely low in sugar and calories and is great for your health, to boot! For a major taste treat, splash this full-bodied dressing on roasted vegetables.

YIELD: about ¼ cup	**PREP:** 5 minutes	**WAIT:** 2 days

¼ cup of extra virgin olive oil

3 tbsp. of white wine vinegar

1 tsp. of prepared mustard

1 garlic clove, peeled and crushed

¼ tsp. of hot-pepper sauce

Salt and freshly ground black pepper to taste

1. Combine all of the ingredients in a jar that has a tight-fitting lid and mix well.

2. Cover and refrigerate until ready to use. Shake vigorously before serving.

3. While this dressing is ready to use immediately, the flavor will be more intense if you let it chill out in the refrigerator for a few days.

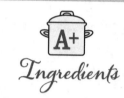

Ingredients

WHITE WINE VINEGAR
Supports heart health

MUSTARD
Fights inflammation

GARLIC
Boosts bone health

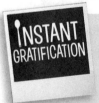
INSTANT GRATIFICATION

Be on the Best-Dressed List

Correction: Make that the best-dressing list! This tasty vinaigrette dressing is worthy of the fanciest five-star restaurant in town. To make it, marinate finely chopped shallots in wine vinegar for 15 minutes. Then whisk it with extra virgin olive oil, add salt and pepper to taste—and modestly accept the applause from around the dinner table!

KITCHEN CAPERS

When you're whipping up a recipe that calls for prepared mustard and you don't have any, don't rush off to the store. Instead, for each tablespoon needed, mix 1 tablespoon of dry mustard with 1 teaspoon each of vinegar, sugar, and water.

CULINARY Q & A

? What's the best way to get mustard stains out of fabric?

! If the spill has just happened, dab it with a half-and-half solution of white vinegar and water. If it has set, soak the area in the same mix. Then wash the item as usual.

CLASSIC BUTTERMILK DRESSING

This tangy dressing, which contains no oil, gained popularity during World War II, when many kitchen staples, including fats and oils, were rationed. Well, it's just as tasty today as it was back then—and it's especially delicious on coleslaw or potato salad.

YIELD: about 1 cup   **PREP:** 5 minutes

2 tbsp. of apple cider vinegar

2 tbsp. of prepared mustard

1 tbsp. of light brown sugar

1 tsp. of paprika

1 tsp. of salt

⅛ tsp. of cayenne pepper

1 cup of buttermilk

1. Mix together the first six ingredients in a pint jar that has a tight-fitting lid.

2. Add the buttermilk, screw the lid on tight, and shake until it is thoroughly combined.

3. Drizzle it over the salad of your choice.

Ingredients

PAPRIKA
Helps drive energy production

CAYENNE PEPPER
Supports metabolism

BUTTERMILK
Soothes acid reflux

Whenever you buy a quart of buttermilk for a recipe, freeze what you don't use in 1-cup portions. That way, the extra portion won't be shoved to the back of the fridge and spoil—and you will always have fresh buttermilk on hand when you need it for another recipe.

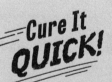

Cure It **QUICK!**

HEALTHY-SKIN DRESSING The dynamic duo of unprocessed apple cider vinegar and raw honey is not only a boon to your internal health. It's also one of the best tools you can use to retain (or regain) the health of your skin—which is, after all, your body's largest organ. This dressing gives you a simple and delicious way to help smooth cellulite, soften your skin, fight blemishes, and generally reduce signs of aging. To make it, mix ¼ cup of unfiltered ACV, 2 tablespoons of raw honey, and 2 tablespoons of water in a blender, along with salt and pepper to taste if you like. With the machine still running, slowly pour in ¾ cup of olive oil. Use the mixture to dress your favorite green salad, splash it onto steamed vegetables, or drizzle it over baked potatoes.

GREEN GODDESS DRESSING

While there are countless variations of green goddess dressing, this is one of the tastiest—and easiest to whip up. Plus, it's loaded with tons of health-boosting ingredients!

YIELD: about 2 cups **PREP:** 10 minutes

1 avocado, peeled, pitted, and chopped

1 scallion (green and white parts), chopped

1 cup of fresh basil

¼ cup of fresh parsley, chopped

¼ cup of extra virgin olive oil

¼ cup of water

Juice of 1 large lemon

2 tbsp. of apple cider vinegar

1 tsp. of honey

½ tsp. of minced garlic

½ tsp. of sea salt

1. Combine the first six ingredients in a food processor, and pulse until mixed.

2. Add the remaining ingredients and blend thoroughly.

3. If the dressing is too thick, add more water a little bit at a time, pulsing after each addition. Refrigerate in a sealed jar for up to 2 weeks.

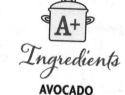

Ingredients

AVOCADO
Supports metabolism

PARSLEY
Fights fatigue

LEMON
Promotes healthy weight loss

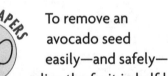

KITCHEN CAPERS

To remove an avocado seed easily—and safely— slice the fruit in half lengthwise. Then firmly jab the pit with the business end of a sturdy knife. Gently twist the blade to dislodge the big seed and lift it out.

CULINARY Q & A

? I've always heard that when you only use half an avocado, the other half will stay fresh longer if you leave the seed in. Is that true?

! Avocados are incredibly nutritious, loaded with healthy fats, potassium, and fiber. So don't let them go to waste! But the key to keeping a cut avocado fresh is not the seed; it's preventing exposure to light and air. Remove the seed, then gently smooth aluminum foil over the cut surface, pressing the foil into the depression where the seed was. You may still see brown spots when you remove the foil, but they are harmless—just scrape them off with a knife.

MUSTARD-TARRAGON MARINADE

This quick and easy blend is well worth trying during the next outdoor grilling season. It's great with chicken, pork, or substantial fish like salmon, swordfish, and halibut.

YIELD: about 1½ cups	PREP: 5 minutes	WAIT: 4–8 hours

1 cup of extra virgin olive oil

¼ cup of Dijon mustard

¼ cup of tarragon white wine vinegar

1 tbsp. of minced fresh tarragon

2 garlic cloves

1. Process all of the ingredients in a blender or food processor until the consistency is smooth.

2. Pour the mixture into a glass or ceramic dish, and set your meat, fish, or poultry into the marinade.

3. Cover the container, and refrigerate for 4 to 8 hours, depending on the size of meat.

4. About 30 minutes before grilling, remove it from the fridge, and let it sit at room temperature.

A+

Ingredients

EXTRA VIRGIN OLIVE OIL
Supports healthy weight loss

WHITE WINE VINEGAR
Boosts heart health

TARRAGON
Helps fight free radicals

When you make a marinade, multiply the recipe if necessary to ensure that your meat, poultry, or fish is fully submerged in the liquid. Otherwise, you will need to turn the pieces several times while marinating.

KITCHEN CAPERS

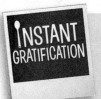

INSTANT GRATIFICATION

Authentic French Dressing

Forget the gooey orange imposter you see at the supermarket! This classic vinaigrette is the real deal, and it couldn't be simpler to make. Using a wire whisk, beat 1 tablespoon of red or white wine vinegar with salt and pepper to taste until the salt dissolves. (If you like, add mustard, crushed garlic, and/or fresh herbs to taste.) Then whisk in ⅔ cup of extra virgin olive oil a drizzle at a time. Use it as a salad dressing, a topping for lightly steamed vegetables, or a dipping sauce for raw veggies or crusty French bread.

BELLINI MARINADE

This light, summery mix was inspired by the Bellini cocktail, the delightful peach and champagne concoction invented at Harry's Bar in Venice—one of Ernest Hemingway's favorite haunts. The sweet-tart blend is fabulous for chicken, fish, or grilled fruit.

YIELD: about 1¼ cups   **PREP:** 5 minutes   **WAIT:** 10 minutes to 2 hours

½ cup of champagne vinegar

½ cup of peach nectar

2 tbsp. of crème de cassis (black currant liqueur)

2 tbsp. of freshly squeezed lemon juice

1 tbsp. of extra virgin olive oil

1 tbsp. of grated lemon zest

½ tsp. of coarsely ground black pepper

½ tsp. of salt

1. Combine all of the ingredients in a small bowl until thoroughly mixed together.

2. Put the poultry, fish, or fruit in a ceramic or glass bowl. Add the marinade, and turn the solids to coat completely.

3. Cover and refrigerate. Wait varies 1 to 2 hours for chicken, 30 to 60 minutes for fish, and about 10 minutes for fruit. Then remove, and grill as desired.

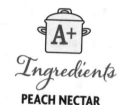

Ingredients

PEACH NECTAR
Boosts kidney function

CRÈME DE CASSIS
Fights inflammation

LEMON JUICE
Helps maintain liver health

 KITCHEN CAPERS Whenever you drain canned peaches, or any other canned fruit, freeze the juice in ice cube trays. That way, you'll have it on hand to add a touch of sweetness—and vitamins—to marinades, dressings, and other recipes.

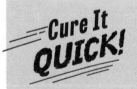 **Cure It QUICK!** **STRIKE BACK AT STROKE** Cold-water fish are famous for their mega-supply of omega-3 fatty acids, which can help dramatically reduce your risk for stroke and other cardiovascular diseases. Well, guess what? Flaxseed oil does exactly the same thing—and just 1 table-spoon of this tasty salad dressing fills your omega-3 quota for 2 ½ days! To make it, mix 2 tablespoons each of flaxseed oil, apple cider vinegar, and water with ½ teaspoon each of sugar and dried tarragon. Add salt and freshly ground pepper to taste, and have at it!

RED WINE MARINADE

Red wine vinegar is loaded with plenty of essential nutrients as well as antioxidants that help reduce cell damage from environmental factors.

YIELD: 2 cups	PREP: 5 minutes	COOK: 15 minutes

¼ cup of olive oil

1 cup of minced onion

2 garlic cloves, minced

½ cup of garlic red wine vinegar

¾ cup of dry red wine

½ cup of water

¼ cup of tomato paste

1 tbsp. of fresh rosemary

1 bay leaf

1. In a heavy, nonreactive skillet, warm the oil over medium heat. Add the onion and garlic, reduce the heat to low, and cook, stirring, until they're softened (about 5 minutes).

2. Stir in the vinegar and cook until it's reduced by half.

3. Add remaining ingredients and simmer for 5 minutes.

4. Once cool, transfer the marinade to a dish, and tuck in beef or lamb. Refrigerate, covered, for at least several hours, until 30 minutes before grilling time.

Some commercial culinary vinegars—particularly red wine and inexpensive balsamic varieties—contain sulfites. So if you're sensitive to those chemicals, read the labels carefully to make sure the brands you choose are all clear.

KITCHEN CAPERS

A+

Ingredients

ONION
Fights inflammation

RED WINE
Maintains healthy blood sugar

TOMATO PASTE
Promotes good skin health

INSTANT GRATIFICATION

New York Minute Marinade

When you're fixin' to grill chicken (maybe for last-minute company) and you need a marinade *now*, this simple trick will save the day: Just mix 1 cup of your favorite vinaigrette dressing with ½ cup of ready-made barbecue sauce—multiplying the ingredients as needed. Pour the mixture over your chicken in a ceramic or glass dish. Toss to coat, and refrigerate, covered, for 30 minutes or so while you and your guests enjoy a pre-dinner cocktail. Then drain the chicken and grill. Baste the chicken with the barbecue sauce as needed.

MADEIRA MARINADE

Tuck this recipe into your arsenal and enjoy it with eye-of-round roast for dinner on a cold winter's night—or charcoal-grilled filets on a warm summer evening.

YIELD: 2 cups	PREP: 15 minutes

1 cup of Madeira wine

½ cup of sherry vinegar

¼ cup of sweet almond oil

¼ cup of chopped shallots

3 garlic cloves, minced

3 whole bay leaves, crumbled

3 whole cloves, crushed

2 tbsp. of roasted almond slivers

1 tbsp. of allspice berries, crushed

1 tbsp. of ground black pepper

1 tbsp. of herbes de Provence, crushed

Kosher or sea salt to taste

1. Combine the wine and vinegar in a nonreactive bowl.

2. Slowly whisk in the oil.

3. Mix in the remaining ingredients. Use the marinade immediately, or refrigerate or freeze it until needed.

KITCHEN CAPERS When a recipe calls simply for "almond oil," use the sweet version. It has a nutty flavor and truly amazing health benefits. On the other hand, bitter almond oil has an unpleasant, pungent flavor and a strange aftertaste—and may even be slightly toxic.

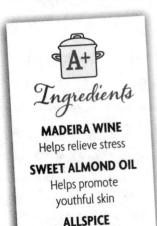

A+
Ingredients

MADEIRA WINE
Helps relieve stress

SWEET ALMOND OIL
Helps promote youthful skin

ALLSPICE
Boosts oral health

CULINARY Q & A

? What exactly is herbes de Provence? And where can I get it?

! This blend of herbs has a warm, woodsy taste and is full of rich antioxidants. You can buy it at any supermarket, or mix up a batch of your own: Combine 4 or 5 crumbled bay leaves; 2 tablespoons each of dried basil and oregano; 1 tablespoon of dried rosemary; and 1 teaspoon each of dried lavender and sage. Store the mixture in a cool spot in an opaque container. It should stay fresh for about a year.

WAKE-UP CALL LEMON MARINADE

This out-of-the-ordinary marinade is made with espresso, which studies show may help regulate blood sugar levels and promote weight loss.

YIELD: 2 cups	PREP: 10 minutes

1 tbsp. of instant, freeze-dried espresso

1 cup of freshly brewed espresso

½ cup of unsulfured molasses

¼ cup of balsamic vinegar

¼ cup of freshly squeezed lemon juice

1 tbsp. of soy sauce

¼ tsp. of ground cardamom

¼ tsp. of red pepper flakes

Thinly sliced peel of 1 lemon

1. Dissolve the instant espresso in the brewed version and cool to room temperature.

2. Mix it and the remaining ingredients together in a nonreactive bowl.

3. Add chicken or pork to a sturdy plastic bag, then pour in your marinade, following the easy Kitchen Capers directions below.

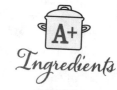

A+ Ingredients

ESPRESSO
Helps maintain liver health

MOLASSES
Boosts sexual health

CARDAMOM
Helps ease asthma symptoms

KITCHEN CAPERS One easy way to apply a marinade is to insert the meat or fish in a sturdy plastic bag, pour in the marinade, and then seal the bag tightly. Then periodically turn the bag so the meat is marinated evenly. To play it safe, put the marinade-filled bag in a shallow pan to catch any leaks.

Cure It QUICK!

COUNTERACT CATARACTS No nutrient can cure cataracts, but studies show that quercetin, a powerful antioxidant, may help delay their formation or slow their development. And dried tea leaves (both green and black) contain more quercetin than any other food. So what does that have to do with marinades? Just this: While there is no specific recommended dosage for cataract avoidance, simply adding 2 tablespoons or so of tea leaves to your favorite marinade recipe will help fend off these dreaded vision foggers—and add a surprising burst of flavor to boot.

HEART-HEALTHY BLUEBERRY MARINADE

This delightfully different marinade is packed with fiber-rich blueberries that can reduce your total cholesterol and decrease your risk of heart disease.

YIELD: about 4 cups	PREP: 5 minutes	WAIT: 8–12 hours

2 cups of blueberries (fresh or frozen)

1 cup of blueberry vinegar

¾ cup of extra virgin olive oil

1 tsp. of dried tarragon

1 tsp. of dried thyme

1 tsp. of shredded fresh mint leaves

½ tsp. of freshly ground black pepper

½ tsp. of salt

1. Combine the berries and vinegar in a small saucepan and boil for 1 minute.

2. Remove from the heat and stir in the remaining ingredients.

3. Let the marinade cool, then pour it over your chosen meat. Refrigerate in a covered container overnight, or for at least 8 hours, before grilling.

4. It's delicious as a marinade for chicken, fish, or beef.

A+ Ingredients

BLUEBERRIES
Support brain health

TARRAGON
Promotes cardiovascular health

THYME
Helps alleviate respiratory problems

KITCHEN CAPERS To save leftover fresh herbs, chop and spoon them into ice cube trays—one tablespoon per cube. Cover with water and freeze. Then drop a cube or two right into whatever soup, stew, casserole, or sauce you're cookin' up.

CULINARY Q & A

? What do I do when a recipe calls for dried herbs and I only have fresh ones on hand—or vice versa? There's some kind of substitution formula, isn't there?

! When you're substituting fresh herbs for dried, the basic rule is to use double the amount, but this is not a clear-cut rule, since the intensity of flavor can vary. Your best bet is to let your taste buds be your guide. Start with less, then add more until the flavor is to your liking.

MEXICAN MARINADE

Give south-of-the-border flavor to chicken, pork, or beef with this mighty marinade.
Just add tortillas and all the fixin's and you'll have the tastiest tacos around!

YIELD: about 1¾ cups	PREP: 5 minutes	WAIT: 4–12 hours

¾ cup of garlic apple cider vinegar

¾ cup of minced onion

⅓ cup of fresh hot green pepper, cored, seeded, and minced

3 tbsp. of minced fresh cilantro

2 garlic cloves, minced

1 tsp. of salt

1. Mix all of the ingredients together in a glass or ceramic dish.

2. Add the meat of your choice, and let it sit, tightly covered, in the refrigerator for 4 to 12 hours (see "Call on a Solo Performer," below, for details).

3. Remove 30 minutes before grilling or roasting. Then, cook to your desired doneness, and serve.

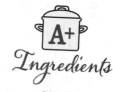

Ingredients

ONION
Fights coughs and colds

HOT GREEN PEPPER
Helps manage blood pressure

CILANTRO
Supports cardiovascular health

The rule of thumb for marinating any kind of meat or seafood is to soak it, tightly covered, in the refrigerator for 4 to 12 hours. Always remember to use a nonreactive dish, preferably glass or ceramic, and remove it from the fridge about 30 minutes before grilling time.

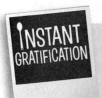

Call On a Solo Performer

To tenderize even the toughest kind of meat, simply marinate it in vinegar for 4 to 12 hours (the tougher the meat, the more time in the "drink" it'll need). Start with 4 hours, and then check the texture. If the meat still feels tough to the touch, let it sit for longer. Check back periodically until it is tender. Any kind of vinegar will do the softening job, but to add enticing flavor, go with an herb- or fruit-infused type.

COFFEE-MOLASSES MARINADE

Attention, coffee lovers! Are you ready for a pick-me-up? This surprising bold mix will give pork spareribs or chicken breasts a delicious java jolt.

YIELD: 2 ¼ cups	PREP: 5 minutes	COOK: 5 minutes

1 cup of strong coffee

½ cup of garlic red wine vinegar

¼ cup of Dijon mustard

¼ cup of unsulfured molasses

1 tbsp. of Worcestershire sauce

1. Combine all of the ingredients in a nonreactive pan and bring to a boil over medium heat.

2. Reduce the heat to low and simmer for about 2 to 3 minutes.

3. Cool to room temperature before transferring to a glass or ceramic dish. Add the meat, making sure all sides are coated with the marinade.

4. Refrigerate, tightly covered, for 4 to 8 hours, depending on the size of the meat.

A+ Ingredients

COFFEE
Helps support brain function

DIJON MUSTARD
Fights inflammation

MOLASSES
Boosts sexual health

KITCHEN CAPERS

If you have granite countertops in your kitchen, use caution when you are making marinades, dressings, or anything else that contains vinegar. It (or any other acidic substance) can damage the granite's protective sealant and it can also dull the finish.

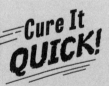
Cure It QUICK!

GIVE YOUR IMMUNE SYSTEM A BOOSTER SHOT
Your body relies on beta-carotene to fend off health woes ranging from cold and flu viruses to other more deadly diseases. Apricots rank among the top sources of beta-carotene, and this sweet-and-sour sauce is a delicious, fast way to tap into that protective power. To make it, puree four peeled and quartered apricots in a food processor, then blend in ½ cup of water, 2 tablespoons each of sugar and honey, and 1 tablespoon of lemon vinegar. Serve it immediately, or cover and refrigerate until you're ready to (for example) drizzle it over fresh peaches, ice cream, or angel food cake.

LUSCIOUS LEMON-ADE

If you love fish, then this marinade has your name written all over it. It's the perfect complement to firm, oily fish like salmon, halibut, or swordfish.

YIELD: 1 cup   **PREP:** 5 minutes   **COOK:** 10 minutes

½ cup of extra virgin olive oil

¼ cup of minced shallots

1 garlic clove, minced

¼ cup of minced fresh parsley

3 tbsp. of lemon thyme white wine vinegar

2 tbsp. of minced fresh lemon thyme

1. Warm the oil in a heavy, nonreactive skillet over medium heat.

2. Toss in the shallots and garlic, reduce the heat to low, and cook until softened, about 5 minutes.

3. Add the remaining ingredients and simmer for an additional 2 minutes.

4. Remove from the heat, let cool, and transfer to a glass or ceramic dish. Insert your fish pieces, and refrigerate, tightly covered, for 4 to 8 hours.

KITCHEN CAPERS

To rid your kitchen of unpleasant aromas caused by foods like garlic, onions, or fish, add ½ cup of white vinegar to a quart of water, and let it simmer (not boil) on the stove. Before you know it, the bad odors will be gone, baby, gone!

A+

Ingredients

EXTRA VIRGIN OLIVE OIL
Supports weight loss

PARSLEY
Promotes strong bones

LEMON THYME
Helps ease muscle pain

CULINARY Q & A

? I love salmon, but removing all those tiny bones seems all but impossible. Is there some trick to make it easier?

! You bet! First of all, add a pair of tweezers or needle-nose pliers to your kitchen collection just for bone-removing purposes. Second, to zero right in on the offending slivers, drape each fillet, flesh side up, over a large, curved bowl that's turned upside down. The bones will stick out of the fish so you can pluck 'em right out.

SAM HOUSTON'S ROOTIN' TOOTIN' BBQ SAUCE

General Sam Houston is best known as a military hero, president of the Republic of Texas, and, later, the state's first governor. But he was also an accomplished cook. According to numerous historical records, Sam created this recipe, and he whipped it up frequently. It's equally tasty on barbecued ribs, steaks, chops, or grilled chicken.

YIELD: about 4 cups	**PREP:** 10 minutes	**COOK:** 25 minutes

3 tbsp. of vegetable oil

¼ medium yellow onion, grated

2 garlic cloves, minced

1 cup of ketchup

¼ cup of lemon juice

¼ cup of Worcestershire sauce

2 tbsp. of apple cider vinegar

2 tbsp. of brown sugar

2 tsp. of paprika

1 tsp. of hot-pepper sauce

4 dried chile pequins, crumbled, or 1 tbsp. of chili powder

1 tbsp. of dry mustard

2 tsp. of water

Salt and black pepper to taste

1. Heat the oil in a medium-size pot on medium-low. Add the onion, stirring for 5 minutes.

2. Add the garlic and continue to stir for another 60 seconds. Stir in the next eight ingredients until they're thoroughly blended.

3. Mix the mustard with the water to form a smooth paste, and stir it into the pot.

4. Bring the contents to a boil, then turn the heat down to low, cover the pot, and simmer for 10 minutes.

5. Remove the lid and stir. Then replace the lid and cook for another 10 minutes.

6. Add salt and pepper, then brush the sauce onto the meat of your choice.

A+ Ingredients

KETCHUP
Boosts eye health

WORCESTERSHIRE SAUCE
Enhances digestion

CHILE PEPPERS
Clear head congestion

KITCHEN CAPERS

You can freeze just about any sauce or marinade. Pour the liquid into tight-sealing freezer bags, and lay them flat. Once the contents have frozen solid, stand the slim, trim packages straight up like file folders. They should keep all their tasty goodness for at least three months.

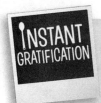

Last-Minute Marinade

Here's an almost-instant marinade for barbecued chicken pieces: Whirl 1 ½ cups of lemon vinegar, 2 crushed garlic cloves, ⅓ cup of extra virgin olive oil, 1 tablespoon of soy sauce, and 10 black peppercorns in a blender. Pour the marinade into a nonreactive baking dish, insert the chicken, and turn the pieces to coat both sides. Cover and refrigerate for 30 to 60 minutes. Remove it from the fridge about 30 minutes before cooking.

CULINARY Q & A

? When a recipe tells you to marinate something "overnight," just how long does it really mean?

! "Overnight" in cookbook jargon means a minimum of four hours, or longer if you'd like. Most marinades can go 24 hours or more with no problem at all. And sometimes, as with game or tough cuts of beef, longer is better. In cases where more precise timing is important, recipes will typically specify the optimum number of hours.

FRESHEN UP FAST!

The very same vinegar that removes unpleasant smells from the air can also eliminate food aromas from other odor collectors in your kitchen—namely these:

Odoriferous Surface	Your Action Plan
Cutting boards and wooden countertops	Simply wipe the surface with a sponge dampened with white vinegar. L'eau de garlic, onion, or fish will be a goner before you can say "goodbye!"
Plastic bowls or food-storage containers	Soak a slice of bread in vinegar, tuck it into the bowl or container, and cover the top tightly. Let it sit overnight, then toss out the bread, wash the item in soapy water, and it should smell as fresh as a daisy. If any slight odor lingers, repeat the process.*
Your hands	Sprinkle a little salt on your skin, and add a few drops of vinegar. Rub your "paws" together, then rinse with clear water, and wash your hands as usual.

* This trick also removes built-up food odors from lunch boxes and garbage cans.

SWEET-AND-TANGY BARBECUE SAUCE

This healthy homemade barbecue sauce is full of essential nutrients. It's perfect for beef, pork, or poultry, or even as a topping for baked potatoes.

YIELD: 2½ cups	**PREP:** 5 minutes	**COOK:** 15 minutes

1 cup of ketchup

½ cup of orange juice

⅓ cup of molasses

¼ cup of balsamic vinegar

Juice of 2 limes

2 tbsp. of brown sugar, lightly packed

1 ½ tbsp. of minced ginger

1 tbsp. of chili powder

½ tsp. of salt

1. Mix all of the ingredients together in a saucepan over medium heat.

2. Simmer for 15 minutes, stirring occasionally.

3. Remove the pan from the heat and let the sauce cool to room temperature before using. Store the sauce, covered, in the refrigerator, where it will keep for about three weeks.

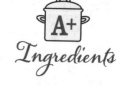

Ingredients

ORANGE JUICE
Helps fight free radicals

MOLASSES
Promotes skin health

LIME JUICE
Supports digestion

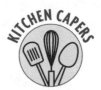
KITCHEN CAPERS

Any basting sauce that contains sugar, honey, molasses, or juice should be applied *after* the food is partially cooked. Otherwise, the sauce will burn before the vittles are done!

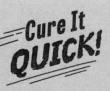
Cure It QUICK!

DELICIOUS DIABETES DODGER Numerous studies show that adding ½ to 1 teaspoon of cinnamon to your diet every day could be enough to help control your blood sugar levels and avoid type 2 diabetes, which is rapidly reaching epidemic proportions across our country. This sauce is one scrumptious way to get your daily dose. To make it, combine ¼ cup of sugar, 1 ½ tablespoons of water, 1 tablespoon of butter, ½ tablespoon of cinnamon, and 1 teaspoon of balsamic vinegar in a small microwave-safe container and microwave it on high for two minutes. Immediately drizzle the sauce over baked apples or fruit salad. **Note:** *If you already have either type 1 or type 2 diabetes, consult your doctor before you start dosing yourself with cinnamon—or anything else!*

SASSY BOURBON BASTING SAUCE

Apple cider vinegar is a health miracle in a bottle! And it lends intense flavor to this zesty sauce. Try it on chicken or ribs at your next backyard barbecue.

YIELD: about 2 cups   **PREP:** 5 minutes

1 cup of bourbon

1 cup of ketchup

¼ cup of apple cider vinegar

2 tsp. of Worcestershire sauce

½ tsp. of prepared mustard

2 garlic cloves, minced (optional)

Salt and freshly ground black pepper to taste

1. Whisk all of the ingredients together in a medium-size bowl.*

2. Brush the chicken or ribs with a thin coating of the sauce before putting them over the coals. Then baste several times as the meat cooks.

3. Drizzle the remainder onto your entrée just before you serve it up.

   * *You can either use the sauce immediately, or cover and refrigerate it until cooking time.*

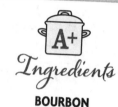

A+ Ingredients

BOURBON
Supports healthy weight loss

APPLE CIDER VINEGAR
Enhances digestion

WORCESTERSHIRE SAUCE
Boosts your mood

KITCHEN CAPERS

Commercial basting brushes can cost a pretty penny. So forget 'em! Instead, start a collection of natural-bristle paintbrushes in various sizes. Wash them with soap and water after each use, and store them, handles down, in an attractive container that you keep close at hand.

INSTANT GRATIFICATION

Baked Ham Glaze in a Flash

Nothing dresses up a baked ham like this quick glaze. To make it, simply whisk 1 cup of brown sugar, ⅓ cup of molasses, 3 tablespoons of apple cider vinegar, and 2 teaspoons of dry mustard in a small bowl. Several times during the last 45 minutes of baking, brush the ham with the sauce and the baking juices.

GINGERY MANGO BARBECUE SAUCE

This spicy winner uses the Marvelous Mango Vinegar on page 20. Give it a try the next time you grill chicken, ribs, or shrimp. You and your guests will love it!

YIELD: about 2 cups	**PREP:** 5 minutes

1 cup of ketchup

1 cup of raw honey

¾ cup of dark soy sauce

½ cup of Marvelous Mango Vinegar

1 tbsp. of finely grated ginger

1 tbsp. of minced garlic

1. Whisk all of the ingredients together in a bowl or large jar.

2. Cover tightly with a non-metallic lid and refrigerate for up to 3 weeks. Use it as you would any other barbecue sauce.*

* Don't use very high heat with this sauce or it's likely to burn; stick with the medium-high range or below.

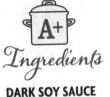

A+
Ingredients

DARK SOY SAUCE
Helps slow formation of free radicals

MANGOES
Boost libido

GINGER
Helps relieve inflammation

To add oodles of oomph to your barbecued creations, baste the meat using a brush made from sprigs of fresh parsley, sage, rosemary, and thyme tied onto the handle of a wooden spoon.

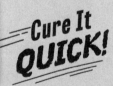

DELICIOUS VISION INSURANCE The leading cause of blindness in people over age 65 is age-related macular degeneration (ARMD). One secret to battling this dreaded disease is to eat plenty of dark, leafy greens, which contain lutein and zeaxanthin. These antioxidants strengthen your eyes' macula (a tiny spot in the center of your retina, which is critical for straight-ahead vision). One of the most potent sources of these vision guardians is kale, the star of this tasty sauce. To make it, mix 2 cups of kale, ¼ cup each of unfiltered apple cider vinegar and water, and 2 tablespoons of dry mustard in a blender or food processor. Enjoy this eye-protecting topper on chicken, fish, baked potatoes, or pasta. It also makes a delicious dip for crackers, corn chips, or raw veggies.

BASIL CREAM SAUCE

The fresh herbs in this creamy treat are full of folate as well as vitamins K, A, and C!
Try it drizzled on steamed vegetables or poured over grilled chicken or fish.

YIELD: about 2 ½ cups **PREP:** 5 minutes

1 cup of fresh basil

1 cup of fresh parsley

1 cup of pine nuts, toasted

8 oz. of cream cheese, at
room temperature

½ cup of freshly grated
Parmesan cheese

¼ cup of basil white
wine vinegar

¼ cup of extra virgin
olive oil

¼ cup of plain yogurt

1 tsp. of hot-pepper sauce

½ tsp. of salt

1. Combine all of the ingredients in a blender or food processor and process until smooth.

2. Serve immediately, or refrigerate and bring the sauce to room temperature before serving.

KITCHEN CAPERS Don't freeze Basil Cream Sauce or any recipe that contains sour cream, cream cheese, mayonnaise, or yogurt. In freezing temperatures, those ingredients tend to separate. While the taste may not change, the texture could be less than satisfactory.

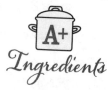

A+

Ingredients

BASIL
Fights bacteria

PINE NUTS
Boost energy

YOGURT
Fends off colds
and allergies

CULINARY Q & A

? It seems that every recipe I read that includes pine nuts says to toast them. What is the best way to do this?

! Pine nuts are great for vision and can boost your energy, too! To toast a small amount, set a small skillet over medium heat for a minute or so. Then add the nuts and toss them every few seconds to make sure they don't burn. They should be perfectly toasted in a minute or two.

For larger quantities, spread the nuts in a single layer on a heavy baking sheet. Bake at 350°F for about three to five minutes, or until they're golden in color and have a nutty aroma. Rotate the pan about halfway through so the nuts cook evenly.

CRAB SAUCE

This unique—but highly versatile—sauce pairs beautifully with shellfish, artichoke hearts, boiled potatoes, hard-boiled eggs, or cold or grilled fish.

YIELD: about 1 ½ cups   **PREP:** 10 minutes

2 tbsp. of white wine vinegar

1 cup of mayonnaise

2 tbsp. of freshly squeezed lemon juice

1 tbsp. of Dijon mustard

2 garlic cloves, minced

1 scallion (white and light green parts), minced

½ cup of canned flaked crab meat

1 tsp. of soy sauce

Salt and freshly ground pepper to taste

1. In a medium-size mixing bowl, beat the vinegar into the mayonnaise.

2. Whisk in the lemon juice, mustard, garlic, and scallion.

3. Stir in the crab meat and soy sauce, and season with salt and pepper to taste.

4. Serve at room temperature for best results.

KITCHEN CAPERS

To freeze sauce in individual portions, fill a muffin tin with silicone liners and fill each one with sauce, leaving ⅛ inch of room for expansion on top. Then pop the tin into the freezer. When it's frozen, "unwrap" the nuggets and transfer them to a freezer container.

A+

Ingredients

SCALLIONS
Boost immunity

CRAB MEAT
Enhances blood circulation

SOY SAUCE
Fights harmful bacteria

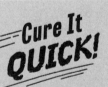

Cure It **QUICK!**

"BEET" HIGH BLOOD PRESSURE Beets are true superstars when it comes to maintaining healthy blood pressure. And this simple sauce is one of the best—and tastiest—ways to add them to your diet. To make about 2 cups, combine 1 cup of beets, 1 cup of grated horseradish (fresh or preserved in vinegar), ¼ cup of garlic or chili red wine vinegar, and 1 teaspoon of sugar in a nonreactive bowl. Mix thoroughly. Taste and add more vinegar or sugar if desired. Put the mixture in a glass jar with a tight-fitting lid, and refrigerate for 3 to 4 hours before using. This sauce goes with chicken, pork, or roast beef—either cooked or in a cold sandwich.

BÉARNAISE SAUCE

This French classic might seem fancy, but it's as easy to make as any other sauce. Try it on steak, spooned atop poached eggs, spread on fish, or drizzled over roasted potatoes.

YIELD: about 1–1 ½ cups   **PREP:** 20 minutes

¼ cup of dry white wine

¼ cup of white wine vinegar

1 tbsp. of dried tarragon

1 tbsp. of minced shallots

3 egg yolks

¼ tsp. of freshly ground black or white pepper

2 sticks of unsalted butter

2 tbsp. of minced fresh tarragon

Salt and pepper to taste

1. Combine the first four ingredients in a small saucepan and cook over medium heat until the liquid is reduced to about 2 tablespoons. Cool and strain into a bowl through a fine sieve or coffee filter.

2. In the top of a double boiler,* whisk the egg yolks until they're thickened. Add in the vinegar mixture and the pepper until the mixture is warm and thick enough that you can see the bottom of the pan between strokes and a light cream forms on the wires of your whisk.

3. Melt the butter in a separate pan, let it cool slightly, and then skim off the light foam that forms on top of the butter.

4. Add the melted butter (minus any solids at the bottom), 1 tablespoon at a time, to the egg mixture. Whisk continuously, making sure that each spoonful of butter is blended in before adding more.

5. Add the tarragon and season with salt and pepper to taste. Serve warm.

   * Or use a stainless steel bowl set over a pan with 2 inches of simmering water in it.

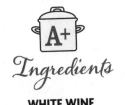

A+

Ingredients

WHITE WINE
Helps support healthy bones

EGG YOLKS
Boost heart health

TARRAGON
Enhances digestion

You can keep béarnaise sauce warm until serving time in one of two ways: Either turn off the heat under the water and keep the sauce in its container on top, or remove the bowl from the pan, and gently warm it over simmering water just before serving.

KITCHEN CAPERS

FRESH TOMATO & BASIL SAUCE

This no-cook pasta sauce is so easy to prepare! And it's packed with lycopene-rich tomatoes, which can help to reduce the risk of contracting deadly diseases.

YIELD: 4–6 servings	**PREP:** 20 minutes	**WAIT:** 1 hour

2 lbs. of fresh, ripe tomatoes, blanched, peeled, and chopped

1 cup of chopped fresh basil leaves

3 tbsp. of white wine (preferably sherry) vinegar

3 oz. of capers, drained and rinsed

Salt and freshly ground black pepper

1 cup of extra virgin olive oil

1. Combine the tomatoes and basil, and let them stand, covered, at room temperature for an hour or so.

2. Mix in the vinegar, capers, salt, and pepper.

3. Cook and drain your pasta* and toss it with the olive oil. Add the tomato sauce, toss again, and serve.

   * *This sauce goes best with angel hair or other thin, string-type pasta.*

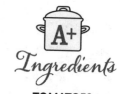

Ingredients

TOMATOES
Support cardiovascular health

BASIL
Helps maintain healthy vision

CAPERS
Help increase bone density

Fresh Tomato & Basil Sauce (above) is just as scrumptious as a topping for grilled chicken, baked potatoes, or almost any kind of quiche. In any of these cases, add the olive oil just after step 2, and mix well before using.

KITCHEN CAPERS

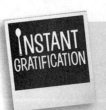

Pasta Sauce—on the Double!

When you need to dress up some linguine, fettuccine, or ravioli—*right now*—here's how to do it: Mix a container of high-quality, refrigerated basil or kale pesto with grape tomatoes, a teaspoon or so of minced garlic from a jar, and a tablespoon of wine vinegar (either plain or herb-infused). You'll have a five-star fine-dining experience in five minutes flat!

CAPONATA SAUCE

This Italian classic comes straight from Sicily, where they *really* know pasta—and where folks routinely live healthy, happy, and active lives well into their senior years.

YIELD: 6–8 servings	PREP: 20 minutes	COOK: 20 minutes

2 medium eggplants, diced

⅓ cup of extra virgin olive oil

1 can (16 oz.) of diced tomatoes, drained

1 medium onion, chopped

2 celery ribs, chopped

1 bell pepper (red, yellow, or orange), diced

Salt to taste

¾ cup of black olives

2 tbsp. of slivered almonds

3 tbsp. of sugar

½ cup of red wine vinegar

1. In a large saucepan, sauté the eggplant in the oil until softened. Remove with a slotted spoon and set aside.

2. Add the tomatoes, onion, celery, and pepper to the pan, and sauté until the onion becomes transparent.

3. Add salt to taste, and mix in the olives, almonds, and eggplant.

4. In a small bowl or measuring cup, dissolve the sugar in the vinegar. Pour the blend into the pan, and stir to mix the ingredients.

5. Cover, and simmer for 10 minutes. Pour the sauce over pasta, and enjoy!

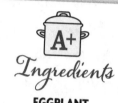

A+ Ingredients

EGGPLANT
Aids weight-loss efforts

CELERY
Helps fight free radicals

OLIVES
Help support healthy bones

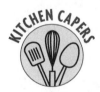

KITCHEN CAPERS

Leftover Caponata Sauce (above) is a delicious salad topping. Toss it with arugula, a bit of extra virgin olive oil, and red wine vinegar, and dig in!

CULINARY Q & A

? My grandma used to always add salt to eggplant to make it less bitter. Is that step really necessary?

! No. Most varieties of eggplant on the market today have had the bitterness bred out of them, so there's no salt needed. Plus, here's a bonus—they are an excellent source of vitamins and minerals across the board, too!

SUN-DRIED TOMATO PESTO

If you've only had the premade sun-dried tomato pesto from the grocery store, do yourself a favor and give this DIY version a try. You'll never use the packaged stuff again!

YIELD: 4 servings   **PREP:** 20 minutes

4 oz. of sun-dried tomatoes

¼ cup of chopped pine nuts

3 tbsp. of chopped onion

2 tbsp. of chopped fresh basil

2 tbsp. of chopped fresh parsley

1 tbsp. of chopped garlic

⅓ cup of crushed tomatoes

¼ cup of balsamic vinegar

¼ cup of red wine

1 tbsp. of tomato paste

½ cup of extra virgin olive oil

½ cup of freshly grated Parmesan cheese

1. Put the sun-dried tomatoes in a bowl, cover them with warm water, and let sit for 5 minutes, or until tender.

2. In a food processor or blender, combine the sun-dried tomatoes, pine nuts, onion, basil, parsley, and garlic until well blended.

3. Add the crushed tomatoes, vinegar, red wine, and tomato paste. Process again.

4. Pour the mix into a bowl. Stir in the olive oil and Parmesan cheese, and season with salt to taste.

Keep a new wooden spoon from absorbing food odors: Before the first use, soak it overnight in apple cider vinegar. The next morning, dry it off and your next batch of cookies won't taste like pesto!

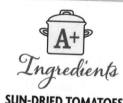

A+ Ingredients

SUN-DRIED TOMATOES
Help prevent anemia

ONIONS
Boost immunity

PARMESAN CHEESE
Regulates blood pressure

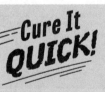

Cure It QUICK!

HAVE A (HEALTHY) HEART Cooked tomatoes, garlic, and extra virgin olive oil are all renowned for fighting off heart disease—and other serious illnesses, too. This quick and easy sauce is a tasty way to enjoy the benefits: Sauté 3 minced garlic cloves in ½ cup of olive oil until lightly golden. Add a 16-ounce can of diced tomatoes (drained) and 2 ½ teaspoons of dried rosemary. Cook on the stove for about 12 minutes. Then, remove the sauce from the heat, stir in 2 teaspoons of balsamic vinegar, and toss it with your favorite pasta!

TIMELY TRADE-OFFS

Uh oh! You are ready to whip up a delicious meal, but find that you are out of one key ingredient—vinegar! What do you do now? Well, there's no need to get your apron in a twist. Just reach for this handy chart of go-to substitutes! (And here's another tip: You might want to make a copy of it and tuck it into one of your favorite cookbooks, so you can always find it at a moment's notice.)

AWOL Vinegar	Pinch Hitter (per 1 tablespoon)
Apple cider	1 tablespoon of either lemon or lime juice or 2 tablespoons of white wine
Balsamic	1 tablespoon of either brown rice or Chinese black vinegar *or* ½ teaspoon of sugar per tablespoon of apple cider or (preferably) red wine vinegar
Champagne	1 tablespoon of either white wine or rice vinegar*
Herb vinegar	1 tablespoon of either wine, rice, or apple cider vinegar plus 1 or 2 teaspoons of chopped fresh herbs
Malt vinegar	1 tablespoon of either lemon juice or apple cider vinegar
Raspberry vinegar	1 tablespoon of sherry vinegar
Red wine vinegar	Equal parts of white vinegar and red wine
Sherry vinegar	1 tablespoon of white wine vinegar *or*, if you don't need the acidic property of vinegar, 1 tablespoon of red or white wine
White vinegar	1 tablespoon of either lemon or lime juice
White wine vinegar	1 tablespoon of rice vinegar

* *Champagne vinegar is very mild, so don't substitute any stronger type.*

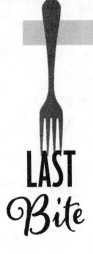

DRESSING, MARINADE, & SAUCE SECRETS

4 KEYS TO SALAD DRESSING SUCCESS

Whether you're making a simple oil and vinegar blend or a multiple-ingredient creation, this trio of tips will ensure the best possible results:

1. The magic word is *quality*. Any dressing—or sauce—is only as good as the ingredients it's made from, so always use the best ones you can find.

2. Think "last-minute marvel." For most salads, you want to apply the dressing at the last minute. Otherwise, the vinegar will soak the greens, and they'll become unpleasantly limp and soggy. The two exceptions: marinated-vegetable salads and "wilted" salads, in which a heated dressing is designed to soften up the leafy greens (some fine examples of both are coming up in Chapter Three).

3. While there are exceptions (as noted in the relevant recipes), most dressings are at their peak of flavor if you make them just before serving time.

4. To save cleanup time, don't make your salad dressing in a mixing bowl. Instead, whisk the ingredients together in the bottom of your serving bowl. Then add your greens and other salad components and toss them thoroughly.

CULINARY Q & A

? I've learned the hard way that the wine vinegars and other flavored types my supermarket sells are sorely lacking in flavor. But I don't have the time—or frankly, the inclination—to make all the kinds I like to use in cooking. Aren't there good commercial vinegars I can buy somewhere?

! You bet there are! In fact, flavored "craft vinegars" have become downright trendy, for both cooking and mixing in cocktails. Specialty food shops and small online retailers sell so many different kinds it makes your head swim. Just search for "buy flavored vinegars [name of your town]" and up will pop scads of suppliers—both web-based and local brick-and-mortar versions—where you can buy top-quality flavored vinegars (and oils, too).

INTENSIVE CARE FOR HARD-WORKING CUTTING BOARDS

Day after day, cutting boards pick up food residue and odors galore. That's especially true when you're working with pungent marinade and sauce ingredients like onions, garlic, and hot peppers. Here are two simple ways to get rid of them both:

The slower version. After you use the board for the last time at night, spray it with full-strength vinegar. Overnight, the potent acid will work its cleansing magic. Come morning, rinse the board with clear water, and you'll be good to go.

Faster action. Give the board a good rubdown with baking soda. Then spray the surface with full-strength vinegar (the mix will bubble up for a moment or so and then subside). Let it sit for 10 minutes, and then rinse.

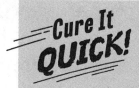

ANTI-ASTHMA MARINADE Since as far back as the 1600s, medical gurus have been touting the miraculous lung-clearing prowess of what is essentially garlic marinated in a vinegar-honey mixture. Taking this potent syrup consistently just may keep you free of asthma symptoms. To make it, put the peeled cloves of three garlic bulbs in a nonreactive pan with 2 cups of water, and simmer until the garlic cloves are soft and there is about 1 cup of water left in the pan. Using a slotted spoon, transfer the garlic to a jar that has a tight-fitting lid. Add 1 cup of apple cider vinegar and ¼ cup of raw, organic honey to the water in the pan, and boil the mixture until it's syrupy. Pour the syrup over the garlic in the jar, put the lid on, and let it sit for at least eight hours. Then every morning on an empty stomach, swallow one or two garlic cloves along with 1 teaspoon of the syrup.

CUSTOMIZE YOUR BARBECUE SAUCE

When there's no time to make barbecue sauce, a splash of vinegar will perk up a jar of the store-bought stuff lickety-split. But don't stop there. Depending on what you have on hand, you can give the mix even more down-home flavor. For example, toss in minced garlic, green pepper, and onion; red pepper flakes or hot sauce; Worcestershire or soy sauce; horseradish or spicy brown mustard; minced red or green tomatoes; or a dollop of honey, molasses, or brown sugar.

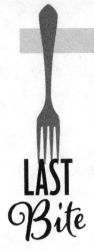

LAST Bite

KEEP GARLIC AT THE READY

In theory, fresh, dried garlic will keep for up to several months in a cool, dark place. But real life conditions being what they are, those bulbs often go belly-up before their time. The simple solution: Preserve your garlic, whether it is homegrown or store-bought, in vinegar. If you do, it will keep for up to a year in the refrigerator. And unlike the stuff you buy in jars at the supermarket, it will retain its full fresh flavor, no problem. Here's the ultra-easy preservation procedure:

1. Break the garlic heads apart, peel the cloves, and put them in a large mixing bowl filled with cool water.

2. Clean the cloves with your fingertips to remove any dirt, and cut off any brown spots using a small paring knife.

3. Transfer the cleaned garlic to a colander or large strainer. Rinse the cloves thoroughly, and put them into small, sterilized glass jars. (Half-pint canning jars, with either plastic or clamp-style glass lids are perfect.)

4. Bring white vinegar* to a boil in a large nonreactive pot. Immediately pour the vinegar over the garlic and close the jar lids tightly.

5. Let the jars sit until they reach room temperature, and then stash them in the refrigerator. Or, if you prefer, process them in a hot-water bath or pressure canner, and store them at room temperature (see page 144 for the simple details).

Roughly 1 cup of vinegar for each half-pint jar should be plenty, but it's always smart to err on the side of caution and boil a little more than you think you'll need.

Even if you don't have toddlers at home—or grandbabies—it's a smart idea to have a plastic sippy cup easily accessible in your kitchen. Why? It's an ideal tool for making and dispensing salad dressings! Just add all the ingredients to the cup, put your thumb over the spout, and shake until the ingredients are emulsified. Then drizzle the dressing through the spout onto your salad.

KITCHEN CAPERS

CULINARY Q & A

? I've always heard that eggs yolks are fattening and unhealthy. But now there seems to be conflicting opinions. Is this really true?

! Absolutely not! That relic of the fat-phobic days has been debunked big-time. Now we know that eggs are packed with nutrients that are essential for good health. For older adults, egg yolks are especially valuable for two reasons: One, folks of a certain age often have a mild iron deficiency, which can lower their energy level. That, in turn, can lead to less physical activity. Egg yolks provide this essential mineral in a more absorbable form than iron supplements can. Two, a single egg yolk contains about 40 IUs of vitamin D, which teams up with calcium to promote bone health and decrease the risk for fractures and osteoporosis.

PRESERVE FRESH HERBS: A THIRD OPTION

If you grow your own herbs or routinely buy them in quantity, you know that drying and freezing are both excellent ways to preserve your bounty. But did you know that you can also do the job with vinegar? Here's all there is to it:

- Loosely pack sterilized jars with the fresh herbs (one type per jar unless you want to create specific combos).

- Pour in enough warmed vinegar to cover the tops by 1 inch, making sure that all of the leaves are immersed.

- Store the jars at room temperature, away from light and sources of heat, and use the herbs in the same quantities as dried herbs. They should stay in fine fettle for several years.

Note: *Basil and tarragon are especially good candidates for vinegar storage.*

SOAK BEFORE YOU MIX

When you're adding dried herbs to a salad dressing or other cold mixture, give them a flavor boost by mixing them with just enough hot water to moisten the herbs. Then set them aside for about 15 minutes before using. You'll be amazed at the difference it makes!

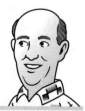

Chapter Three

Scrumptious
Salads

In Chapter Two, you found hordes of ways to use vinegar in marinades, sauces, and—of course—salad dressings. But that was just the beginning! Here, you'll learn how to put this miraculous taste treat to work in salads ranging from simple appetizer courses to hearty main-dish creations. The roster includes new takes on classic recipes like potato salad and coleslaw, as well as off-beat—and surprisingly delicious—combos you've probably never thought of before.

KALE & YUKON GOLD POTATO SALAD

This hale and hearty salad is jam-packed with color, flavor, and five-star nutrition. Serve it as a main dish or as a side and enjoy the leftovers the next day.

YIELD: 6 servings   **PREP:** 10 minutes   **COOK:** 25 minutes

1 lb. of petite Yukon Gold potatoes, halved

¼ cup of extra virgin olive oil, divided

1 shallot, halved and sliced

¾ lb. of asparagus, trimmed and cut into 1-inch pieces

7 cups of chopped green curly kale (1-inch pieces), with tough ribs and stems removed

¼ cup of plain Greek yogurt

¼ cup of white balsamic vinegar

Salt, freshly ground black pepper, and sugar to taste

½ cup of chopped scallions

¼ cup of chopped walnuts

3 tbsp. of Gorgonzola cheese (more or less to taste)

1. Toss the potatoes with 1 tablespoon of the oil and half of the shallot slices.

2. Spread evenly on a baking sheet, set it in the upper third portion of the oven, and roast for 15 minutes at 450°F.

3. Add the asparagus and roast for 10 minutes, or until the potatoes are golden brown and tender.

4. While the vegetables are roasting, boil the kale in 1 inch of water, tossing constantly with tongs, until the kale is bright green and slightly wilted. Drain off the excess water.

5. To make the dressing, combine the yogurt and vinegar with the remaining olive oil and shallot slices using a blender or small food processor. Add salt, pepper, and sugar to taste.

6. Toss the potatoes, asparagus, and kale with the dressing in a serving bowl, and top with the scallions, walnuts, and cheese.

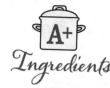

A+

Ingredients

YUKON GOLD POTATOES
Help calm anxiety

ASPARAGUS
Promotes healthy brain function

KALE
Helps support immune system

KITCHEN CAPERS Never use hand-painted dishes to serve a salad with a vinegar-based dressing. Vinegar will corrode the paint, which could ruin your treasured dishes, and could also release harmful toxins into the food.

CULINARY Q & A

? How can I prolong the life of my fresh herbs?

! It's easy! First, untie the herbs and immerse them in cool water, shaking gently to dislodge any debris. Clip off any broken or browned leaves. Gently shake off the excess water, but don't use a salad spinner; it'll bruise the leaves. Next, put the stems in a container of water, with the leaves just above the rim. Cover the leaves loosely with a plastic bag and place in the fridge (unless it's basil, then leave uncovered and keep at room temperature, where it will stay fresh for up to a month). Change the water when it looks murky, and snip off the bottoms of any stems that start to decay.

CHILLED-HERB LIFE SPAN

Most common herbs will keep their fresh, tasty, and health-giving goodness if you follow the refrigeration game plan described in the Culinary Q & A (at left).

Herb	Life Expectancy
Cilantro	2 weeks
Mint	1 month
Oregano	1 month
Rosemary	6 weeks
Sage	1 month
Tarragon	2 weeks
Thyme	6 weeks

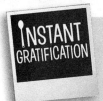

INSTANT GRATIFICATION

Super Food—Super Fast

Kale has earned kudos from coast to coast for its astounding ability to help detoxify your system, boost weight loss, protect your immune system, improve your vision, and help fight deadly diseases—and that's just for starters. Here's an ultra-quick way to put that firepower to work: Remove the stems from a bunch of Tuscan kale, tear the leaves into bite-size pieces, and put them in a nonreactive bowl. Using your fingers, massage 2 teaspoons of sea salt or kosher salt into the kale and let it sit for 5 minutes. Add 4 peaches (pitted and sliced), ¼ cup of extra virgin olive oil, ¼ cup of sherry vinegar, 3 ounces of feta cheese, and a pinch of crushed red pepper flakes. Toss to coat the ingredients evenly, and divide your super salad into four portions before serving.

FRENCH CARROT SALAD

This simple, tasty salad is a classic in southern France, and for good reason: Besides tasting sweet and delicious, it delivers a full load of carrots' health-giving benefits for your lungs, liver, blood, and digestive system. Plus, the parsley boosts your kidney and adrenal functions, and the mint helps eliminate bad bacteria in your body.

YIELD: 4–6 servings   **PREP:** 10 minutes

1 lb. of carrots, grated

2 tbsp. of extra virgin olive oil

1 tbsp. of lemon vinegar

1 garlic clove, finely chopped (optional)

Pinch of sea salt

3 tbsp. of finely chopped fresh flat-leaf parsley

1 tbsp. of chopped fresh mint

1. In a large mixing bowl, toss the carrots, oil, vinegar, garlic, and salt together.

2. Transfer the salad to a serving bowl or to individual bowls.

3. Whichever serving style you choose, sprinkle the parsley and mint on top.

A+

Ingredients

CARROTS
Keep skin healthy

PARSLEY
Promotes strong bones

MINT
Aids digestion

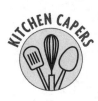

KITCHEN CAPERS

Flat-leaf parsley holds its own in a dressed salad. It's also the easiest kind to chop. Rinse it thoroughly in cold water and spin it dry. It'll stay fresh and crisp in a salad spinner for several days. For easy chopping, pull the leaves from the stalks and mass them into a pile.

CULINARY Q & A

? I've noticed carrots in unusual colors showing up at our local supermarket. Are they interchangeable in recipes, or do they all taste different?

! Yes, there is some flavor variation among the different colors, but it's extremely subtle, which means that any type or color of carrot will work just fine interchangeably. You can even add several different colored carrots to make a recipe especially festive. Try it with the French Carrot Salad recipe, above!

MALTY MUSTARDY COLESLAW

Cabbage is one of the world's healthiest foods, full of vitamins K, C, and B$_6$, plus potassium, calcium, fiber, and folate. And malt vinegar further amps up the nutrition!

YIELD: 8 servings	PREP: 15 minutes	WAIT: 1 hour or more

1 head of shredded green cabbage

1 head of shredded red cabbage

1 large carrot, coarsely grated

1 small red onion, thinly sliced

1 cup of mayonnaise

½ cup of malt vinegar

¼ cup of coarse-grain mustard

2 tbsp. of sugar

Juice of 1 lemon

1. Combine the first four ingredients in a large bowl.

2. In a smaller bowl, whisk together the mayonnaise, vinegar, mustard, sugar, and lemon juice to make the dressing.

3. Toss the slaw with the dressing, and season to taste with a dash of salt and pepper.

4. Cover and refrigerate for at least an hour before serving.

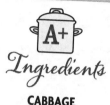

A+ Ingredients

CABBAGE
Fights inflammation

MAYONNAISE
Enhances digestion

MALT VINEGAR
Promotes a healthy heart

KITCHEN CAPERS

If you have trouble digesting raw onions, just marinate them in sherry vinegar for an hour or so before you add them to a salad or sandwich.

Cure It QUICK!

LOWER STROKE RISK? Medical studies have shown that simply getting 20 milligrams of zinc each day can greatly enhance your recovery from a stroke. What's more, you don't need to take supplements. You can easily get your quota or more simply by eating plenty of zinc-rich foods, like the lentils in this super-quick salad. To make it, rinse and drain a 19-ounce can of lentils. Then mix them in a bowl with ½ cup of chopped red onion, 2 tablespoons of chopped cilantro, and 1 tablespoon of chopped basil. Toss the ingredients with your favorite vinaigrette dressing, and you'll be on the fast track to recovery!
Note: *Other plentiful sources of zinc include plain yogurt, lean meat, oysters, and crab.*

SPINACH SALAD WITH ONIONS & ORANGES

We all need iron in our diets to maintain the oxygen supply in our blood. Spinach, onions, and red wine vinegar are all rich in that essential mineral, plus other vital nutrients, too. This salad is a simple, delicious way to help meet your quota.

YIELD: 4 servings	PREP: 10 minutes

5-6 cups of baby spinach

1 cup of mandarin oranges, drained

½ cup of chopped red, Vidalia®, Texas Sweet, or Walla Walla onions

2 tbsp. of red wine vinegar

1 tbsp. of orange marmalade

⅓ cup of extra virgin olive oil

1. Arrange the spinach leaves on four plates, and distribute the orange sections and onions among them.

2. Whisk the vinegar and marmalade together. Gradually add the oil as you continue to whisk.

3. Pour the dressing over the salad, serve it up, and add salt and pepper to taste.

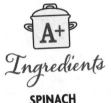

A+ Ingredients

SPINACH
Promotes healthy vision

ORANGES
Help maintain kidney health

ONIONS
Fight inflammation

KITCHEN CAPERS

To liven up limp spinach, or any other kind of salad greens, add 1 teaspoon of white or apple cider vinegar to a pan of water, and let the greens soak in it for 15 minutes. They'll be as fresh and crisp as new!

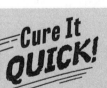
Cure It QUICK!

DANDY DANDELION DETOX SALAD Believe it or not, the humble (some would say noxious) dandelion ranks in the top tier of foods that help fight toxins in your body by ramping up the action of your liver—your body's major detoxifying organ. To put this surprisingly tasty superpower to work for you, simply mix fresh, young dandelion greens with a dressing made from 1 cup of olive oil, ⅓ cup of apple cider vinegar, and salt and freshly ground black pepper to taste. **Note:** *You can buy organically grown greens in specialty-food shops and farmers' markets. If you pick your own supply from a yard or a vacant lot, make sure the area has not been exposed to high levels of airborne pollutants and has not been treated with any chemicals!*

IF YOU CAN'T BEAT 'EM, EAT 'EM!

Dandelion greens aren't the only weeds that make fine additions to salads or to many of the soups, stews, and casseroles you will find in upcoming chapters. Here is a small sampling of other delicious weed winners.

Tasty Weed	Part(s) to Eat	Flavor	How to Enjoy It
Chickweed	Leaves and stems	Mild spinach	Toss in salads; add to soups or stews.
Chicory	Young leaves and roots	Tangy and bitter	Toss leaves in salads; boil or bake young roots and use as you would potatoes.
Pigweed	Leaves and seeds	Mild leaves; nutlike, crunchy seeds	Toss young leaves in salads or use on sandwiches; use older leaves in cooked dishes; sprinkle ripe black seeds on sweet breads, muffins, or cookies.
Purslane	Leaves and stems	Sweet-and-sour	Toss in salads.
Queen Anne's lace (a.k.a. wild carrot)	Roots	Mild carrot	Chop and add to salads or soups.
Shepherd's purse	Basal leaves	Peppery	Chop and add to salads.

Note: *Some of these plants can cause allergic reactions if you consume large quantities. So enjoy them as occasional treats, not as part of your daily diet. And avoid anything that's been treated with chemicals.*

SPINACH-APPLE SALAD

Here's a nugget of nutritional trivia for you: The synergistic combo of spinach and apples delivers a jolt of energy to your body and also helps ease any pain in your muscles or joints. But you don't have to be tired or aching to enjoy this scrumptious salad.

YIELD: 4 servings	PREP: 15 minutes

2 apples, cored and diced

4 tbsp. of freshly squeezed lemon juice, divided

3 tbsp. of extra virgin olive oil

2 tbsp. of raw honey

1 tbsp. of unprocessed apple cider vinegar

8 cups of baby spinach leaves

Salt and ground black pepper to taste

2/3 cup of crumbled goat cheese

1/2 cup of walnuts

1. Toss the apples with 2 tablespoons of the freshly squeezed lemon juice.

2. Whisk the remaining juice with the oil, honey, and vinegar.

3. Combine the spinach, apples, and dressing, and divide among four bowls. Season with a dash of salt and pepper to taste.

4. Top with the cheese and nuts, and dig in!

A+

Ingredients

APPLES
Help ease joint pain

GOAT CHEESE
Promotes skin health

WALNUTS
Boost your mood

KITCHEN CAPERS Whenever you've served a salad—or any other menu item—that leaves oily, greasy, or sticky residue on your dishes, add 1/2 cup of vinegar to the washing-up water. Whether you do the job by hand or in the dishwasher, the vinegar will cut right through the stubborn stuff.

CULINARY Q & A

? Is goat cheese better for me than the kind made from cow's milk?

! In many ways, yes. Cheese made from goat's milk has some major feathers in its cap. First, it has less than half the sodium of "regular" cheese. It's also richer in vitamins D, K, and the whole B group, and has a greater concentration of calcium. Finally, it's extremely low in lactose, which makes it an ideal choice for lactose-intolerant cheese lovers.

BROCCOLI & MUSHROOM SALAD

For maximum impact, put this salad together about an hour before you intend to serve it, so all the flavors have time to mix and mingle. Then just re-toss, and dig in!

YIELD: 6 servings   **PREP:** 40 minutes

¼ cup of white wine vinegar

2 tbsp. of extra virgin olive oil

1 tbsp. of lemon vinegar

2 tsp. of minced fresh thyme

2 scallions with tops, thinly sliced

2 garlic cloves, minced

Salt and freshly ground black pepper to taste

2 cups of broccoli florets (either fresh or frozen)

2 cups of sliced mushrooms

1. Make the dressing by whisking the first seven ingredients together in a small bowl. Let sit for about 30 minutes so the flavors can blend.

2. Steam the broccoli until it's just tender-crisp—about 3 minutes. Dip it in cold water to stop the cooking and set the color. Drain and put in a medium-size bowl.

3. Add the mushrooms, pour on the dressing, and toss to coat thoroughly. Serve salad at room temperature.

A+ Ingredients

GARLIC
Fights cold and flu germs

BROCCOLI
Helps relieve allergy symptoms

MUSHROOMS
Support healthy weight loss

KITCHEN CAPERS Whenever you steam vegetables, add 2 tablespoons of vinegar to the water. It will ensure that the veggies retain more color and vitamins and also eliminate any unpleasant odors.

INSTANT GRATIFICATION

Easy Beet & Onion Salad

You can whip this salad up in a flash, then let it sit while you fix the rest of your meal—or get ready for your guests to arrive. Drain a 29-ounce can of sliced beets and put them in a bowl. Add 1 large red onion, sliced and separated into rings, and top that with ⅛ teaspoon of garlic salt, a pinch of oregano, and salt and freshly ground black pepper to taste. Combine 2 tablespoons of extra virgin olive oil, 1 tablespoon of red wine vinegar, and ½ teaspoon of sugar in a bottle. Pour the dressing over the salad, and chill it in the refrigerator for at least an hour before serving.

RED BEANS & RICE SALAD

Red beans and rice are as much a part of New Orleans as riverboats and Dixieland jazz. Well, here's that Crescent City classic in salad form. Try it— one bite will have you tappin' your toes and clappin' your hands for more.

YIELD: 4 servings	PREP: 20 minutes	WAIT: 3–4 hours

½ lb. of turkey sausage in casings

1 cup plus 3 tbsp. of garlic red wine vinegar

1 can (15 or 16 oz.) of red beans, drained and rinsed

1 cup of cooked brown rice

½ cup of diced red pepper

½ cup of peeled, seeded, and diced cucumber

¼ cup of diced celery

¼ cup of thinly sliced scallions

1 tbsp. of extra virgin olive oil

1 tbsp. of minced fresh thyme

2 tsp. of coarse-grain mustard

1 garlic clove, minced

½ tsp. of hot-pepper sauce

Salt and freshly ground black pepper to taste

1. Combine the sausage and 1 cup of the vinegar in a nonreactive pan, and bring to a boil over medium heat.

2. Cover, reduce the heat to low, and simmer for 5 minutes, or until the sausage is thoroughly cooked. Remove the sausage from the pan, and cut it into 1-inch pieces.

3. In a large nonreactive bowl, mix together the sausage with the beans, rice, red pepper, cucumber, celery, and scallions.

4. In another bowl, whisk together the 3 tablespoons of vinegar and the remaining ingredients. Pour over the bean mixture, and toss until all ingredients are well coated.

5. Cover and refrigerate for 3 to 4 hours before serving to allow the flavors to blend.

A+ Ingredients

TURKEY SAUSAGE
Supports red blood cell function

RED BEANS
Aid weight loss

THYME
Helps relieve asthma

KITCHEN CAPERS Once they're past babyhood, some vegetables, including cucumbers, kale, lettuce, carrots, and broccoli, can be somewhat coarse, fibrous, or stringy. The easy solution: Before you use them in a salad, sprinkle them with vinegar. It'll soften them right up!

BLACK BEAN SALAD

Besides being absolutely scrumptious, this nutrient-packed salad is a superstar addition to a heart-healthy diet. It makes an especially snazzy side dish, but it is also delicious on its own, served with warm, crusty French bread.

YIELD: 4–6 servings   **PREP:** 15 minutes   **WAIT:** 3 hours

2 cans (15 or 16 oz. each) of black beans, drained and rinsed

1 cup of cherry tomatoes, quartered

½ cup of cooked corn

½ cup of diced sweet red pepper

½ cup of diced sweet yellow pepper

½ cup of thinly sliced scallions

¼ cup of minced fresh cilantro

2 tbsp. of diced jalapeño pepper

¼ cup of sherry vinegar

2 tbsp. of dry sherry

2 tbsp. of extra virgin olive oil

1 tbsp. of minced fresh marjoram

1 tsp. of coarse-grain mustard

½ tsp. of ground cumin seeds

½ tsp. of hot-pepper sauce

1. Combine the first eight ingredients in a large nonreactive bowl.

2. Whisk the remaining ingredients together in a small nonreactive bowl to make the dressing.

3. Pour the dressing over the bean mixture and toss to coat thoroughly.

4. Cover and refrigerate for at least 3 hours so the flavors can blend.

KITCHEN CAPERS To rinse canned beans without damaging them, set the can upside down in the sink, and use a can opener to punch three small holes in the bottom. Flip the can over, remove the top, and hold the open can under cool, gently running water, letting it flow over the beans for several seconds. Then just pour the beans directly into your dish!

INSTANT GRATIFICATION

How Sweet It Is!

Here is an ultra-quick and healthy salad idea: Add roasted sweet potato slices (maybe left over from last night's dinner) and pecans to a plateful of mixed baby greens and top it with balsamic vinegar.

A+

Ingredients

BLACK BEANS
Help maintain healthy blood pressure

CORN
Promotes eye health

SHERRY
Fights coughs and colds

SWEET POTATO SALAD

Sweet potatoes are delicious and healthy in any dish. But this easy, versatile salad will quickly become a year-round favorite—guaranteed to be the hit at any party!

YIELD: 8–12 servings   **PREP:** 10 minutes (including cook time)

3 large sweet potatoes (about 1 lb.), peeled and cut into bite-size cubes

¼ cup of extra virgin olive oil

2 tbsp. of apple cider vinegar

2 tbsp. of Dijon mustard

¼ cup of diced onion

½ rib of celery, thinly sliced

½ small red bell pepper, diced

1. Boil the sweet potatoes in a covered pan until they're just tender enough to pierce with a fork (about 8 to 10 minutes—no longer!).

2. While the potatoes are cooking, mix the oil, vinegar, and mustard in a small bowl to make the dressing.

3. Drain the potatoes into a large bowl, and toss them with the onion, celery, bell pepper, and dressing. Add salt and pepper to taste.

Ingredients

SWEET POTATOES
Fight inflammation

CELERY
Supports liver health

RED BELL PEPPER
Promotes eye health

KITCHEN CAPERS

When you're cooking potatoes or sweet potatoes for use in salads, add a spoonful of vinegar to the cooking water. The taters will stay nice and firm—just the way you want them.

CULINARY Q & A

? What is the difference between sweet potatoes and yams?

! Although their names are often used interchangeably, yams and sweet potatoes belong to completely different plant families. Yams have a white flesh and are rarely found in most grocery stores, except for some ethnic markets, while the orange-fleshed veggies that you may see labeled "yams" at your local grocery store are actually sweet potatoes. Sweet potatoes also contain triple the amount of beta-carotene, which converts to vitamin A in the body and is important for a healthy immune system and normal vision.

SPICY RICE SALAD

This lively mix delivers a major jolt of delicious health power. The brown rice provides a rich dose of whole-grain fiber, while the black currants offer up a boatload of vitamins, minerals, and antioxidants. The pistachios give your heart a big boost, and the array of spices helps protect you against woes ranging from cold viruses to dreaded diseases.

YIELD: 4 servings	**PREP:** 60 minutes	**WAIT:** 3–4 hours

1 ½ cups of water

1 tsp. of salt

¾ cup of long-grain brown rice, uncooked

1 tbsp. of minced fresh ginger

½ cup of dried black currants*

Boiling water

¼ cup of extra virgin olive oil

¼ cup of finely chopped red onion

¼ cup of toasted pistachios

3 tbsp. of sherry vinegar

½ tsp. of ground allspice

¼ tsp. of ground cinnamon

¼ tsp. of ground nutmeg

* Or substitute red zante currants (a variety of raisin), which are commonly sold in supermarkets.

1. Bring the water and salt to a boil in a saucepan over medium-high heat. Stir in the rice and ginger and return to a boil. Cover, reduce the heat to low, and simmer for 45 minutes, or until the rice is cooked.

2. Put the currants in a small, heat-proof bowl and cover with boiling water. Let them sit for 20 minutes, then drain.

3. Combine the currants and rice with the remaining ingredients in a large nonreactive bowl, and toss everything together until thoroughly coated.

4. Cover, and put in the refrigerator for 3 to 4 hours before serving. Then toss one more time, and enjoy!

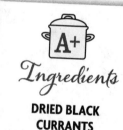

A+

Ingredients

DRIED BLACK CURRANTS
Promote brain function

PISTACHIOS
Aid weight loss

CINNAMON
Boosts metabolism

KITCHEN CAPERS When you're shopping for pistachios, look for ones with slightly opened shells. These are easier to open, and the gap indicates mature, ripe nuts. To toast them quickly, remove the shells and heat the nuts in a skillet over medium heat, stirring constantly to prevent scorching.

QUICK CUCUMBER SALAD

Rice vinegar is a staple in many traditional Asian dishes, but it also makes an excellent addition when tossed with tasty fresh cucumber in this super salad.

YIELD: 6 servings   **PREP:** 10 minutes

3 cups of peeled, thinly sliced seedless cucumbers

3 tbsp. of rice vinegar*

2 tsp. of dark sesame oil

1 tsp. of sugar

½ tsp. of salt

2 tbsp. of chopped dry-roasted, unsalted peanuts

2 tbsp. of chopped green onion

* *Japanese rice vinegar has a light, delicate taste. For a robust flavor, use a Chinese variety.*

1. Combine the first five ingredients in a bowl, and then toss until the cucumber slices are thoroughly coated.

2. Transfer the mixture evenly to salad plates to serve, and sprinkle with the peanuts and chopped green onion to garnish. Then dig right in!

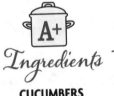

A+

Ingredients

CUCUMBERS
Boost immunity

SESAME OIL
Supports oral health

PEANUTS
Help support weight loss

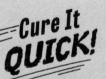

Cure It
QUICK!

THE SALAD THAT COULD SAVE YOUR LIFE
And it couldn't be simpler to make. Slice an avocado, and top it with a dressing made from balsamic vinegar and extra virgin olive oil (the exact proportions are your call). This treat is a great health booster because avocados contain both beta-sitosterol and glutathione. Beta-sitosterol inhibits the absorption of cholesterol from your intestines into your bloodstream, which can cut your risk of heart disease. It can also reduce inflammation, boost immunity, and may hinder the development of diseases. Glutathione is a powerful antioxidant that boosts the immune system, encourages a healthy nervous system, helps slow the aging process, and may help prevent heart disease, as well as other serious issues.

CABBAGE-APPLE SLAW

Remember the Ravishing Rose Hip Vinegar recipe (see page 21) in Chapter One? Well, it's the perfect addition to this out-of-the-ordinary slaw. And if you've never tried the tangy-sweet combo of cabbage and apples, you're in for one humdinger of a taste treat!

YIELD: 4 servings   **PREP:** 15 minutes   **WAIT:** 1 hour

2 cups of shredded green cabbage

2 cups of shredded red cabbage

½ cup of mayonnaise

¼ cup of sour cream

2 tbsp. of rose hip vinegar*

½ tsp. of celery seed

½ tsp. of kosher or sea salt

⅛ tsp. of freshly ground black pepper

1 large sweet apple, unpeeled, cored, and sliced into thin slivers

2 tbsp. of finely chopped fresh flat-leaf parsley

* Or substitute apple cider vinegar.

1. Combine the green and red cabbage in a large bowl and set aside.

2. In a medium bowl, whisk the next six ingredients to create the dressing, and then stir in the apple.

3. Pour the dressing over the cabbage and toss gently until thoroughly coated.

4. Cover and refrigerate for at least an hour. Then sprinkle the parsley on top just before serving.

KITCHEN CAPERS No sour cream? No worries! In a blender, mix 1 cup of cottage cheese, ¼ cup of milk, and 1 teaspoon of vinegar until creamy. You may like the DIY version so much that you'll never go back to the store-bought stuff!

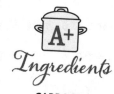

A+

Ingredients

CABBAGE
Promotes good digestion

ROSE HIP VINEGAR
Enhances skin health

APPLES
Support heart health

CULINARY Q & A

? I can never manage to slice avocados neatly for my salads. Is there an easy, no-fail trick to it that I haven't discovered?

! Yep! Just cut the fruit in half lengthwise, all the way around the pit. Lift off the top half, and remove the seed. Cut the flesh of each half into strips or chunks, then gently lift each piece out of the skin with a pointy spoon.

BROCCOLI-NUT SALAD

Your family and guests will shout, "More, more!" when they taste this guaranteed crowd pleaser. (Just don't tell any kids in the crowd that it's also one of the healthiest collections of food that you could put on your plate!)

YIELD: 6–8 servings   **PREP:** 15 minutes   **COOK:** 15 minutes

2 bunches of fresh broccoli florets, cut into bite-size pieces

1 lb. of bacon, cooked crisp and crumbled

1 cup of golden raisins

1 cup of pecan pieces*

¼ cup of thinly sliced red onion

1 cup of mayonnaise

½ cup of sugar

¼ cup of white wine vinegar

Or substitute your favorite nuts.

1. Mix the first five ingredients together in a large bowl and set aside.

2. In a small bowl, mix the remaining ingredients until well blended to make the dressing.

3. Pour the dressing over the broccoli mixture in a serving bowl, and toss gently. Then serve, and enjoy!

A+

Ingredients

BROCCOLI
Supports liver health

RAISINS
Fight tooth decay

PECANS
Aid weight loss

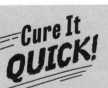

KITCHEN CAPERS

To stop onion tears in their tracks, just sprinkle vinegar generously over the surface of the cutting board before you start slicing the bulb. Besides reducing the flow of the onion's tear-generating chemicals, the vinegar will minimize the onion odor on the board, too.

Cure It QUICK!

ROAST CALORIES FAST Trying to shed pounds? If so, then the Tuscan Panzanella recipe (at right) has your name written all over it. The reason: Red, yellow, and orange bell peppers can boost your metabolic rate, thereby ramping up your body's calorie-burning power. Granted, your quick fix does need to marinate for a while, but you can put it together in a flash—if you have a stash of roasted peppers all ready to go (see the Culinary Q & A box, at right).

TUSCAN PANZANELLA

This classic bread salad has long been a favorite in Tuscany. With its delicious mix of garlic, tomatoes, basil, roasted red peppers, it's easy to see why!

YIELD: 4–6 servings   **PREP:** 35 minutes   **WAIT:** 30 minutes

1 loaf of stale Italian bread

1 cup of extra virgin olive oil

2 garlic cloves, peeled and mashed

4 tbsp. of red wine vinegar

Sea salt and ground black pepper

1 lb. of ripe red plum tomatoes, blanched and quartered

4 bell peppers (red and yellow), roasted, peeled, and cut into strips

½ cup of pitted black olives

5 tbsp. of capers

3 oz. of anchovies

1 bunch of fresh basil, thinly torn

1. Chop the bread into pieces, and put it in a large nonreactive bowl.

2. In a small spouted bowl, mix the oil with the garlic and 2 to 3 tablespoons of the vinegar.

3. Pour the mix over the bread. Season it with salt and pepper, and stir. Add more vinegar if desired.

4. Mix in the remaining ingredients. Let the combination sit for 30 minutes to develop full flavor, then serve.

A⁺ Ingredients

BELL PEPPERS
Boost eyesight

BLACK OLIVES
Help relieve allergies

ANCHOVIES
Aid in maintaining heart health

KITCHEN CAPERS The salty taste of anchovies can be overwhelming. So to reduce the harshness, simply soak them in milk for about 30 minutes. Then pull them out, dry them off, and toss them into your salad!

CULINARY Q & A

? I have always been intimidated by any recipes that call for roasted peppers. What is an easy way I can prepare them?

! Cut a small slit near the stem of each pepper. Broil or grill the peppers until the skin has blackened. Seal them in ziplock bags to steam for about 15 minutes. Remove stems, cores, and seeds, and scrape off skins. Chop and use as needed.

POTATO & ARTICHOKE SALAD

Serve up this fresh—and highly healthy—take on potato salad at your next outdoor cookout. It pairs well with any grilled meat, and as an added bonus, it's full of essential nutrients and antioxidants, too.

YIELD: 10–12 servings	PREP: 45 minutes	WAIT: 3–24 hours

1 ½ lbs. of new potatoes

⅔ cup of plain yogurt

½ cup of mayonnaise

1 tbsp. of lemon vinegar

1 ½ tsp. of dried tarragon

1 tsp. of sharp prepared mustard

2 garlic cloves, minced

Salt and black pepper to taste

1 can (13 ¾ oz.) of artichoke hearts, drained and quartered

1 cup of frozen baby peas

1 cup of thinly sliced celery

½ cup of pitted and halved black olives

4–6 scallions with tops, finely snipped

3 tbsp. of minced fresh parsley

Fresh tarragon for garnish

Paprika for garnish

1. Bring a large pot of water to a boil. Add the potatoes and cook just until fork tender (20 to 25 minutes). Drain and set aside.

2. While the potatoes are cooking, make the dressing by whisking the yogurt and mayonnaise together in a small bowl. Add the vinegar, dried tarragon, mustard, and garlic, and whisk again. Season to taste with the salt and pepper.

3. When the potatoes are cool enough to handle, cut them into bite-sized cubes and put them in a large bowl.

4. Mix in all the remaining ingredients, except for the garnish. Pour the dressing on top, and toss to coat thoroughly. Cover and refrigerate for at least 3 hours and up to 24 hours.

5. Sprinkle the fresh tarragon and paprika on top and serve.

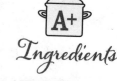

A+ Ingredients

ARTICHOKE HEARTS
Help support liver health

CELERY
Maintains healthy blood pressure

BLACK OLIVES
Fight free radicals in body fat

KITCHEN CAPERS When a recipe calls for fresh garlic, use garlic vinegar instead. One teaspoon of it is equivalent to a small garlic clove. Make your own supply to keep on hand with the easy recipe in Chapter One (see "Herbal Vinegar All-Stars" (on page 15), or simply use 12 garlic cloves per quart of white or red wine vinegar.

New Life for Old Potato Salad

If you have a hankering for cooked spuds, and you've got leftover potato salad in the refrigerator, you're in luck! Simply preheat your oven to 425°F (or plug in your toaster oven). Then put the salad into a cast-iron skillet, and bake it for about 30 minutes, shaking the pan every 10 minutes or so to loosen it up, until the potatoes are golden brown. Then spoon the mix onto a plate and dig in!

CULINARY Q & A

? It always seems that when I'm in a hurry to make a salad or other recipe, I don't have all the types of herbs it calls for. Are there any good substitution guidelines?

! Yes, and they couldn't be simpler: You can substitute mild-flavored herbs like parsley and chives for any other kind at any time. Or, you can also use dried herbs in place of fresh, or vice versa. See the Culinary Q & A box on page 48 for the right formula.

COLOR UP FOR HEALTH!

Here's a stunning factoid for you: Each year, the average American eats more than 130 pounds of potatoes. If you're one of those spud lovers, that gives you an easy—and delicious—way to power up your health. How? Just swap at least part of your white-potato intake for the more colorful types that contain two valuable nutrients. The winners below (and others) are turning up in more and more local supermarkets and farmers' markets—so toss 'em in your cart!

Colorful Spuds	Powerful Nutrients	Superstar Varieties
Pink, red, blue, and purple	Anthocyanins—the same phytonutrients that give many berries their potent antioxidant kick	Mountain Rose, Rose Gold, All Red, Ruby Crescent, All Blue (a.k.a. Purple Marker), Purple Viking
Yellow	Carotenoids that give a rocket boost to essential vitamin A action	Yukon Gold, Saginaw Gold, Yellow Finn, Carola, Charlotte

PESTO POTATO & PEA SALAD

If you like pesto, you'll love this vinegar-spiked version served with vitamin-rich Yukon Gold potatoes. For the utmost in flavor, prepare this salad at least 4 hours ahead of time.

YIELD: 4–6 servings	PREP: 35 minutes	WAIT: 4–24 hours

½ cup of freshly grated Parmesan cheese

¼ cup of firmly packed, coarsely chopped fresh basil leaves

2 tbsp. of balsamic vinegar

2 tbsp. of red wine vinegar

½ tsp. of salt

¼ tsp. of ground black pepper

¾ cup of extra virgin olive oil

10 medium Yukon Gold potatoes (about 2 lbs.), unpeeled

2 celery ribs, cut into ⅛-inch-thick slices

1 cup of frozen baby peas, thawed

1. To make the pesto, mix the first six ingredients in a blender, gradually adding the olive oil until the combination is smooth.

2. Bring a large pot of water to a boil. Add potatoes and cook, uncovered, until they can be pierced with the tip of a knife (about 20 minutes).

3. Drain the potatoes and rinse under cold water until cool enough to handle. Cut into ½-inch-thick slices and put them in a medium-size bowl.

4. Add the celery, peas, and ¾ cup of the pesto. Toss, cover, and refrigerate for at least 4 hours.

5. Toss with the remaining pesto, and season to taste with salt and pepper. Serve chilled.

KITCHEN CAPERS

To clean blenders and small appliances, wipe the surface with a soft cloth that's dampened with white vinegar. Buff dry with another cloth. Never spray vinegar on the casing; it could seep inside and damage internal parts.

A+

Ingredients

BASIL
Fights inflammation

YUKON GOLD POTATOES
Help maintain strong bones

BABY PEAS
Boost immune system

Cure It QUICK!

RAISE YOUR GLASS TO RED! Red wines contain antioxidants that help to heal and protect your body. They also help to ward off diseases, including heart problems and lung disease. So pour yourself a glass a couple times a week to enjoy the benefits, or simply try the Pesto Potato & Pea Salad (above) for a dose of red wine vinegar!

PATRIOTIC POTATO SALAD

When the new potatoes start rolling in—whether you dig 'em up from your own garden or buy 'em at the farmers' market—here's a dandy way to celebrate: Just run Old Glory up the flagpole, and serve this red, white, and blue salad.

YIELD: 4–6 servings   **PREP:** 30 minutes

2 lbs. of small blue, red, and white potatoes

½ cup of dry rosé wine

⅔ cup of extra virgin olive oil

⅔ cup of minced fresh parsley

½ cup of thinly sliced scallions or shallots

6 tbsp. of white wine vinegar

2 tbsp. of minced fresh summer savory, rosemary, and/or chervil

4 tsp. of Dijon mustard

Salt and freshly ground black pepper to taste

1. In a saucepan, cook the potatoes in boiling water until just fork tender—about 20 minutes (don't overcook!), and drain.

2. Cut them into ¼-inch-thick slices, put in a bowl, and sprinkle with wine.

3. In a small bowl, combine the remaining ingredients to make the dressing, and mix well.

4. Toss the potatoes with the dressing, and serve warm or chilled.

Ingredients

BLUE AND RED POTATOES
Help healthy digestion

WHITE POTATOES
Support brain health

ROSÉ WINE
Promotes cardiovascular health

KITCHEN CAPERS If you're not certain that the rosé you're about to choose is dry, ask an expert wine shop clerk for guidance. Contrary to what you may have heard, you cannot tell a sweet rosé from a dry one simply by glancing at the color of the wine or checking the label for the alcohol content.

CULINARY Q & A

? Is there any way to get rid of white, cloudy spots on stainless steel saucepans and pots? They won't come off in the dishwasher or with any cleanser I've tried.

! Those unattractive (but harmless) splotches are mineral deposits left after boiling hard tap water. Simply wipe them with a half-and-half solution of white vinegar and warm water. Repeat the process periodically.

CALIFORNIA COBB SALAD

This salad was born when Bob Cobb, owner of the renowned Brown Derby restaurant, threw it together for a friend, who showed up unexpectedly for a late-night meal.

YIELD: 4 servings   **PREP:** 10 minutes

2 cups of bite-size chunks of cooked chicken

4 slices of bacon, cooked crisp and crumbled

2 hard-boiled eggs, finely chopped (a generous ½ cup)

3 cups of torn romaine lettuce leaves

1 cup of torn curly endive leaves

1 cup of watercress leaves (about 1 bunch)

3 scallions, thinly sliced

1 large avocado, chopped

1 large tomato, chopped

¼ cup of crumbled blue cheese

⅔ cup of balsamic vinaigrette

Freshly ground black pepper

1. Cook the chicken, bacon, and eggs if you don't already have these on hand.

2. Toss the lettuce, endive, and watercress together in a bowl.

3. Place the next three ingredients on top of the greens, and sprinkle the blue cheese on top.

4. Toss the salad with the vinaigrette, top with black pepper, and serve.

A+

Ingredients

CHICKEN
Maintains healthy blood pressure

WATERCRESS
Boosts immunity

AVOCADO
Encourages deep, restful sleep

KITCHEN CAPERS Instead of cooking chicken for the recipe above, pick up a rotisserie chicken at the supermarket. Just pull the meat off the bones, and freeze any extra in recipe-size portions, so you'll always have some on hand.

Cure It QUICK!

HAVE A (HEALTHY) HEART According to cardiac health pros, tomatoes are one of the most heart-healthy foods of all. So are broccoli, spinach, and walnuts—so let's put them together! Just mix 1 cup of fresh broccoli florets, 1 cup of torn spinach leaves, ½ cup of sun-dried tomatoes, and ½ cup of chopped walnuts in a bowl, and toss it all with red wine vinaigrette dressing (another heart-pleasing champ). Add salt and pepper to taste, and serve!

FEED-A-HUNGRY-BUNCH SALAD

This substantial salad rose to fame during World War II, when it was a major go-to recipe for serving at meetings and working parties for wartime public service groups.

YIELD: 12 servings	PREP: 30 minutes	COOK: 30–40 minutes

1 lb. of macaroni

2 qts. of water

1 tsp. of salt

¼ cup of apple cider vinegar

⅓ cup of mayonnaise

2 tbsp. of light corn syrup

¼ tsp. of ground black pepper

2 cups of diced cooked ham

1 cup of chopped celery

¼ cup of chopped pimento

¼ cup of chopped scallions

3 cups of salad greens

2 tomatoes, cut into wedges

1. Boil the macaroni in salted water until tender (about 12 minutes). Drain, reserving ½ cup of the liquid.

2. Immediately combine the macaroni and vinegar in a large bowl, and set aside.

3. In another bowl, mix the mayonnaise, corn syrup, and pepper. Gradually stir in the cooking liquid you saved. Add the macaroni, ham, celery, pimento, and scallions. Cover and refrigerate until chilled.

4. Put the greens on a platter and spoon the macaroni mixture into the center, and arrange the tomato wedges around the outside.

A+ Ingredients

MACARONI
Supports weight loss

HAM
Boosts immunity

SALAD GREENS
Help relieve anxiety

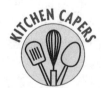

KITCHEN CAPERS Don't confuse corn syrup with high-fructose corn syrup (HFCS), which is being blamed for scads of rampaging health woes. Classic corn syrup is perfectly safe to consume—in moderation, of course.

CULINARY Q & A

? I love to use boiled ham in salads, but it often makes the mixture taste overly salty. Is there any way to avoid that?

! There is—and it's easy! Simply add 2 tablespoons of either white or apple cider vinegar to the water that you boil the ham in. It'll draw out some of the salty taste and perk up the flavor to boot!

AGE-DEFYING EGG SALAD

Eggs rank high on the list of the world's healthiest—and most youth-enhancing—foods. This is one of the easiest ways to enjoy the good taste and bountiful benefits of hen fruit.

YIELD: 1 serving	PREP: 10 minutes	WAIT: 20 minutes

2 eggs

½ tbsp. of mayonnaise

½ tbsp. of prepared mustard

1 tsp. of balsamic vinegar

4–6 grape tomatoes, halved

½ tbsp. of diced red onion

Salt and ground black pepper to taste

1. Hard-boil two eggs, or grab two eggs that have already been hard-boiled. Separate the yolks from the whites.

2. Mash the yolks and mix them with the mayonnaise, mustard, and vinegar in a bowl until blended.

3. Stir in the tomatoes and onion. Chop the egg whites, and fold into the mix. If necessary, add more mayonnaise, mustard, and/or vinegar for moisture. Season to taste with the salt and pepper.

4. Sandwich the mixture between two slices of whole-grain bread, or enjoy it on its own.

A+ Ingredients

MAYONNAISE
Boosts heart health

GRAPE TOMATOES
Support a healthy immune system

RED ONION
Helps balance blood sugar

KITCHEN CAPERS

While vinegar is renowned as a kitchen-cleaning star, it does have its limits. If you're cleaning up a raw egg spill, it'll only make the problem worse. Vinegar will permanently set in fabric stains left by eggs, ice cream, butter, milk, grease, and more. So use traditional cleaners for those jobs.

CULINARY Q & A

? What's the best way to peel the shell from a hard-boiled egg without gouging the egg white? I always have trouble!

! Here's an easy trick: First, tap the egg against the counter, then roll the egg gently back and forth. Keep doing so until the egg's shell is cracked all over. Find the end of your egg that has a small pocket of space between the white and the shell, and start peeling there. The shell will come off in neat strips every time.

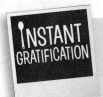

Turkey Bird Dinner Take 2

The day after you enjoy a roasted turkey for dinner, grab any leftovers, and turn them into this quick, easy, and ultra-healthy salad. In a medium-size bowl, mix 2 cups of diced turkey with 1 cup of seedless grapes, ½ cup of chopped pecans, ¼ cup of chopped fresh parsley, 2 sliced celery ribs, 3 tablespoons of mayonnaise, and 2 teaspoons of balsamic or apple cider vinegar. This salad, spooned between two slices of hearty, whole-grain bread, makes one of the tastiest sandwiches you could ever ask for. You can also eat it by itself or even wrapped in lettuce leaves. This recipe makes two to four servings, but you can multiply the ingredients to suit the amount of turkey and the number of hungry mouths you have on hand.

LET'S HEAR IT FOR HEN FRUIT!

The humble egg is one of the healthiest foods you can add to a salad—or consume in any other way. That's especially true for aging adults. The reason: As we get older, our appetites tend to shrink, so it's important to make sure that everything going into our bodies benefits the bottom line in some way. And each egg is a neatly "wrapped," versatile, and easily digestible package containing seven essential assets.

Anti-Aging Nutrient	How It Helps Your Bottom Line
Choline	Boosts memory and cognition and helps reduce chronic inflammation, which has been linked to Alzheimer's disease
Iron	Drives energy production
Protein	Essential for timely tissue repair and renewal (including efficient wound healing)
Selenium	Important for maintaining a strong immune system and proper thyroid function
Tryptophan	Converted by your body into mood-lifting and sleep-inducing serotonin
Vitamin B_{12}	Essential for red blood cell production
Vitamin D	Joins with calcium to promote bone health and decrease the risk for fractures and osteoporosis

BELGIAN ENDIVE & FENNEL SALAD

This crisp, substantial salad is perfect for the cold days of winter. The offbeat veggies offer up a flavorful surprise—and boatloads of disease-fighting nutrients.

YIELD: 4 servings   **PREP:** 10 minutes

4 heads of red Belgian endive,* broken into pieces

1 fennel bulb, thinly sliced

8 oz. of mustard greens, roughly torn into pieces

1 pear,** cored and thinly sliced

6 tbsp. of extra virgin olive oil

4 tbsp. of white wine vinegar

2 tsp. of whole-grain mustard

Sea salt and freshly ground black pepper

1 tbsp. of chopped fresh flat-leaf parsley

1 tbsp. of slivered almonds, toasted

* Or substitute radicchio.

** Or substitute a crisp apple.

1. Arrange the endive pieces on a serving plate, and add the fennel, mustard greens, and pear.

2. Whisk the extra virgin olive oil, white wine vinegar, whole-grain mustard, salt, and pepper together to make the dressing, and pour it over the salad.

3. Sprinkle the parsley and almonds on top to garnish. Then serve!

A+ Ingredients

BELGIAN ENDIVE
Maintains digestive health

MUSTARD GREENS
Help fight free radicals

PEARS
Aid weight loss

KITCHEN CAPERS

When your mustard, ketchup, or mayo has dwindled to less than the amount called for in a recipe, dribble a spoonful of vinegar into the container, and shake it hard. There's a good chance that the vinegar will add just enough liquid to get you what you need.

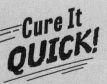

Cure It QUICK!

LOSE THE BLUES SALAD Feeling down in the dumps? Just mix up an easy green salad that has a vinegar-based dressing, like the one above—or use leftover potato salad—and mix some borage flowers into it. These pretty blooms are surefire cheerer-uppers. Besides being a mood lifter and a taste treat, borage packs a good supply of calcium and potassium. (For more on edible flowers, see "Looks Good Enough to Eat!" on page 103.)

A-TAD-TOO-EARLY HONEYDEW SALAD

Whether you grow melons in your garden or buy them at the market, it's hard to know for sure when they're fully ripe. When you have a honeydew that's underripe, don't compost it—toss it into this sensational salad. (The firm texture makes this salad such a treat.)

YIELD: 6 servings   **PREP:** 15 minutes

4 cups of cubed, slightly underripe honeydew melon

1 cup of diced celery

1 cup of finely diced sweet red pepper

1 cup of toasted walnuts

4 tbsp. of lime juice

½ cup of extra virgin olive oil

4 tbsp. of minced fresh parsley

2 tbsp. of white wine vinegar

2 tsp. of honey

Salt and freshly ground black pepper to taste

1. Toss the first five ingredients together in a large salad bowl and set aside.

2. Whisk the remaining ingredients together, and pour over the melon mixture. Toss to coat.

3. Serve immediately, or cover and refrigerate until serving time.

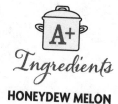

A+

Ingredients

HONEYDEW MELON
Hydrates your body

WALNUTS
Boost your mood

LIME JUICE
Promotes healthy digestion

KITCHEN CAPERS To toast walnuts, shell them and spread them in a single layer on a baking sheet. Bake at 350°F, stirring once or twice, until lightly browned and fragrant (10 to 12 minutes).

CULINARY Q & A

? How can I easily tell if a honeydew melon is ripe before I purchase it, and is there a way to make it ripen at home?

! Melons will not ripen off the vine, so look for the following signs when you're buying. The outside of a honeydew should be dull looking and pale in color; a shiny or green exterior is a sign that it's underripe. Next, check the end where the vine was attached. It should feel slightly soft and have a sweet fragrance. Finally, try tapping the melon with the palm of your hand. If you hear a hollow sound, it's ripe. Otherwise, give it a pass.

PERFECTLY PLEASING PINEAPPLE SALAD

There's no salad that's easier or more versatile than this refreshing winner. The mildly tangy dressing will complement just about any entrée. Plus, tossing in a handful or two of rotisserie chicken chunks would make it a meal in itself.

YIELD: 6 servings	**PREP:** 10 minutes	**WAIT:** 30 minutes

1 can (8 oz.) of unsweetened pineapple slices

1 tbsp. of extra virgin olive oil

1 tbsp. of raw honey

1 ½ tsp. of apple cider vinegar

1 ½ tsp. of soy sauce

6 cups of torn romaine lettuce

½ cup of thinly sliced red onion

1. Drain the pineapple, reserving the juice. Cut the slices in half and set aside.

2. Pour the oil, honey, vinegar, soy sauce, and reserved juice into a jar with a tight-fitting lid to make the dressing. Shake vigorously to blend thoroughly, and refrigerate for at least 30 minutes.

3. Combine the lettuce, onion, and pineapple in a serving bowl. Drizzle with the dressing and toss to coat.

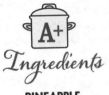

A+ Ingredients

PINEAPPLE
Boosts immunity

RAW HONEY
Promotes memory

ROMAINE LETTUCE
Helps build
healthy bones

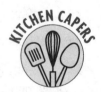

KITCHEN CAPERS

Don't discard the outer leaves of romaine lettuce. Just wash them to remove all the grit. The reason: The outer leaves have the highest concentration of phytonutrients and antioxidant properties.

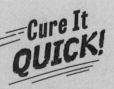

Cure It QUICK!

BERRY DELICIOUS BRAIN BOOSTER Scientific studies show that eating berries regularly can improve your memory, enhance general brain function, delay cognitive aging, and possibly reduce your risk of developing Parkinson's disease. Here is one simple and scrumptious way to enjoy that gray-cell firepower: Gently mix 1 cup each of raspberries and blueberries with a dozen large strawberries (all washed and dried). Add ¼ cup of sparkling red wine, 4 tablespoons of sugar (more or less to taste), and 2 teaspoons of balsamic vinegar. Stir to mix, cover, and refrigerate for two to three hours before serving. (This recipe makes approximately four servings.)

FROZEN CUCUMBER SALAD

A frozen salad?! Yes, indeed. This tasty concoction is perfect for summertime, plus it's packed with B vitamins from the cucumbers, which are known to help ease feelings of anxiety and can reduce the damaging effects of stress.

YIELD: 4 servings	PREP: 20 minutes	WAIT: 24 hours

7 cups of thinly sliced cucumber

3 medium onions, thinly sliced

1 green pepper, chopped

1 red pepper, chopped

2 cups of sugar

1 cup of apple cider vinegar

1 tbsp. of salt

1 tsp. of celery seed

1. Mix all of the ingredients thoroughly in a large bowl.

2. Cover and refrigerate for 24 hours.

3. Transfer the mixture, including the liquid, to a container,* and freeze for up to 3 months or so.

4. To serve, simply defrost, either in the refrigerator or at room temperature.

   * Or use four single-serving containers.

A+ Ingredients

CUCUMBER
Promotes healthy skin

GREEN PEPPER
Supports nervous system health

CELERY SEED
Enhances the quality and duration of sleep

KITCHEN CAPERS

If you're freezing leftovers or made-ahead meals, store them in rectangular or square containers with flat lids. They'll stack neatly, and they'll nestle right into the corners of your freezer, giving you lots of room for other foods!

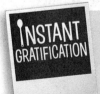

INSTANT GRATIFICATION

Italian Summer Salad

Celebrate summer with this quick and easy classic! Slice a couple of red, ripe, fresh-from-the-vine tomatoes. Alternate and overlap them on a platter with thin slices of fresh mozzarella cheese. Sprinkle chopped fresh basil leaves on top, followed by kalamata olives. (The quantities depend on the size of your platter and the crowd you're feeding, but the more you use of each ingredient, the better.) Drizzle a balsamic vinaigrette over the top, and season with salt and pepper. Let the salad sit for 15 minutes at room temp before serving.

CROWD-PLEASING MEDITERRANEAN ORZO SALAD

The balsamic vinegar in this salad provides you with a huge helping of antioxidants that can repair damage caused by free radicals and protect the body from harmful diseases.

YIELD: about 20 servings   **PREP:** 30 minutes

- ¼ cup of balsamic vinegar
- 1 tsp. of brown mustard
- 1 tsp. of salt
- ½ tsp. of ground black pepper
- ½ cup of extra virgin olive oil
- 16 oz. of orzo pasta (a.k.a. risoni), cooked, drained, and cooled to room temperature
- 1 cup of pitted kalamata olives, chopped
- 4 scallions, chopped
- 2 roasted red peppers, seeded and chopped
- 1 medium summer squash, diced (¼-inch pieces)
- 1 medium zucchini, diced (¼-inch pieces)
- ½ red onion, minced
- ½ lb. of feta cheese, crumbled

1. To make the dressing, whisk the vinegar, mustard, salt, and black pepper together in a small bowl. Slowly add the olive oil while stirring. Set aside.

2. In a large bowl, combine the remaining ingredients. Add the dressing and cheese, toss to coat well, and serve.

3. If you aren't planning to serve the salad right away, cover and refrigerate.

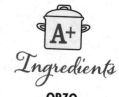

A+

Ingredients

ORZO
Boosts your energy

ZUCCHINI
Helps maintain heart health

FETA CHEESE
Aids weight loss

KITCHEN CAPERS If you chill a dressed salad, always taste it before serving—even if it was fine before it went into the fridge. After a while, the flavors absorb into the salad, and it may need additional seasonings.

CULINARY Q & A

? Every time I make a pasta salad I follow the recipe perfectly, but it comes out bland. What am I doing wrong?

! Nothing! When you add sauce or dressing to chilled pasta, some of the flavor can be absorbed. To combat this, simply add more vinaigrette dressing. You'll also be adding extra essential nutrients as a bonus!

TOMATO-WATERMELON SALAD

Watermelon is mostly water, but it also contains a boatload of lycopene, vitamins, antioxidants, and amino acids! Put it to work in this unique summer salad.

YIELD: 4 servings	PREP: 30 minutes	WAIT: 3 hours

3 tbsp. of apple cider vinegar

2 tbsp. of extra virgin olive oil

Freshly ground black pepper to taste

4 cups of diced seedless watermelon

2 cups of halved cherry tomatoes

1 scallion, chopped

½ English cucumber, diced

½ cup of crumbled feta cheese

¼ cup of chopped fresh mint

1 tbsp. of chopped fresh cilantro

1. In a small bowl, whisk the vinegar, oil, and pepper together to make the dressing, and set aside.

2. Combine the remaining ingredients in a large bowl until mixed well.

3. Add the dressing to the mixture and toss to coat thoroughly.

4. Cover and put in the refrigerator for about 3 hours before serving.

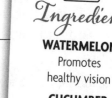

A+
Ingredients

WATERMELON
Promotes healthy vision

CUCUMBER
Boosts hydration

MINT
Supports digestion

Fruits like strawberries, blueberries, and raspberries add a burst of flavor—and a health boost—to green salads. Fresh pineapple and citrus fruits team up well with dark, leafy greens, such as spinach and kale.

KITCHEN CAPERS

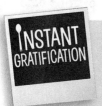

INSTANT GRATIFICATION

Blue on Blue Salad

If you like blueberries and blue cheese, you'll love this nourishing treat. To make six servings, mix 4 cups of your favorite lettuce mixture, torn into bite-size pieces; 1 cup of fresh blueberries; and 1 cup of diced blue cheese. Toss it with ½ cup of vinaigrette dressing. White wine, apple cider, and balsamic vinegars all make delicious toppers, or make your dressing using blueberry vinegar. Buy it from a craft-vinegar supplier, or make your own with the recipe for Berry Lovely Vinegar on page 18. Use 1 cup of fresh blueberries for every 2 cups of white wine vinegar.

WHITE BEAN & PASTA SALAD

White beans are full of disease-fighting dietary fiber and protein.
Whip them up with pasta in this hearty salad, and you won't be sorry.

YIELD: 4 servings   **PREP:** 20 minutes

½ lb. of penne or other short pasta

⅓ cup of extra virgin olive oil

¼ cup of chopped fresh flat-leaf parsley

2 tbsp. of red wine vinegar

1 garlic clove, minced

Salt and freshly ground black pepper to taste

1 can (16 oz.) of cannellini beans, drained and rinsed

4 scallions, finely chopped

1 cup of shredded radicchio

¼ cup of black olives

1. Cook the pasta for 7 to 10 minutes, until it's tender but firm. Drain, rinse under cold water, and transfer to a large mixing bowl.

2. When the pasta has cooled slightly, add the oil, parsley, vinegar, garlic, salt, and pepper. Toss well, and cool to room temperature.

3. Add the last four ingredients, toss to combine thoroughly, and serve.

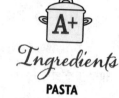

A+

Ingredients

PASTA
Helps sustain energy

CANNELLINI BEANS
Promote good skin health

RADICCHIO
Maintains healthy blood sugar

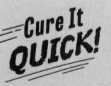

KITCHEN CAPERS This vinegar trick keeps an open jar of olives fresh longer. Every time you remove olives, pour in enough white vinegar to cover the remaining ones, and screw the lid back on. They should stay good to eat for several months beyond their expiration date.

Cure It QUICK!

EASE YOUR ACHIN' BACK SALAD You don't need to have a sore back to enjoy this delicious salad—but if you do, this recipe could soothe it. For a single serving, spread 1 cup of fresh baby spinach leaves on a plate. Mix ½ cup of cooked chicken pieces with ½ cup of drained canned pineapple chunks and ¼ cup of sliced red onion, and put it onto the greens. Top with 2 or 3 tablespoons of balsamic vinaigrette dressing. **Note:** *While all the ingredients will help ease discomfort, the superstar is the pineapple. The fruit is rich in bromelain, a powerful enzyme that helps reduce inflammation from muscle and joint conditions.*

SUMMER VEGETABLE-RICE SALAD

When summer's bounty comes rolling in—whether it comes from your own garden or your local farmers' market—serve it up in this scrumptious salad. You won't find an easier way to deliver bushels of flavor and a major load of health-giving nutrition.

YIELD: 4 servings	PREP: 25 minutes	WAIT: 3-4 hours

2 cups of long-grain brown rice, cooked

1 cup of cherry tomatoes, halved

½ cup of diced summer squash

½ cup of peas, cooked

¼ cup of thinly sliced celery

¼ cup of thinly sliced green onion

¾ cup of sour cream

3 tbsp. of herbal vinegar

2 tbsp. of minced fresh herbs

1. Combine the first six ingredients in bowl.

2. Mix the remaining ingredients together to make the dressing.* Pour it over the rice mixture, and toss until everything is coated.

3. Cover and refrigerate for several hours before serving, so the flavors can blend.

   * *This tastes best when the herbs and vinegar are of the same type.*

Ingredients

BROWN RICE
Promotes good digestion

SUMMER SQUASH
Supports bone health

PEAS
Boost immunity

Just before you add rice or pasta to boiling water, drop in a spoonful of vinegar. It'll reduce the starch content—thereby making your rice fluffy, and keeping your spaghetti, rigatoni, or lasagna from clumping while it's boiling. It'll be ready right away for your sauce or dressing.

INSTANT GRATIFICATION

Orange It Great?!

When you need a quick, healthy treat, these almost-instant fruit cups are just the ticket. To make four servings, cut two oranges in half. Scoop out the insides, dice each section, and put the pieces in a bowl. (Don't throw out the orange rinds). Chop an apple, and mix it with the orange bits. Add some sliced seedless grapes, and toss the mix with 4 tablespoons of Fruity Vinaigrette Dressing (page 34). Then scoop everything into the hollowed-out orange peels, and serve!

NASTURTIUM & ARUGULA SALAD

"Sing" an ode to spring by serving up this ultra-simple salad! The bright red, orange, and yellow flowers and lilypad-lookalike leaves are a healthy addition to any main course.

YIELD: 4 servings	PREP: 10 minutes

2 cups of young nasturtium leaves

2 cups of young arugula leaves

12 nasturtium flowers, pistils removed*

2 tbsp. of apple cider vinegar

1 tbsp. of finely chopped chives

1 small garlic clove, minced

1 tsp. of raw honey

4 tbsp. of extra virgin olive oil

Salt and freshly ground pepper to taste

* While the pistils are harmless, they have a bitter taste that some don't like.

1. Combine the nasturtium leaves, arugula leaves, and nasturtium flowers in a bowl.

2. In another bowl, make the dressing by whisking the vinegar, chives, garlic, and honey together. Still whisking, slowly add the olive oil.

3. Season the dressing with salt and pepper, and lightly toss the leaves and flowers with it.

A+ Ingredients

ARUGULA
Enhances athletic performance

NASTURTIUMS
Fight cold and flu germs

CHIVES
Promote sound, restful sleep

Although nasturtiums are highly nutritious, they (like a number of other herbs) can be harmful to pregnant women or nursing mothers. So don't serve them to anyone in either of those categories!

KITCHEN CAPERS

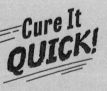

Cure It QUICK!

STOP A COLD IN ITS TRACKS! We all know that chicken soup packs prodigious cold-fighting power. Well, nasturtium leaves can actually stop trouble before it starts. Just wash a small handful of the leaves and dry them thoroughly (in a salad spinner if possible). Then toss them with a dressing of apple cider vinegar and extra virgin olive oil. Almost before this hasty-tasty salad reaches your tummy, those nasty germs will be history!

CULINARY Q & A

? I love using raw nasturtiums in salads. Are they also good for cooking, and what dishes do they work particularly well in?

! They sure are! The stems add an especially flavorful touch to any vegetable soup. Simply chop the stems, blanch them, and toss 'em in at the end of the cooking time. For an added touch of color and flavor, float a few of the colorful flowers on top of each serving bowl. Nasturtiums—and other flowers—are also tasty in stews and omelets, and they give an eye- and taste-bud-pleasing jolt to dips served with crackers or raw vegetables.

LOOKS GOOD ENOUGH TO EAT!

Just as a lot of vegetables look as good as they taste, plenty of flowers taste as good as they look. Here's a handful of blooms that can go right from the garden to your salad plate. These also work well in infused vinegars.

Edible Flower	Part to Use	Flavor
Bachelor's buttons (*Centaurea cyanus*)	Whole flowers	Cucumberish
Borage (*Borago officinalis*)*	Flowers (with hairy sepals removed); young leaves	Delicate cucumber with hints of melon
Nasturtium (*Tropaeolum majus*)	Flowers, leaves, and stems	Peppery and mustardy with undertones of honey; akin to watercress
Scented geraniums (*Pelargonium* spp.)	Flowers	Matches the scent— for example, apple, chocolate, lemon, orange
Stock (*Matthiola incana*)	Florets	Warm, spicy

* See Lose the Blues Salad on page 94.

CELERIAC, FENNEL, & APPLE SALAD

This bright, crisp, finely cut combo makes a mighty fine partner for hearty soups, stews, and meats on cold winter evenings. Plus, it gives your health a boost!

YIELD: 4–6 servings   **PREP:** 20 minutes

2 cups of water

3 tbsp. of apple cider vinegar, divided

1 celeriac (a.k.a. celery root), de-stemmed, peeled, and cut into quarters

1 fennel bulb, stem and bottom removed

1 medium apple, cored

½ medium red onion, peeled

1 tbsp. of apple cider

1 tbsp. of Dijon mustard

1 tsp. of raw honey

¼ cup of extra virgin olive oil

Salt and freshly ground black pepper to taste

1. Pour the water and 1 tablespoon of the vinegar into a medium-size bowl.

2. Cut the celeriac, fennel, and apple crosswise into very thin slices. As you finish each batch, toss the slices into the water and vinegar mixture to keep the flesh from turning brown. Then slice the onion in the same way (no need to give it the non-browning treatment).

3. In a small bowl, mix the remaining vinegar with the cider, mustard, and honey. Slowly drizzle in the oil, whisking until the dressing is emulsified. Add the salt and pepper.

4. Drain the vegetables, dry them well, and put them in a large bowl, along with the onion. Then gradually add the dressing, tossing until the slices are coated but not drenched.

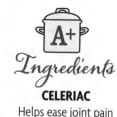

Ingredients

CELERIAC
Helps ease joint pain

FENNEL
Promotes brain function

APPLE CIDER VINEGAR
Helps ease asthma symptoms

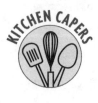

KITCHEN CAPERS It's almost impossible to get all the honey out of a measuring spoon or cup—unless you use this simple trick: Before you pour the honey from its container, run water into your measuring implement, then empty but don't dry it. The sweet stuff will glide right out—no muss, no fuss!

WILD RICE & GINGER BALSAMIC SALAD

Wild rice is not even related to "regular" rice. Rather, it's a grass that's native to North America. It's more flavorful than the "real deal" and full of fiber and energy-boosting minerals to boot—which makes it an excellent base for a salad like this winner.

YIELD: 4 servings   **PREP:** 35 minutes

1 cup of wild rice, uncooked

6 tbsp. of sunflower oil

1 tbsp. of balsamic vinegar

1 tbsp. of chile oil

2 tsp. of lemon juice

1-inch piece of fresh
   ginger, minced

1 yellow bell pepper, cored,
   seeded, and sliced

1 bunch of scallions, sliced

Lettuce leaves to serve

1. Wash the rice in cold water until the water runs clear. Boil rice in salted water, over medium-low heat. Simmer, uncovered, for 20 minutes. Turn off the heat, and let the rice steam for 10 minutes.

2. Mix sunflower oil, vinegar, chile oil, lemon juice, and ginger in a bowl. Then pour the mixture over the rice. Stir in the peppers and scallions.

3. Arrange the lettuce leaves on plates, and spoon the rice mixture on top.

Ingredients

WILD RICE
Enhances digestion

SUNFLOWER OIL
Maintains healthy cholesterol levels

BALSAMIC VINEGAR
Supports weight loss

KITCHEN CAPERS Wild rice can be used in place of either white or brown rice in any recipe. Just remember that it takes longer to cook than the "genuine" article, so adjust the timing accordingly.

CULINARY Q & A

? I used to cook perfect rice every time on a gas stove, but it never turns out right on my new electric stove. Should I give up and buy a rice cooker?

! Nope. Don't waste your money. Just try this slick trick with your electric stove: Turn on two burners: one set on high heat, the other on low. Start your rice and water on the hotter burner. When the water boils, immediately move the pot to the burner that's set on low. This easy maneuver simulates the quick temperature change that's required for perfect rice.

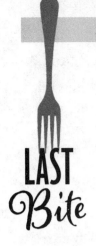

LAST *Bite*

TIMELY TIPS FOR TERRIFIC SALADS

The difference between good salads and great ones lies in the details—if you follow these tips, yours will always be the latter:

Pair the right greens with the right dressing. Tender greens, like arugula, Bibb, or oakleaf lettuce (or mixed baby greens), demand a light, only mildly acidic dressing that will not weigh down their leaves and overwhelm their flavor. A light vinaigrette suits them perfectly. Save the stronger-flavored dressings, such as Caesar, blue cheese, and green goddess, for sturdier greens, like romaine or iceberg lettuce, and more substantial ingredients, like tomatoes and olives.

Use top-quality, in-season ingredients. While you can find excellent salad greens at any time of the year, don't even think of using (for example) fresh tomatoes, peas, or corn when they're out of season. They won't be anywhere near their peak of flavor or nutritional value (more about that coming up in Chapter Six).

Always dry salad greens thoroughly before dressing them. When they're wet, the flavor of the dressing is washed away. Try using a salad spinner—it's hands down the best tool for the drying job.

Only dress what you expect to be eaten at one sitting. Undressed salad will keep in the fridge for a day or two, but with dressing added, that same salad can turn into a gooey mess.

Think "Less is better." You can always add more dressing if you need to. But if you overdo it, there's no turning back, so start with a small amount first. Then go from there.

Leftover chicken, ham, fish, and bean salads make great—and fast—sandwich fillings. All you need to do is split a pita pocket open and fill 'er up with the goodies. Or put them on top of a tortilla and roll it up. In either case, add chopped tomato, fresh lettuce, and/or shredded cheese if you like, and you're good to go.

KEEP RICE ON ICE

Without a doubt, rice makes a terrific addition to salads and other dishes. There is just one problem: The good (a.k.a.) non-instant kind takes a long time to cook, which makes it inconvenient for weeknight dinners. And the pre-cooked frozen rice at the supermarket is expensive. The simple solution: Freeze your own supply at home. All you need is a rimmed sheet pan, plastic freezer bags in either gallon or quart size, a measuring cup or other scoop, and (of course) just-cooked rice. Then:

1. Run both the pan and the scoop under cold water, and shake off the excess. Don't dry the items, though —the moisture will keep the rice from sticking to the surface.

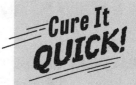

Cure It QUICK!

HEAD OFF A SUGAR CRASH The next time you serve pasta—or order it at your favorite Italian restaurant—make sure your side salad is doused with a good dose of balsamic vinegar. Thanks to the Trebbiano and Lambrusco grapes that it's made from, balsamic vinegar contains compounds that help keep your blood sugar from spiking, thereby preventing the sudden fatigue (a.k.a. sugar crash) that can set in a few hours after you've consumed foods that are high in carbohydrates. **Note:** *This ploy is especially important for runners who load up on carbs before a big race!*

2. Scoop the just-cooked rice from its pot onto the pan, spread it out evenly, and let it cool for 10 minutes or so at room temperature.

3. Transfer the rice into the bags. Use your hands to spread and flatten the rice so it forms an even layer in the bag. Squeeze out as much air as possible before sealing each bag and adding a date label.

4. Lay the filled bags flat in one or more stacks on a clean, dry sheet pan, and set it in the freezer until the rice is frozen (about two hours). Then, for more efficient storage, stand the bags straight up like file folders, either separately or in a single, larger zippered bag. The contents should stay fresh and tasty for three months or so.

To reheat the frozen rice, simply transfer it to a microwave-safe container (no need to thaw first). Cover and cook on full power in 1-minute increments until the rice is hot. Use it immediately or let it cool, as needed.

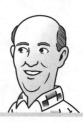

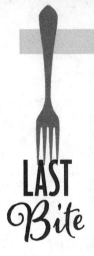

PRACTICAL POINTERS FOR PERFECTLY PLEASING PASTA SALADS

Pasta salad is one of the most versatile dishes of all. It's great for large or small crowds for lunch or hot-weather dinners. You can mix any kind of pasta with fresh or lightly cooked vegetables, as well as meat, cheeses, herbs, and just about any kind of sauce. Pasta salad is also a great way to use up leftovers. But to ensure your fair share of "oohs and aahs" from around the dining table, keep these guidelines in mind:

- While you can use any kind of pasta in a salad, short noodles combine better with other cut-up ingredients to create a consistent texture. Excellent choices include bow ties (farfalle), corkscrews (fusilli), quill shapes (penne and pennette), shells (conchiglie), and wheels (rotelle).

- After draining the pasta, rinse in cold water to stop the cooking process.

- For the best flavor, add the dressing when the pasta is warm or at room temperature. If the noodles are cold, they won't absorb enough of the dressing's flavor. If they're hot, they'll absorb too much dressing and turn soggy.

- Most pasta salads don't fare well in the refrigerator for any length of time, so it's best to prepare them the day you intend to serve them.

- Whenever you refrigerate a pasta salad, let it reach room temperature before serving.

- Just before serving, toss the salad with two large spoons. That way, any dressing that settles on the bottom of the bowl will be thoroughly combined with all of the solid ingredients.

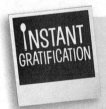

Baked Pasta Pronto

Whenever you make a pasta salad with a vinaigrette dressing, double the recipe and refrigerate the extra servings. The next day, slide the salad into a baking dish, mix in wine or chicken broth as needed to add moisture, and bake at 350°F for about 20 minutes. Top it with shredded cheese, and put it back into the oven just long enough to melt the cheese. Then dig in and eat hearty!

CULINARY Q & A

? I like to buy a head of lettuce from the farmers' market, instead of prewashed, cut-up versions at the supermarket. But it always seems to go bad before I can use it all. What's the best way to keep it fresh?

! There are several methods, but this one works like a charm: Fill a large bowl or clean sink with tepid water. Separate the individual leaves from the head and rinse them thoroughly. Then lift them out of the water, leaving any dirt behind. Repeat the process if necessary, using clean water—some lettuce accumulates a lot of grit at the base of the leaves. Whirl the leaves in a salad spinner until they're thoroughly dry, then roll them up in paper towels or lint-free kitchen towels. Store the leaves, still wrapped up, in plastic bags or a large covered container and put either in the refrigerator. As long as the lettuce is completely dry, it should keep well for several days.

PREP PRODUCE EARLY

Prepping salad ingredients in advance is a major time saver. Unfortunately, when you peel and slice certain fruits and vegetables, though, they almost immediately start to turn brown. Potatoes, apples, and pears are especially prone to changing color quickly. The simple solution: Put the pieces in a bowl, cover them with cold water, and add 1 to 2 tablespoons of vinegar (either white or apple cider will do). There is just one minor catch: Although the produce will stay fresh in your refrigerator for several days, it will start to lose water-soluble vitamins after a couple of hours—so the sooner you use it, the better! (Or pop the produce in the freezer to help it last longer.)

A TOUCH OF GARLIC

Do you love the flavor a garlic vinaigrette gives a salad but find the raw stuff overpowering? If so, try this trick: Instead of mixing garlic into the dressing, slice a clove and rub the cut side over your salad bowl. When you add the greens and toss them with the dressing, it will pick up the garlic juice. The result: a tantalizing taste of garlic without the sharp pungency of the minced version.

Chapter Four

Perfect
Pickles
& Condiments

Of all of vinegar's culinary uses, one of the best known—and most relied upon—is its invaluable contribution to making pickles and condiments of all kinds. In this chapter, we'll zero in on some remarkable recipes for pickled vegetables and fruits, as well as scrumptious and health-giving sandwich spreads, relishes, and chutneys.

BREAD & BUTTER PICKLES

These are classic all-American pickles, and they are a snap to make! Plus, this homemade, preservative-free version will beat store-bought brands hands down.

YIELD: about 2 quarts	PREP: 10 minutes	WAIT: 8–12 hours

1½–2 lbs. of pickling cucumbers, cut into ¼-inch slices

1½ tbsp. of pickling salt

1 large onion, thinly sliced

1 cup of granulated sugar

1 cup of white vinegar

½ cup of apple cider vinegar

1½ tsp. of mustard seeds

½ tsp. of celery seed

⅛ tsp. of turmeric

1. Toss the cukes and salt in a bowl, and cover. Let the bowl rest in the fridge for 90 minutes, then rinse off the salt. Add the onions to the bowl. Set aside.

2. Combine the remaining ingredients in a saucepan, and bring the mixture to a simmer over medium heat.

3. Stir to dissolve the sugar, then pour the hot mixture over the vegetables, and let them sit at room temp for at least 60 minutes.

4. Cover and refrigerate for 8 to 12 hours. Store the pickles in airtight, sterilized jars in the refrigerator for up to 4 weeks.

When you're making pickles or condiments to keep for any length of time, use commercial vinegars, all of which have an acidity level of at least 5 percent. For anything that will be used within a week or so, it's fine to use DIY vinegars because the acidity content is a moot point.

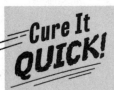
KITCHEN CAPERS

A+
Ingredients

CUCUMBERS
Boost immunity

MUSTARD SEEDS
Help ease asthma symptoms

CELERY SEED
Maintains healthy blood pressure

Cure It **QUICK!** **GIVE HEARTBURN THE HEAVE-HO** With a dill pickle! This homemade version will help do the trick quickly—without the unhealthy additives found in most commercial products. Chop five cucumbers into 1-inch squares and put in a heat-proof bowl with 15 sprigs of fresh dill. Set the bowl aside. Put 1 cup of white wine vinegar in a pan over medium heat, and add 12 whole black peppercorns, ¼ cup of sugar, and 1 teaspoon of salt. Cook until the sugar and salt dissolve. Add 4 peeled and quartered garlic cloves and bring to a boil. Remove from the heat and pour the hot mixture over the cukes. Let stand for 35 minutes and then dig in!

CULINARY Q & A

? I've just started making my own pickles and condiments. How can I store them, so they will last for the longest-possible length of time?

! Anything that contains vinegar and sugar should keep just fine in the fridge or in a cool, dark place (like a kitchen cabinet that's away from the stove or other heat sources) for three to four months—or for whatever length of time the recipe stipulates. When you plan to store your creations at room temperature for any longer than that, use the water-bath canning method of food preservation that's explained in full in "For the Long Haul" on page 144. The process doesn't take long, and it's worth going the extra mile to keep your stash of tasty treats fresh for months—or even years—longer!

TROUBLESHOOTING PICKLES

Pickling foods is just like anything else in life: The more you do it, the better results you will have. While you're learning the ropes, use this handy guide to diagnose any potential problems that might crop up:

If the Pickles Are:	The Problem Is:
Tough	You used too much salt.
Shriveled	You used too much sugar.
Tough and shriveled	You used too much vinegar.
Soft	Not enough salt was added.
Dark, and the liquid is cloudy	You used table salt containing starch and usually iodine, which causes this problem. Use pickling salt instead.
Hollow	The cucumbers were not fresh enough.
Off-color	Either the water has a high mineral content, or you used a copper kettle.
Slippery	The pickles didn't spend enough time in the brine solution.
Mushy	The pickles were cooked too long.

PICKLED CHARD COOLERS

Before summertime, make up a batch of these ultra-simple pickles and keep them in the fridge. They'll cool you down fast when the weather turns steamy and will also give you a healthy dose of probiotics that'll help keep your digestive system running smoothly.

YIELD: about 3 quarts   **PREP:** 15 minutes   **WAIT:** 1 week

1 bunch of Swiss chard stalks

2 cups of hot water

1 cup of unfiltered apple cider vinegar

3 tbsp. of raw honey

3 tbsp. of sriracha hot sauce

1. Cut the stalks about an inch shorter than the depth of the jars, and pack them in tightly.

2. Mix the remaining ingredients together in a bowl, stirring until the honey dissolves.

3. Pour the mixture over the stems so they're completely covered. Close the jars tightly, and store them in the refrigerator for at least a week so the flavor can develop fully. They'll keep in the fridge for up to a year as long as the stems are completely covered with vinegar at all times.

A+ Ingredients

SWISS CHARD
Promotes brain function

APPLE CIDER VINEGAR
Enhances weight loss

HOT SAUCE
Boosts metabolism

If you see bubbles in pickled or canned food—whether homemade or store-bought—it means that the jar contains either air or bacteria, and the contents are not safe to eat. So toss them in the trash, and sterilize the jar before you use it again, even for dry storage.

KITCHEN CAPERS

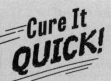

Cure It QUICK!

COOL IT—NOW! As odd as it may seem, hot, spicy foods actually cool your body in two ways: They boost blood circulation, and they cause you to sweat, which releases excess heat from your system. Any kind of hot pickled vegetables are perfect for this job, but what do you do when you have none on hand? Just whip up a batch of these almost-instant coolers: Toss about 2 cups of thinly sliced zucchini, cucumber, or yellow summer squash in a bowl with ½ teaspoon of salt and let it sit for 15 minutes. Drain, and add 1 tablespoon of vinegar, 1 teaspoon each of sugar and extra virgin olive oil, 2 mashed garlic cloves, ½ teaspoon of hot-pepper flakes, and ¼ teaspoon of cayenne pepper. Mix well, and dig in! (Makes four servings.)

EASY SPICY DILL PICKLES

If you've got a fresh crop of cucumbers growing in the backyard garden, this single-quart recipe has your name written all over it: It lets you pickle your harvest in small batches as the cukes ripen, and none of them will go to waste.

YIELD: 1 quart   **PREP:** 20 minutes   **WAIT:** about 6 weeks

4 cups of 3- to 4-inch cucumber slices (sliced lengthwise)

1 bunch of fresh dill, chopped

2 garlic cloves

2 slices of fresh ginger

2 allspice berries

2 whole peppercorns

⅔ cup of white vinegar

¼ cup of cold water*

¼ cup of sugar

3 tsp. of pickling salt

* Use more as needed.

1. Pack the cucumber slices into a 1-quart canning jar. Add the dill and spices, and set aside.

2. Combine the remaining ingredients, in a bowl, and stir until the sugar and salt are completely dissolved.

3. Pour the syrup mixture over the cucumbers, leaving ½-inch headspace. Add more water if needed to cover the cukes.

4. Seal the jar and process for 15 minutes according to the directions in "For the Long Haul" (see page 144). Leave the pickles for at least 6 weeks to develop their full flavor.

KITCHEN CAPERS Always sterilize jars (and lids) that you use for any pickles or condiments: Fill jars with boiling water, and let sit for 10 minutes, then empty. Wait until they're room temperature, before pouring in the contents.

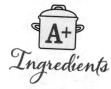

A+

Ingredients

CUCUMBERS
Boost immunity

DILL
Promotes healthy sleep

GARLIC
Supports bone health

CULINARY Q & A

? Exactly what is the difference between salad cucumbers and pickling cucumbers? Are they interchangeable in recipes?

! Cucumbers that are bred to be used for pickling generally have thin skins, which allows the pickling solution to better penetrate and flavor the flesh. They're also short and squat. Salad cukes have thicker skins and grow long and thin. Both can be used for pickling, but make sure the ones you buy don't have a wax coating, which prevents the vinegar from penetrating the skin.

WATERMELON RIND PICKLES

Don't throw away the watermelon rind. Instead put it to work in this recipe! The rind contains healthy, blood-building chlorophyll and more amino acids than even the pink flesh.

YIELD: about 1 quart	PREP: 20 minutes	WAIT: 8 hours

1 lb. of watermelon rind, cut into 1- by 2-inch chunks

5 ¼ cups of water, divided

3 tbsp. of pickling salt

1 ¾ cups of sugar

1 ½ cups of apple cider vinegar

½ tsp. of ground cinnamon

¼ tsp. of ground allspice

⅛ tsp. of ground nutmeg

3 whole cloves

1. With a potato peeler, trim the pink flesh and outer green skin from the thick, white melon rind.

2. Bring 5 cups of the water and the salt to a boil. Add the rind, reduce the heat, and simmer for 5 minutes. Remove from heat, and strain into a bowl.

3. In another pan, mix the remaining ingredients and ¼ cup of water. Bring to a boil, stirring until the sugar has dissolved.

4. Pour the liquid over the rind and let it cool to room temp. Cover the bowl and refrigerate for 8 hours before serving. The pickles will keep in the fridge for up to 4 weeks.

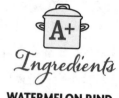

Ingredients

WATERMELON RIND
Boosts immunity

CINNAMON
Fights inflammation

ALLSPICE
Enhances digestion

KITCHEN CAPERS For a variation on the recipe above, try using the rind of cantaloupe or pumpkin instead. These two gems also make delightfully delectable pickles.

INSTANT GRATIFICATION

Pickle the Melon, Too

After you've made watermelon rind pickles, remove the seeds from the melon, cut it into bite-size chunks, and turn it into these pretty pink pleasers. To make about 6 pints of pickles, combine 1 quart of water, 1 pint of white vinegar, 2 cups of sugar, and ¼ cup of pickling or kosher salt in a pan, and bring the mixture to a boil. In the meantime, put a few fresh dill sprigs into sterilized canning jars, and fill the remaining space with melon. Pour the hot vinegar mixture over the fruit and herbs, and seal the jars. When slightly cooled, refrigerate for at least eight hours.

PICKLED SLICED ONIONS

If more folks knew the benefits of onions, they wouldn't mind having smelly breath! Onions are linked to healthy blood sugar, cold and flu relief, and lowered inflammation.

YIELD: about 2 quarts	PREP: 25 minutes	WAIT: 1 week

1 ½ tsp. of whole black peppercorns

1 ½ tsp. of whole mustard seeds

1 bay leaf

3 cups of malt vinegar*

2 lbs. of sweet or red onions, sliced and separated into rings

* Malt is a traditional choice but any type of vinegar will work.

1. Simmer the spices in the vinegar for 20 minutes, and then strain them out.

2. Blanch the onion rings in a pot of boiling water for 20 seconds. Strain, and let the onions sit until they're cool enough to handle.

3. Pack them firmly into sterilized glass jars, and pour in the warm, strained vinegar so the onions are covered.

4. Put the lids on, and stash jars in the fridge for at least a week to develop the onions' flavor. If fully covered with vinegar, they'll keep for at least a year in the refrigerator.

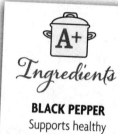

A+

Ingredients

BLACK PEPPER
Supports healthy bone development

BAY LEAVES
Help calm anxiety

ONIONS
Fight colds

KITCHEN CAPERS Figuring out how many fruits or vegetables of any kind will fit into a canning jar is not an exact science. So always make sure that you have a few more jars and lids than you think you'll need, all sterilized and ready to go—just in case.

CULINARY Q & A

? I've tried every trick I've ever heard for cutting onions without tears, but my eyes still gush like a waterfall every time I start chopping. Do you have any ideas?

! Given your state of dire sensitivity, it's time for desperate measures: Whenever you need to cut or peel onions, wear snug-fitting swim goggles. You might look a little silly wearing them on dry land, but you'll feel a lot more comfortable!

ONE-DAY-WONDER MIXED PICKLES

This merry medley needs to cure for only 24 hours, so it's ideal when you want a relatively quick but impressive dish for a barbecue, family reunion, or potluck supper.

YIELD: 2 quarts   **PREP:** 35 minutes   **WAIT:** 24 hours

2 cups of cauliflower florets

2 cups of trimmed green beans, cut into bite-size pieces

2 cucumbers, sliced

2 small red bell peppers, cut into slivers

1 ½ cups of sugar

1 cup of white vinegar

1 tbsp. of pickling salt

1 tsp. of celery seeds

1 tsp. of mustard seeds

1 tsp. of whole black peppercorns

1. Steam the cauliflower and beans until tender-crisp (about 10 minutes). Submerge them in cold water to stop the cooking. Drain and let the veggies cool to room temperature.

2. In a large bowl, mix the cauliflower and beans with the cucumbers and bell peppers. Set aside.

3. Combine the remaining ingredients in a pan. Boil, then reduce the heat and simmer, stirring constantly until the sugar and salt are dissolved.

4. Pour the liquid over the veggies, cool to room temperature, then cover the bowl. Refrigerate for at least 24 hours before serving.

Ingredients

CAULIFLOWER
Supports cardiovascular health

GREEN BEANS
Enhance sound sleep

RED BELL PEPPERS
Promote eye health

Invite friends to pickle, freeze, or can your summer bounty assembly-line style. Everyone will go home with tasty goodies and warm memories to savor through the winter.

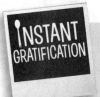

Quick & Easy Refrigerator Pickles
When you want enough classic pickles to feed a crowd—this recipe is perfect: Wash and de-stem 50 small (4-inch) cucumbers. Then slice them into quarters lengthwise and put them in a 3-gallon crock. Mix 3 cups of sugar, ½ cup of pickling salt, and 1 tablespoon of mustard seed in 1 gallon of apple cider vinegar, stirring until the sugar and salt are dissolved. Pour the mixture over the cucumbers. Cover them with a plate, and top the plate with something heavy so the cukes remain immersed in the liquid. Tuck the crock into the fridge, and let the pickles ripen for four days before serving.

PICKLED CHERRY TOMATOES & FENNEL

The contrasting flavors of cherry tomatoes and fennel deliver a one-of-a-kind kick that teams up for a tasty topping for grilled steak, pork, or chicken.

YIELD: 8 servings	**PREP:** 15 minutes	**WAIT:** 6–24 hours

¾ cup of water

½ cup of rice vinegar*

2 tsp. of sugar

Pinch of ground cinnamon

Pinch of ground cloves

1 fennel bulb, trimmed, cored, and cut into 1 ½- by ⅓-inch strips

1 pint of cherry tomatoes, halved

* Or substitute white wine or sherry vinegar.

1. Combine the water, vinegar, sugar, cinnamon, and cloves in a shallow nonreactive dish.

2. Add the fennel and the tomatoes, cover the mixture, and put in the refrigerator for at least 6 hours.

3. After 6 hours, give it a taste. If you'd like a bolder flavor, let the mixture steep in the fridge for a bit longer. Otherwise, proceed to step 4.

4. Drain, and serve this salad lightly chilled.

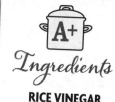

A+

Ingredients

RICE VINEGAR
Fights free radicals

FENNEL
Maintains healthy blood pressure

CHERRY TOMATOES
Promote healthy vision

KITCHEN CAPERS

There's no limit to the kinds of veggies or fruits that you can pickle. The key is to use ones that are young, firm, and uniformly sized. Avoid any that are damaged, sprouting, or showing signs of dampness.

CULINARY Q & A

? I have seen sweet anise at the grocery store, and it looks exactly the same as fennel I've seen elsewhere. Are they the same thing?

! No. In supermarkets, fennel is often mislabeled "sweet anise," and that's a shame because people who don't like the taste of licorice avoid it for that reason. Actually, the flavor of fennel is sweeter and more delicate than that of anise, and becomes even more so when it's cooked. By the way, all parts of the fennel plant are edible—and tasty—including the stems and the soft, fragrant leaves. Plus, it can help maintain bone strength, boost skin health, and promote a healthy immune system.

PICKLED PUMPKIN

This unique recipe is simple to make but full of flavor! And pumpkin
is packed with fiber, potassium, and vitamin C to boost heart health.

YIELD: 2 ½ pints	PREP: 1 hour	WAIT: 2 weeks

3 cups of apple cider vinegar

2 cups of sugar

2 cups of water

20 whole black peppercorns

15 whole cloves

10 allspice berries

2 cinnamon sticks, crushed

1 bay leaf

8 cups (about 3 lbs.)
of cubed pumpkin

1. Combine the first three ingredients in a large pot and heat to dissolve the sugar.

2. Put all the spices in a muslin spice bag, or tie them tightly in a piece of cheesecloth. Add the spice pouch and pumpkin to the pot. Bring to a boil, then reduce the heat to a simmer.

3. Cook until the pumpkin pieces are translucent and fork-tender (30 to 40 minutes). Then ladle them into sterilized canning jars. Cover with the liquid, leaving ½-inch headspace, and prepare for pantry storage (see "For the Long Haul" on page 144).

4. Let the pickles cure for at least 2 weeks before eating.

A+ Ingredients

BLACK PEPPERCORNS
Promote heart health

ALLSPICE BERRIES
Help relieve pain

PUMPKIN
Promotes weight loss

KITCHEN CAPERS

Small sugar pumpkins, which have a sweet taste, are especially good for the recipe above. But any kind will do. Just don't use a Halloween pumpkin! They're big in size but not in flavor.

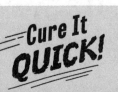

Cure It QUICK!

LIVE LONGER AND BETTER Eating just one or two garlic cloves a day can help boost your immunity, control blood sugar, and reduce your risk of developing heart disease. Whip up this pickled garlic with a sweet variety like 'Creole Red' or 'Spanish Roja'. Mix ¾ cup of white vinegar, 2 tablespoons of sugar, and ¼ teaspoon each of black peppercorns, cumin seed, and hot chili flakes in a saucepan. Boil, then add 1 cup of peeled garlic cloves, return to a boil, and simmer, uncovered, for two minutes. Pour the mix into a sterilized jar, cover, and cool to room temperature. Refrigerate for at least 24 hours. It'll keep for 30 days.

PURPLE EGGS & PICKLED BEETS

The comic novelty of violet eggs paired with beets has "reformed" generations of vegetable-phobic children. But you don't have to be in the under-10 set to enjoy the flavor, color, and health-giving clout of this classic duo.

YIELD: 8–10 servings   **PREP:** 10 minutes   **WAIT:** 24–48 hours

6 cups of diced cooked beets

6–12 hard-boiled eggs, peeled

2 cups of water

1 ½ cups of sugar

1 ½ cups of white or white wine vinegar

20 whole cloves

5 allspice berries

1 cinnamon stick

1. Put the beets and eggs in a large glass or ceramic jar.

2. Combine all the remaining ingredients in a pan. Bring to a boil, then reduce the heat to medium-low, simmer for 5 minutes, and pour the mixture over the beets and eggs.

3. Refrigerate the jar for 1 to 2 days before eating. The eggs will keep for 1 week; the beets for 2 weeks.

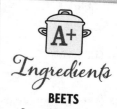

Ingredients

BEETS
Boost heart health

EGGS
Support memory and cognition

CLOVES
Promote restful sleep

KITCHEN CAPERS

When you're boiling eggs, add 2 tablespoons of vinegar per quart of water before you turn on the heat. It'll keep the shells from cracking and also make the boiled eggs easier to peel.

CULINARY Q & A

? I keep hearing all kinds of hoopla about beet greens. Are they really as good for me as they're cracked up to be?

! They sure are! In fact, according to recent studies, beet greens rank among the healthiest foods of all. Just make sure you choose and care for them correctly to make the most out of them. When you shop for beet greens, look for those that are crisp and brightly colored. Once you've made your choice and returned home, immediately snip off the greens; otherwise, they'll leach moisture from the bulbs. Then wash the greens, blot them dry with paper towels, and refrigerate them in a plastic bag until you're ready to use them. They will keep for about three days.

SPICED PICKLED EGGS

These nutritious nuggets are delicious when sliced and served atop a salad of chicken and mixed greens—or simply as a healthy snack. They also work perfectly when you're making deviled eggs for a party platter.

YIELD: 12 eggs	**PREP:** 10 minutes	**WAIT:** 10 days

12 small hard-boiled eggs, peeled

1 small onion, thinly sliced

3 cups of white or white wine vinegar

1 tbsp. of raw honey

1 tsp. of allspice berries

1 tsp. of whole cloves

½ tsp. of coriander

1 bay leaf

1 cinnamon stick

¼-inch slice of ginger

1. Put the eggs and onion in a wide-mouthed jar or crock.

2. Combine the remaining ingredients in a nonreactive pan and bring the mixture to a boil. Reduce the heat and simmer for 5 minutes.

3. Pour the hot liquid over the eggs and onion.

4. Cover the jar or crock, and refrigerate it for at least 10 days before serving. The eggs will keep for up to 2 months in the refrigerator.

KITCHEN CAPERS When you've got both raw and hard-boiled eggs in the fridge, it's hard to tell them apart. One way: Add a little balsamic vinegar to the water when you boil them. The vinegar will tint the shells so you know which is which.

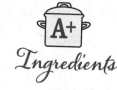

A+ Ingredients

EGGS
Promote skin health

ONION
Boosts immunity

RAW HONEY
Helps healthy digestion

INSTANT GRATIFICATION

Pickled Cheese, If You Please

Believe it or not, pickled feta cheese is delicious as an omelet filling or served with crackers. To make it, rinse 7 ounces of feta cheese, pat it dry, and cut it into ½-inch cubes. Put a layer of cubes on the bottom of a sterilized 1-pint canning jar, and top the cheese with a layer of chopped fresh thyme. Repeat the layers until the jar is nearly full. Then whisk 7 ounces of white wine vinegar with 1 teaspoon of raw honey, and pour the mix over the cheese until the jar is full. Refrigerate for at least 24 hours before eating.

SPICED PEACHES

These sweet-and-spicy, make-ahead gems are the perfect way to put peaches to work. A treasure trove of essential minerals, peaches are low in calories and high in vitamin C, which can help protect your body from infection and disease.

YIELD: 6 peaches	**PREP:** 20 minutes	**WAIT:** 8–48 hours

18 whole cloves

6 firm, ripe peaches, peeled

2 cups of apple cider vinegar

2 cups of sugar

½ cup of brandy

4 cinnamon sticks, broken

KITCHEN CAPERS Select all peaches for pickling when they are fully ripe and their skins have a rosy-pink blush. The best time for peaches is at the height of summer.

1. Push 3 cloves into the flesh of each skinless peach. Set the peaches aside.

2. Combine the remaining ingredients in a pan. Bring to a simmer over low heat, stirring to dissolve the sugar, and continue to simmer for 5 minutes.

3. Drop the peaches, one or two at a time, into the simmering syrup. Poach them until the flesh is tender when pierced with the tip of a knife (about 5 minutes). Remove the peaches from the syrup, and put them in a deep glass bowl or crock.

4. Pour the hot syrup over the peaches, covering completely. Cool them to room temperature, cover, and refrigerate for at least 8 hours. Serve chilled.

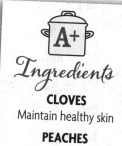

A+
Ingredients

CLOVES
Maintain healthy skin

PEACHES
Help calm anxiety

BRANDY
Boosts cardiovascular health

CULINARY Q & A

? I've seen recipes that want you to peel peaches, but I find that difficult to do without gouging the fruit. Is there a trick that makes it easier?

! There sure is—and it couldn't be simpler. Just bring a large pot of water to a boil. Drop the peaches into the boiling water, turn off the heat, and let the fruit sit for two to three minutes. Then, using a slotted spoon, take the peaches out of the drink and slip the skins off. That's all there is to it! By the way, this trick also works just as well to peel apricots and nectarines.

PICKLED PLUMS & CHERRIES

Plums can help increase the amount of energy-boosting iron your body can absorb from food, while cherries have been linked to relieving insomnia and joint pain.

YIELD: 12 servings	PREP: 30 minutes	WAIT: 2 days

1 lb. of plums (red or black), pitted but not peeled, and cut into wedges

2 cups of halved, pitted sweet cherries

2 garlic cloves, crushed

4 bay leaves

1 ½ cups of sugar

1 cup of red wine vinegar

¼ cup of balsamic vinegar

1 tbsp. of pickling salt

1 tsp. of mustard seeds

½ tsp. of fennel seeds

½ tsp. of ground cinnamon

½ tsp. of ground cloves

¼ tsp. of ground ginger

1. Toss the plums, cherries, and crushed garlic cloves in a large bowl, and set aside.

2. Boil the remaining ingredients in a pot, stirring continuously. Reduce the heat, simmer, and stir until the sugar and salt dissolve.

3. Pour the liquid over the fruit mixture, cover, and refrigerate for 2 days before you serve. Store, covered, in the fridge for up to 2 months.

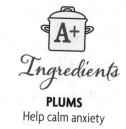

Ingredients

PLUMS
Help calm anxiety

CHERRIES
Improve brain function

BALSAMIC VINEGAR
Promotes skin health

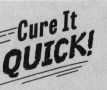

KITCHEN CAPERS If you don't have a cherry pitter, the tip of a veggie peeler or pointed knife will work. So will an extra-large paper clip. Just straighten one end and use the other end as a hook.

Cure It QUICK! **ROUT OUT GOUT!** Cherries can help clear toxins from your body and clean your kidneys, putting them at the top of the pain-relief list. Each day, add cherries to your diet, or try them pickled: Stir 2 cups of water, 1 cup of sugar, and ¾ cup of balsamic vinegar in a pan over medium heat until the sugar has dissolved. Bring the mixture to a boil and add 1 ¼ pounds of pitted cherries. Reduce the heat to low and simmer for 10 minutes. Transfer the cherries to jars with a slotted spoon (about five half-pint jars). Cook the vinegar mixture for another 5 minutes on high. Then ladle it over the cherries, leaving ½ inch of space at the top. Screw on lids, refrigerate, and let sit for a few days. They'll keep for two to three months.

SPICED PRUNES WITH EARL GREY TEA

Earl Grey tea is known to help with digestion and digestive system problems and provides other health benefits. The aromatic liquid also gives soups and sauces a tasty kick.

YIELD: 6 cups	PREP: 40 minutes	WAIT: 2 weeks

2 lbs. of prunes

3 ⅔ cups of cold, pre-brewed Earl Grey tea

1 ¼ cups of white wine vinegar

1 cup of sugar

16 allspice berries

6 whole cloves

1 cinnamon stick, broken in half

1. Pour the tea over the prunes. Cover and let soak for 6 to 24 hours, then transfer contents to a pan. Bring to a boil and simmer until the prunes are tender (15 to 20 minutes).

2. Using a slotted spoon, move the fruit to warm, sterilized jars, filling them to within ½ inch of the tops.

3. Add the remaining ingredients to the pan. Stir constantly over low heat until the sugar has dissolved. Boil until it has reduced and thickened (2 to 3 minutes).

4. Pour the liquid over the prunes, until completely covered, and ensure that the spices are evenly divided among the jars.

5. Seal the jars, add labels, and store in a cool, dark place for at least 2 weeks before using.

KITCHEN CAPERS

For pickling or any other purpose, look for prunes that are slightly soft and somewhat flexible. The skin should be bluish black and free of blemishes.

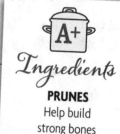

A+ Ingredients

PRUNES
Help build strong bones

TEA
Aids weight loss

CINNAMON
Freshens breath

CULINARY Q & A

? How can I get rid of the marks left by cranberries and other colorful foods on my stainless steel pots and pans?

! Pour in enough white vinegar to cover the marks, and let it sit for 30 minutes. Wash the pot with hot, soapy water and rinse with cold water. For burnt-on food, mix 1 cup of vinegar in enough water to cover the stains (if they're near the top of a large pot, add another cup or so of vinegar). Bring the liquid to a boil, and after five minutes, remove from heat. When cool, wash the pot as usual.

PICKLED GRAPES WITH ROSEMARY & RED PEPPER

These colorful, spicy-tart treats make a perfect addition to an appetizer platter. Or add them to chicken, potato, or mixed green salads. You'll love the rich, complex flavors.

YIELD: 4 pints	**PREP:** 10 minutes	**WAIT:** 1 hour

3 cups (about 1 lb.) of seedless green grapes

3 cups (about 1 lb.) of seedless red grapes

6 fresh rosemary sprigs, divided

2 cups of white wine vinegar

1 cup of water

3 garlic cloves, peeled and thinly sliced

2 tbsp. of kosher or coarse sea salt

2 tsp. of sugar

½ tsp. of dried crushed red pepper

1. Pack the grapes into four 1-pint canning jars. Add 1 rosemary sprig to each jar.

2. Mix the rest of the ingredients and the remaining rosemary sprigs in a pan and bring to a boil. Remove from the heat and discard the rosemary.

3. Pour the hot vinegar mixture over the grapes. Cover the jars loosely and let the contents cool to room temperature. Chill for at least 1 hour before serving. Store in the refrigerator for up to a week.

 KITCHEN CAPERS Use an old-fashioned rubber jar opener when peeling garlic cloves. Just put the cloves in the center of the opener and roll them around for a minute or so. The skins will slip right off.

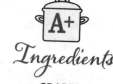 **A+**

Ingredients

GRAPES
Soothe Inflammation

ROSEMARY
Helps relieve stress

WHITE WINE VINEGAR
Maintains healthy glucose levels

 INSTANT GRATIFICATION

Pickled Fruit in a Flash

This brine is perfect for pickling fruit. Combine ½ cup of white balsamic vinegar, ¼ cup of sugar, and 2 teaspoons of kosher salt in a saucepan over high heat. Bring to a boil, then remove from the heat. Let the mixture cool, stirring occasionally. Put your fruit in a sterilized 24-ounce jar. Pour the brine over the fruit, seal, and refrigerate for 24 hours before serving. **Note:** *Try these combos: 1 pound of strawberries and 2 rosemary sprigs; 1 pound of chopped honeydew melon and 2 thyme sprigs; or 1 pound of sliced peaches and 2 mint sprigs.*

HEALTHY HOMEMADE KETCHUP

Store-bought ketchup is generally high in sodium, high-fructose corn syrup, and other undesirable additives. This DIY version is more flavorful, healthier, and easy to make!

YIELD: 1½ quarts   **PREP:** 20 minutes   **COOK:** 2½ hours

10 lbs. of ripe tomatoes, finely chopped

1 large red, Vidalia®, Walla Walla, or Texas Sweet onion, finely chopped

1 cup of apple cider vinegar

1 cup of packed brown sugar

2 tbsp. of salt

1 tsp. of baking soda

1 tsp. of cayenne pepper

1 tsp. of ground allspice

1 tsp. of ground cinnamon

¼ tsp. of ground nutmeg

1. Cook the tomatoes and onion in a saucepan over medium heat for 30 minutes, or until the veggies are soft.

2. Remove from the heat and force the mixture through a strainer, including as much pulp as possible. Pour it back into the pan and reheat it.

3. Add the remaining ingredients and simmer, stirring occasionally, until the blend is thick (about 2 hours).

4. Ladle the ketchup through a funnel (see Kitchen Capers, below) into sterilized bottles and store them in the fridge, where the ketchup will stay at its peak of flavor for about 1 month.

 KITCHEN CAPERS Use a wide-mouthed funnel when making ketchup or other condiments. It'll help you fill bottles or jars easily.

 **A+ Ingredients**

TOMATOES
Support heart health

RED ONIONS
Boost immunity

NUTMEG
Helps relieve pain

CULINARY Q & A

? I've heard that cooked tomatoes are actually better for you than fresh, uncooked ones. Is that really true?

! Yes. Cooked tomatoes have more lycopene, a powerful antioxidant shown to lower the risk of disease and illness. Consuming just 25 milligrams of lycopene a day can lower your cholesterol at rates comparable to those of prescribed statin drugs. **Note:** *Beta-carotene, which boosts your vision and the overall health of your eyes, is also higher in cooked tomatoes than in raw ones.*

MUSHROOM KETCHUP

As you can see from this unique variation, tomato ketchup is far from the only topping in town. This version stars fresh mushrooms, which contain essential nutrients that contribute to cardiovascular health and regulate blood pressure.

YIELD: 4 or 5 half-pint jars	PREP: 30 minutes	COOK: 1–2 hours

3 lbs. of mushrooms, thinly sliced

2 tbsp. of kosher or sea salt

1 cup of chopped onion

1 cup of mixed-herb sherry vinegar*

2 garlic cloves, minced

1 small hot red pepper, cored, seeded, and chopped

2 tbsp. of raw honey

1 tbsp. of chopped fresh marjoram

1 tbsp. of chopped fresh parsley

1 tbsp. of chopped fresh thyme

½ tsp. of ground allspice

½ tsp. of ground ginger

¼ tsp. of ground cloves

1 bay leaf

* See the recipe for Elegant Herbal Vinegar on page 12.

1. Mix the mushrooms and salt in a nonreactive bowl. Cover and let stand at room temperature for 24 hours, stirring occasionally.

2. Puree the mixture in a food processor or blender, then pour it into a nonreactive pot. Set aside.

3. Combine the remaining ingredients, except the bay leaf, in a food processor or blender, until smooth.

4. Add the puree to the mushroom mixture in the pot and stir to mix thoroughly. Add the bay leaf.

5. Bring to a boil over medium-high heat. Reduce the heat and simmer, uncovered, stirring often, until the ketchup is very thick (1 to 2 hours).

6. Remove the bay leaf and process the ketchup following the directions in "For the Long Haul" on page 144.

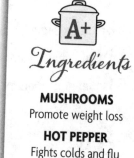

Ingredients

MUSHROOMS
Promote weight loss

HOT PEPPER
Fights colds and flu

MARJORAM
Helps prevent anemia

KITCHEN CAPERS

When handling hot peppers leaves you with a nasty burn, soothe pain by washing your skin with white vinegar. Or, stop trouble from the start by soaking the peppers in vinegar for four hours before you cut into them. It'll neutralize the trouble-causing chemicals in the oil.

BIG APPLE HOT DOG TOPPING

This classic condiment has been a mainstay of New York City hot dog vendors—and their customers—for a century. Don't tell the guys selling red hots on Broadway, but it's just as tasty on hamburgers, turkey burgers, and chicken sandwiches as it is on franks.

YIELD: ½ cup   **PREP:** 5 minutes   **COOK:** about 15 minutes

2 large onions, cut into quarters and thinly sliced (about 2 cups)

⅓ cup of ketchup (store-bought or homemade)

1 tbsp. of apple cider vinegar

1 tbsp. of water

¾ tsp. of sugar

1. Mix all of the ingredients together in a nonreactive pan, and simmer until the onions are translucent (about 15 minutes).

2. Pour the mixture into a container, cover tightly, and store it in the refrigerator.

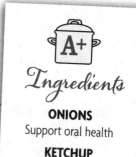

A+

Ingredients

ONIONS
Support oral health

KETCHUP
Boosts eye health

APPLE CIDER VINEGAR
Helps fight free radicals

KITCHEN CAPERS

When you need ketchup now, but you have none on hand, mix 1 cup of tomato sauce with 1 tablespoon of sugar and 1 teaspoon of white vinegar.

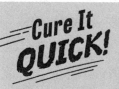

Cure It **QUICK!**

CONQUER COLDS And flu viruses, too! How? Mix up a batch of this marvelous mustard and use it frequently throughout the cold and flu season. Mustard seeds are rich in anti-inflammatory compounds that, consumed regularly, can stop cold and flu symptoms in their tracks. And your own DIY medicine contains more of the active ingredient than common supermarket brands do. To make it, mix 2 cups of dry mustard with ½ cup of water. Whisk in ½ cup each of apple cider vinegar and extra virgin olive oil. Stir in ½ cup of firmly packed brown sugar and a pinch of salt. Then ladle the mixture into small sterilized jars. Screw the lids on tightly and store the jars in the refrigerator for up to two months. (For longer storage, can your "crop" following the instructions in "For the Long Haul" on page 144.)
Note: *This mustard is ultra-hot at first, but the longer it's stored, the milder it gets—without losing any of its potent heroic healing power.*

CRANBERRY KETCHUP

If you only think of ketchup as an accessory to French fries, think again! This cranberry version lends itself especially well to baked ham, pork, or any kind of wild game.

YIELD: about 4 cups	PREP: 20 minutes	COOK: 40 minutes

4 cups of cranberries (fresh or frozen)

2 large onions, minced

1 cup of dry white wine

1 cup of water

3 cups of sugar

2 cups of apple cider vinegar

1 tbsp. of celery seed

1 tbsp. of ground allspice

1 tbsp. of ground cinnamon

½ tbsp. of ground cloves

1 ½ tsp. of freshly ground black pepper

1 tsp. of salt

½ tsp. of dry mustard

1. Put the berries, onions, wine, and water in a large pan. Boil over medium heat until the cranberries pop.

2. Let the mixture cool slightly, then transfer it to a blender or food processor, and puree.

3. Return the pureed mixture to the pan and mix in the remaining ingredients.

4. Reduce the heat to low and simmer, stirring often, until thick (about 30 minutes). Pack the ketchup into hot sterilized jars and prepare for storage (see "For the Long Haul" on page 144).

KITCHEN CAPERS Before using fresh cranberries, discard any stems and shriveled berries. Leave any white cranberries—they're perfectly edible, and they are also sweeter than their red counterparts!

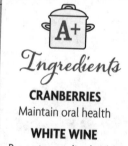

A+

Ingredients

CRANBERRIES
Maintain oral health

WHITE WINE
Promotes cardiac health

APPLE CIDER VINEGAR
Enhances weight loss

INSTANT GRATIFICATION

No Muss, No Fuss Tomato Ketchup

With this quick and easy recipe, there's no need to buy ketchup from the store again! In a nonreactive bowl, combine three 6-ounce cans of tomato paste, 6 tablespoons each of apple cider vinegar and raw honey, ½ teaspoon each of ground cloves and sea salt, and ¼ teaspoon of ground allspice. Whisk until the mix is very smooth, and then stir in enough water to achieve your desired consistency. Refrigerate in a sealed container for up to two weeks.

PEACHY-KEEN SANDWICH TOPPER

This oddball-sounding concoction is actually an old-time recipe for hot dog relish. It is also an absolute match made in heaven for burgers and grilled chicken.

YIELD: 12 half-pint jars	**PREP:** 20 minutes	**COOK:** 2 hours

10 large red tomatoes, peeled and finely chopped

9 peaches, peeled and finely chopped

3 large onions, peeled and finely chopped

2 sweet red peppers, finely chopped

1 ½ cups of apple cider vinegar

1 ½ cups of raw honey

4 tbsp. of mixed pickling spices, tied in a muslin bag

1 tbsp. of pickling salt

1. Combine all of the ingredients in a large pot.

2. Cook the mixture, uncovered, on medium heat until it thickens (at least 2 hours).

3. Remove the spice bag and ladle the relish into sterilized half-pint jars, leaving ½ inch of headspace, and process for 10 minutes, following the directions in "For the Long Haul" on page 144.*

If you don't need your batch to last more than 2 months, halve the recipe and keep it in the fridge.

A+ Ingredients

TOMATOES
Promote brain health

PEACHES
Maintain skin health

APPLE CIDER VINEGAR
Helps balance blood sugar

KITCHEN CAPERS There are many ways to remove the skin from an onion, but this is one of the easiest: Cut the onion in half lengthwise from end to end. Then grab hold of the skin along the cut edge and peel it off. That's all there is to it!

CULINARY Q & A

? It seems like every time I peel and chop large quantities of tomatoes, I wind up with red splotches on my apron and sleeves. How can I get the stains out?

! Saturate the juiced spots with white vinegar, let it sink in, then wash as usual. Make sure the stains are gone before you put clothes in the dryer. If there's any trace of a stain, the heat will cook it into the fabric, and you'll never get it out. Also, be certain that you use only white vinegar for this or any other stain-removal task.

CLASSIC COARSE-GRAIN MUSTARD

Mustard seeds are an excellent source of minerals such as calcium, magnesium, and potassium. And homemade mustard is better than anything you're likely to find on store shelves. This full-bodied blend is truly delicious and is a cinch to make.

YIELD: about 1 ½ cups	**PREP:** 10 minutes	**WAIT:** 48 hours

¼ cup of brown mustard seeds, crushed

¼ cup of yellow (a.k.a. white) mustard seeds, crushed

½ cup of malt vinegar

¼ cup of beer*

Pinch of kosher or sea salt

1 tbsp. of brown sugar

A hearty brown ale is a good choice, but use any kind of beer you fancy.

1. Mix the first five ingredients together in a small nonreactive bowl. Cover the bowl, and let it sit for about 24 hours.

2. Add the brown sugar, and blend the mixture in a blender or food processor until combined.

3. Pour the blend into a sterilized jar, and store it in the refrigerator for at least a day or so before serving, so the flavors can blend. Tightly covered, the mustard will keep for up to 1 month.

A+

Ingredients

MUSTARD SEEDS
Fight skin infections

MALT VINEGAR
Aids weight loss

BEER
Supports bone health

Mustard seeds are flavorless until they're broken open or heated to release their essential oils. So always crush or toast them before using, even if your recipe doesn't specify that step. To toast mustard (or any other) seeds, heat them on medium in a skillet, stirring until they're fragrant.

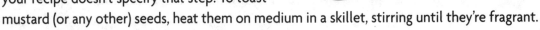

KITCHEN CAPERS

INSTANT GRATIFICATION

A Honey of a Honey Mustard

If you always order honey mustard on sandwiches at your local deli, this easy DIY version is just for you! First, mix 3 tablespoons of dry mustard with 1½ tablespoons of cold water and 1 teaspoon of white or apple cider vinegar to form a thick paste. Add 2 tablespoons of raw honey and 1 tablespoon of canola oil, and whisk until the mixture is very smooth. That's all there is to it!

MIGHTY MARVELOUS MUSTARD

If you're new at the mustard-making game, this super sandwich spread makes a perfect debut recipe. Not only is it easy to make, but its flavor defies description—it manages to be sweet, sour, spicy, and mellow all at once. Try it—you'll love it!

| **YIELD:** about 2 cups | **PREP:** 10 minutes | **WAIT:** 3 days |

⅔ cup of dry mustard

½ cup of dark brown sugar

¼ cup of apple cider vinegar

1 tsp. of lemon juice

1 tsp. of Worcestershire sauce

¼ cup of extra virgin olive oil

Salt and freshly ground
    black pepper to taste

1. Mix the first five ingredients in a blender. With the machine still running, slowly add the olive oil.

2. Taste, add salt and pepper as desired, and whirl briefly to blend everything together.

3. Pour the mixture into a sterilized jar, screw the lid on tightly, and put it in the refrigerator to mellow for three days before using.

KITCHEN CAPERS

To soften brown sugar that's become solidified, put the amount you need in a glass bowl, place a couple of damp paper towels on top of the sugar, and cover the bowl tightly. Microwave it for 30 seconds. If it's still hard, continue to heat for 10-second intervals.

A+

Ingredients

MUSTARD POWDER
Fights colds and flu

APPLE CIDER VINEGAR
Enhances digestive processes

EXTRA VIRGIN OLIVE OIL
Supports weight loss

CULINARY Q & A

? Recently a friend told me that whenever he gets a sudden muscle cramp, he helps treat it with mustard. Is he just pulling my leg?

! Nope. It really can help! Here's how to try it: When you feel a cramp coming on, just swallow a teaspoon of mustard, and chase it down with water. Repeat every two minutes until the twinges stop. The more pure mustard it contains, the sooner you're likely to feel relief, so for that reason, a potent DIY version, like the one in "Conquer Colds" (see page 129), is best. But any kind of mustard will work. Keep small mustard packets with you, and you'll always be prepared on the go!

ANCHOVY MAYONNAISE

Grilled fish all but cries out for this salty, seaworthy sauce. It's also a great dip for fresh raw vegetables. For this purpose, you'll want to multiply the recipe to suit the number of guests. And be sure to make more than you think you'll need because it'll be a big hit!

YIELD: about 1 cup   **PREP:** 15 minutes

½ cup of whole-grain bread crumbs

3 tbsp. of apple cider vinegar

3 anchovy fillets

1 garlic clove

1 large bunch of parsley, coarsely chopped

⅓ cup of extra virgin olive oil

Salt and freshly ground black pepper to taste

1. Soak the bread crumbs in the vinegar for 10 minutes. Squeeze out the excess moisture with your hands and discard the liquid.

2. Puree the crumbs, anchovies, garlic, and parsley in a food processor.

3. With the machine still running, slowly add the olive oil a little at a time. Continue processing until the sauce is thick and creamy.

4. Taste the mixture, and season as desired with salt and pepper. Serve at room temperature.

A+ Ingredients

WHOLE-GRAIN BREAD CRUMBS
Promote healthy digestion

ANCHOVIES
Fight inflammation

PARSLEY
Supports strong bones

KITCHEN CAPERS

Homemade bread crumbs are tastier than store bought, and they're easy to make. Take a loaf of bread (any kind will do), and slice off any part of the crust that is too tough. Then cut the bread into large cubes, toss it into a food processor, and let 'er rip.

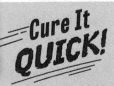

Cure It QUICK!

THANKS FOR THE MEMORIES MAYO Garlic is a star when it comes to boosting your brain cells and your memory. Enjoy the pungent bulb in this mayonnaise (a.k.a. aioli): Process 4 to 10 peeled, crushed garlic cloves (use taste to determine the amount), 2 egg yolks, and a pinch of salt in a blender until smooth. Add 1 ½ to 2 tablespoons of white wine vinegar and process again. With the machine still running, gradually pour in 1 ¼ cups of extra virgin olive oil. If the mixture is too thick, add more vinegar until you have the right consistency. Use the blend as you would any other mayonnaise.

HIGH-SUMMER CORN RELISH

The time to make this traditional relish is at the height of summer, when farmers' markets—and maybe your own garden—are overflowing with just-picked corn. Use your tasty handiwork immediately, or tuck it away to enjoy throughout the winter.

YIELD: about 11 cups   **PREP:** 20 minutes   **COOK:** 15–25 minutes

Kernels from 8 fresh-picked ears of corn (about 5 ½ lbs.)

8 celery ribs, finely chopped

2 green bell peppers, diced

2 red bell peppers, diced

2 medium onions, finely chopped

4 ½ cups of apple cider vinegar

½ cup of sugar

1 tbsp. of mustard seeds

1 tbsp. of salt

4 allspice berries

1. Put all the ingredients in a large pot and stir over low heat until the sugar has completely dissolved.

2. Bring the mixture to a boil, stirring continuously. Reduce the heat and simmer, stirring occasionally, for 15 to 20 minutes, or until the vegetables are tender.

3. Spoon the blend into warm sterilized jars to within ⅛ inch of the tops. The relish should remain fresh for about 3 months stored in a cool, dark place.

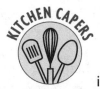

KITCHEN CAPERS When you have more fresh corn than you can use immediately—for corn relish or other purposes—shuck the ears, seal them in freezer bags, and freeze. They should stay in fine shape for up to one month.

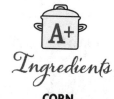

A+

Ingredients

CORN
Helps maintain vision

CELERY
Promotes liver health

BELL PEPPERS
Boost immune system

INSTANT GRATIFICATION

Fast & Easy Relish

A spoonful of this treat will wake up any sandwich, and it's a major crowd pleaser on any buffet table that features cold meats. Mix 4 teaspoons each of grated onion and finely chopped green bell pepper with 3 tablespoons of your favorite prepared mustard; 3 teaspoons each of malt vinegar, olive oil, and sugar; and ½ teaspoon of ground black pepper. Let the mixture sit for at least 30 minutes so the flavors can blend, and serve. This recipe makes about ⅓ cup of relish.

MANGO CHUTNEY

This fruity blend has a sweet-and-savory bite that makes it a perfect companion for seafood, poultry, beef, or pork. It also adds a flavorful jolt to a cold sandwich, and it's delicious when paired with cream cheese on a toasted bagel or English muffin.

YIELD: 6 cups **PREP:** 15 minutes **COOK:** 1 ¼ hours

1 cup of sugar

½ cup of white or apple cider vinegar

2 mangoes, peeled, pitted, and cut into ¾-inch pieces

1 small onion, chopped

¼ cup of golden raisins

2 tbsp. of crystallized ginger, finely chopped

2 garlic cloves, minced

1. Combine the sugar and vinegar in a 6-quart pot, and bring the mixture to a boil, stirring until the sugar has dissolved.

2. Add the remaining ingredients, and simmer, stirring occasionally for 45 to 60 minutes, or until the blend reaches a slightly thickened, syrupy consistency.

3. Pour it into sterilized jars, and store it in a cool, dark place, where it should keep for up to 1 year.

A+

Ingredients

MANGOES
Support eye health

GOLDEN RAISINS
Help promote healthy blood pressure

CRYSTALLIZED GINGER
Fights inflammation

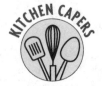

KITCHEN CAPERS

After you open a jar of any chutney or relish, put it in the fridge. It should stay fine for months. If you detect an "off" odor, appearance, or flavor, toss the whole shebang in the trash.

CULINARY Q & A

? Some recipes call for crystallized ginger and others candied ginger. What's the difference? And if it's not available, can I use fresh or ground ginger?

! There is no difference: The terms *crystallized ginger* and *candied ginger* are interchangeable. To make your own version, see "DIY Candied Ginger" on page 145. As for making substitutions, in most recipes you can use either fresh or ground ginger, combined with sugar. Getting the balance just right can be tricky, though. For the substitution process, see "Send in the Candied-Ginger Pinch Hitters" on page 145.

HOME FRONT PICCALILLI

This sweet-and-sour green tomato relish dates back to World War II. The ingredients can vary, so feel free to add or subtract depending on the produce you have on hand.

YIELD: 3–4 pints	PREP: 15 minutes	COOK: 20 minutes

4 cups of chopped green tomatoes

2 cups of chopped green cabbage

2 cups of chopped red bell peppers

1 cup of chopped firm red tomatoes

¼ cup of salt

1 ½ cups of apple cider vinegar

1 cup of packed light brown sugar

1 tsp. of mustard seed

¼–½ tsp. of cayenne pepper

1. Combine the first five ingredients in a bowl. Cover and refrigerate for 8 to 24 hours. Then drain, rinse, and set aside.

2. Put the remaining ingredients in a large saucepan and bring to a boil. Stir in the vegetables and simmer for 20 minutes.

3. Can the relish (see directions in "For the Long Haul" on page 144), and "relish" it for many months to come. Enjoy it spread on sandwiches, or served on the side with cooked meats.

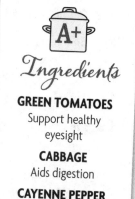

Ingredients

GREEN TOMATOES
Support healthy eyesight

CABBAGE
Aids digestion

CAYENNE PEPPER
Enhances circulation

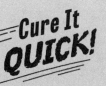

KITCHEN CAPERS If you want to keep green tomatoes unripe for future use, freeze 'em. Just wash them, cut out any bad spots, put them on baking sheets, and slide them into the freezer. Once they're frozen, store them in plastic bags or containers.

Cure It QUICK! **EXCELLENT ULCER ERADICATOR** Help heal and prevent both gastric and duodenal ulcers with this simple pickled red cabbage. Cut a cabbage into quarters, remove the core and outer leaves, and slice each quarter thinly. Toss the slices with 2 tablespoons of salt. Put a plate over the cabbage, top it with a heavy weight, and set aside for 24 hours. When the time's up, put 10 cups of white vinegar and 6 tablespoons of pickling spice in a large nonreactive pot. Boil for six minutes. Pack the cabbage into canning jars (this recipe will fill about eight to ten 12-ounce jars), ladle the hot vinegar mixture on top, and seal the jars. Store them in a cool, dark place at room temperature. They will be ready for action after six days.

FRUIT & TOMATO CHUTNEY

Here's a full-bodied, fruity blend that's tailor-made for grilled pork, chicken, or fish. Keep a supply on hand so you'll be all set for spur-of-the-moment barbecues.

YIELD: about 3 quarts	**PREP:** 30 minutes	**COOK:** 90 minutes

4 lbs. of ripe red tomatoes, peeled, cored, and chopped

5 large tart green apples, peeled, cored, and chopped

1 large onion, diced

2 garlic cloves, minced

1 ½ cups of raisins

1 cup of apple cider vinegar

1 cup of dried apricots, diced

⅓ cup of finely diced crystallized ginger

2 tsp. of salt

1 tsp. of ground cinnamon

Dash of cayenne pepper

1. Combine all of the ingredients in a large stainless steel or enameled iron pot.

2. Cook the mixture over medium heat for 90 minutes, or until very thick, stirring occasionally.

3. Spoon the chutney into hot sterilized jars and prep it for pantry storage. (For directions, see "For the Long Haul" on page 144.)

KITCHEN CAPERS

To peel tomatoes, remove the cores, and drop the tomatoes into boiling water. Wait 30 seconds, then transfer them to a pan of ice water to stop the cooking and release the skins. The peels will slip right off.

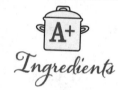

A+

Ingredients

APPLES
Prevent colds

DRIED APRICOTS
Support cardiovascular health

GROUND CINNAMON
Boosts brain function

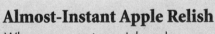

INSTANT GRATIFICATION

Almost-Instant Apple Relish

When you want a quick perker-upper for roast pork or chicken, try this simple recipe. Put 2 tart or sweet-tart apples (peeled, cored, and chopped) in a saucepan with 2 tablespoons of brown sugar and 1 tablespoon of apple cider vinegar. Cook over medium-high heat, stirring for three minutes, or until the sugar has dissolved. Reduce the heat to low and simmer for six minutes, or until the apples are tender. Then serve it up. **Note:** *Although Granny Smith is the most widely available variety, Braeburn, Gravenstein, and Ida Red are all delicious choices.*

APRICOT & ALMOND CHUTNEY

This sweet-and-tangy treat offers a healthy helping of nutrients, thanks to apple cider vinegar. It also goes beautifully with pork, chicken, or fish.

YIELD: about 1 quart	**PREP:** 15 minutes	**COOK:** 70 minutes

1 cup of apple cider vinegar, divided

1 cup of sugar

12 apricots, chopped

2 medium onions, chopped

2 red bell peppers, chopped

1 garlic clove, chopped

1 lemon (including peel), finely chopped

1 orange (including peel), finely chopped

½ cup of raisins

½ cup of sliced crystallized ginger, finely chopped

1 tsp. of salt

½ cup of blanched whole almonds

1 tsp. of ground ginger

1. Pour ¾ cup of the vinegar into a pan. Add the sugar, and stir over low heat until the sugar has completely dissolved. Then bring the mixture to a boil; reduce the heat and simmer for 5 minutes.

2. Add the next nine ingredients to the pan. Simmer over medium heat, stirring frequently, for 30 minutes.

3. Add the almonds, ginger, and remaining ¼ cup of vinegar. Simmer, stirring frequently, for another 30 minutes, or until the chutney has thickened.

4. Spoon the mixture into warm sterilized jars, and store in a cool, dark place for 2 months before eating.

 KITCHEN CAPERS To blanch almonds, put them in a bowl with just enough boiling water to cover them. Wait for one minute, and drain. Rinse under cold water, and pat them dry with a soft cloth or paper towel. Then slip the skins off.

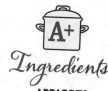

Ingredients

APRICOTS
Help support bone health

ORANGES
Support healthy blood pressure

ALMONDS
Aid weight loss

CULINARY Q & A

? These days, chutney seems to be all the rage among Internet food bloggers. Which one of them invented this fancy concoction?

! Actually, we owe this condiment to British troops in the 18th century. Three factors contributed to its development: the Brits' love of sweet sauces, the presence of foods rarely seen in England, and the need to preserve food with no refrigeration.

NO-WAIT APPLE CRAN-PEARY CHUTNEY

When you're in a hurry to talk turkey, this is the recipe to reach for. That's because, unlike most chutneys, this one doesn't need to cool its heels for weeks before you use it. You can make it up to three days ahead if you want to—or you can serve it immediately.

YIELD: about 3 ½ cups	**PREP:** 25 minutes	**COOK:** 45 minutes

2 cups of apple cider vinegar

1 cup of finely chopped onion

¼ cup of chopped, peeled fresh ginger (about a 2-inch piece)

2 ½ tsp. of finely grated fresh lemon peel

2 ½ tsp. of finely grated fresh orange peel

1 cinnamon stick, broken in half

½ tsp. of dried crushed red pepper

¼ tsp. of ground cloves

1 ¼ cups of packed light brown sugar

1 bag (12-oz.) of fresh cranberries (or frozen, thawed)

1 large apple, peeled, cored, and chopped into bite-size cubes

1 large firm pear, peeled, cored, and chopped into bite-size cubes

1. Combine the first eight ingredients in a large, heavy saucepan. Boil the mix until reduced to 1½ cups (about 10 minutes).

2. Add the remaining ingredients, reduce heat to medium, and stir until the sugar dissolves.

3. Reduce the heat to medium-low. Cover and simmer, stirring occasionally, until the apples and pears are very tender, the berries collapse, and the flavors blend (about 30 minutes). Remove from the heat and discard cinnamon.

4. Using a potato masher (not a food processor!), mash it coarsely.

5. Transfer to a bowl and cool to room temperature before serving. Or cover and put in the fridge for up to 3 days; again bring the chutney to room temperature before serving.

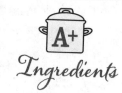

Ingredients

FRESH GINGER
Helps ease joint and muscle pain

CRANBERRIES
Support urinary tract health

PEARS
Boost your energy level

KITCHEN CAPERS Most recipes that use brown sugar call for it to be packed—not simply poured—into a measuring cup. So at shopping time, keep this rule of thumb in mind: A 1-pound bag or box of brown sugar is equivalent to about 2 ½ cups packed.

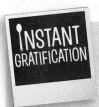
INSTANT GRATIFICATION

Easy Apricot Chutney

Keep this treat on hand to top cream cheese and crackers, to serve with pork or poultry, or to mix into other savory dishes. To make it, combine 1 ½ cups of apricot jam with 1 cup of rice vinegar, ⅓ cup of crushed mustard seed, and 1 tablespoon of minced fresh ginger in a 10- to 12-inch skillet. Bring to a boil, stirring frequently until the mixture is reduced to roughly 2 cups (about eight minutes). Let the chutney cool slightly and serve it up. Or pour the cooled blend into a sterilized jar, cover it tightly, and chill.

CULINARY Q & A

? I like to use a box grater to grate citrus fruits, but a lot of the peel gets stuck in the teeth and wasted. Is there any way around that problem?

! You have two good choices. One is to cover the grater with a piece of wax paper before you start grating the fruit. All of the zest will stay on top of the paper and slide right off when you're finished. Another option is to keep a clean toothbrush on hand expressly for this purpose. When you're finished grating, simply scrape the trapped zest off the toothy surface.

YOUR STATE-OF-THE-FRUIT SELECTION GUIDE

When it comes to ripening patterns, fruits vary considerably. So when you're shopping for fruit to make pickles and condiments, keep these guidelines in mind.

Ripening Style	Fruits That Have It
Never ripen after harvesting	Soft berries, cherries, all citrus fruits, grapes, olives, pineapple, watermelon
Ripen only after harvesting	Avocados
Ripen in color, texture, and juiciness after harvesting, but do not get sweeter	Apricots, blueberries, figs, melon (aside from watermelon), nectarines, passion fruit, peaches, persimmons
Get sweeter after harvesting	Apples, kiwi, mangoes, papayas, pears
Ripen in all ways after harvesting	Bananas

SPICY BLUEBERRY CHUTNEY

This tangy—and eye-catching—blend teams up perfectly with grilled chicken or pork chops, and it's an ideal companion for any kind of curry.

YIELD: 2 cups	**PREP:** 15 minutes	**COOK:** 30 minutes

2 cups of blueberries, fresh or frozen

1 cup of golden raisins

¾ cup of firmly packed light brown sugar

½ cup of balsamic vinegar

½ cup of finely chopped crystallized ginger

⅓ cup of finely chopped onion

1 garlic clove, crushed

1 jalapeño pepper, seeded and finely chopped

Grated zest of 1 large lemon

1 cinnamon stick

⅛ tsp. of ground cloves

⅛ tsp. of ground mace

1. Combine all of the ingredients in a medium-size, heavy-bottomed nonreactive pan. Bring to a boil over high heat, stirring frequently to prevent scorching.

2. Reduce the heat to low and simmer, stirring occasionally, until the mixture is very thick (15 to 20 minutes).

3. Cool to room temperature and serve immediately. Or ladle the hot chutney into sterilized canning jars, let them cool completely, and store them in the fridge for up to 3 months.

KITCHEN CAPERS To remove berry juice stains from your hands, just wash them with a little salt and vinegar! Make sure to scrub well. Then simply rinse your hands. The stains will be gone in a flash!

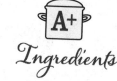

A+

Ingredients

BLUEBERRIES
Boost liver function

JALAPEÑO PEPPER
Fights off coughs and colds

LEMON ZEST
Supports bone health

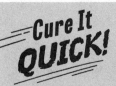

Cure It QUICK!

GUARDIAN ANGEL RELISH The compounds in papayas have been shown to offer angelic protection against truly demonic diseases—as well as against the common cold. And this relish is a delicious way to help meet your fruitful quota. To make four servings, mix 2 diced papayas in a bowl with 1 diced red bell pepper and 1 diced red onion. Add ⅔ cup of red wine vinegar, 1 tablespoon of lime juice, 1 teaspoon of honey, 2 tablespoons of torn fresh cilantro leaves, and a pinch of salt. Stir well, cover, and chill for two hours, stirring several times. Then serve it up!

STRAWBERRY-RHUBARB CHUTNEY

Here's a savory chutney twist on a classic pie flavor that will add pizzazz to everything from grilled meats to a bagel with cream cheese, buttered toast, and even pancakes.

YIELD: 6 servings	**PREP:** 10 minutes	**COOK:** about 15 minutes

4 tbsp. of unsalted butter

½ small onion, diced

1 tsp. of Dijon mustard

½ tsp. of ground allspice

½ tsp. of ground cinnamon

⅛ tsp. of paprika

5 cups of diced, peeled rhubarb stalks (not leaves!)

2 cups of diced fresh strawberries

1 tbsp. of apple cider vinegar

3 tsp. of raw honey

1. Melt the butter in a saucepan over medium-low heat. Add the onion and sauté until tender.

2. Mix in the mustard and spices. Heat, stirring continuously. Add the rhubarb and strawberries; stir until the bubbling subsides. Cook for 10 minutes, mashing with a potato masher often.

3. Once the fruit is soft and broken down, add the vinegar and cook, stirring, for 1 to 2 minutes.

4. Remove from heat and stir in the honey. Serve immediately, or pour it into a sterilized jar and store it, tightly covered, in the fridge.

A+ Ingredients

ONION
Boosts immunity

RHUBARB
Promotes digestive health

STRAWBERRIES
Help protect eyes and skin from sun damage

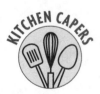

KITCHEN CAPERS

Field-grown rhubarb, which has cherry-red stalks and bright green leaves, is far more flavorful than more common hothouse varieties, which have pink to pale red stalks and yellow-green leaves.

CULINARY Q & A

? I've heard that rhubarb leaves are poisonous. Is that true?

! Eating rhubarb leaves (or flower stems) will make you sick. The severity of the reaction can depend on the variety of rhubarb, the amount swallowed, and the time elapsed between consumption and treatment, as well as the patient's age, weight, and physical condition. Serious poisonings can result in kidney failure. Although deaths are rare, they do happen. So, don't eat any part of a rhubarb plant except the leaf stalks!

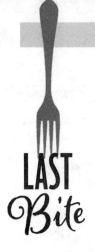

FOR THE LONG HAUL

To store condiments or pickled foods at room temperature almost indefinitely, use the hot-water bath canning method. This may sound intimidating if you've never done it, but don't worry—it's a simple process. Here's all there is to it:

1. Ladle, pour, or pack the prepared ingredients into hot sterilized canning jars, leaving ¼ to ½ inch of space (as specified in your recipe) at the top.

2. Wipe the jar rims with a damp cloth, and attach the lids.

3. Put the jars on a rack in a large, deep pot that's no more than 4 inches larger in diameter than the stove burner.

4. Pour in enough boiling water to cover the lids by 2 inches, and add a tablespoon or two of white vinegar to keep hard-water deposits from forming on the jars' sealers.

5. Cover the pot, bring the water to a hard boil, and boil for 15 minutes (less if specified in your recipe), lowering the heat if necessary to keep the pot from overflowing. Remove the jars and set them on a rack or dish towels to cool.

6. Wipe the jars with white vinegar to remove any food residue. Label them, and then store them in a dry place that's well removed from any heat source, like a furnace, water heater, or hot-water pipes.

7. Wait for the time noted in your recipe before using, so the flavors have a chance to blend. Most pickles take at least six weeks to develop full flavor.

8. Always refrigerate any jar of pickles or condiments after opening.

Note: *Always use either Mason® or Ball® jars that are specifically designed for home canning. Commercial-food jars typically can't handle the necessary heat.*

Apple cider, red wine, and balsamic vinegars give a distinctive flavor boost to pickled fruits and vegetables. There's just one drawback: These dark varieties generally discolor lighter-toned produce like apples, pears, onions, and cauliflower. In these cases, you're better off using distilled white, white wine, sherry, or champagne vinegar.

2 QUICK CANNING TRICKS

When you're canning food, vinegar is a vital asset—regardless of whether it's part of your recipe or not. Here's how to put it to work:

- To prevent hard-water deposits from forming on the jars' sealers, add a tablespoon or two of white vinegar to the canning bath.

- Before you store your jars, wipe the outsides thoroughly with white vinegar. This will remove any food residue that may be on the glass, thereby eliminating the chance of mold forming.

SEND IN THE CANDIED-GINGER PINCH HITTERS

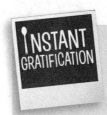

INSTANT GRATIFICATION

DIY Candied Ginger

To make your own candied (a.k.a. crystallized) ginger, peel and chop the amount of fresh ginger that you want to crystallize. For each cup of ginger, make a simple syrup by mixing 1 cup of sugar and 1 cup of water and bringing the mixture to a boil. Add the ginger, reduce the heat, and simmer for 20 minutes. Using a slotted spoon, transfer the ginger to a wire rack (set over a baking sheet so the sticky runoff doesn't mar your countertop). Once the ginger is dry, either use it in your recipe or store it for up to three weeks in the refrigerator.

What do you do when you are whipping up a recipe that calls for crystallized (a.k.a. candied) ginger, and you have none on hand—and no time to rush out and buy any? If you have either fresh or ground ginger on hand, count yourself lucky. Your action plan depends on which version you're using. Here's the deal:

Fresh ginger. Use one-quarter the amount of candied ginger that the recipe calls for, plus sugar to taste. For example, if your recipe calls for ½ cup of candied ginger (8 tablespoons), use 2 tablespoons of grated fresh ginger plus 2 to 4 tablespoons of sugar.

Ground ginger. Because the flavor is much more intense than it is in the fresh version, just about ½ teaspoon of ground ginger is comparable to ½ cup of candied ginger. Mix in sugar as desired—but proceed with caution. (You can always add more, but correcting a too-sweet recipe can be a nightmare.) Your best bet: For each teaspoon of ground ginger, start with 2 tablespoons of sugar and add more as needed.

Chapter Five

Sensational
Soups
& Stews

If the words *comfort food* conjure up thoughts of soups and stews, you've come to the right place. In this chapter, you'll find hearty stews to warm you up on stormy winter nights, chilled soups to cool you down on steamy summer afternoons—and everything in between. And (you guessed it) vinegar plays a leading role in every single one of them.

TOMATO-POTATO-BASIL SOUP

Hands down, our country's two favorite vegetables are tomatoes and spuds. In this satisfying and super-simple soup, that all-American duo teams up with sweet basil, which is one of our best-loved, most-used—and easiest-to-grow—herbs.

YIELD: 4 servings	**PREP:** 20 minutes	**COOK:** 30 minutes

1 lb. of tomatoes, peeled, seeded, and diced

¾ lb. of potatoes, peeled and diced

3 cups of chicken or vegetable stock

1 medium onion, diced

⅓ cup of basil vinegar

¼ cup of minced fresh basil

1 tsp. of salt

½ tsp. of freshly ground black pepper

1. Combine the first five ingredients in a large nonreactive pot. Cover it, and bring the mixture to a boil over medium heat.

2. Reduce the heat to low, and simmer for 30 minutes, or until the potatoes are very soft.

3. Pour the soup into a blender, and puree. Stir in the basil, salt, and pepper, and serve it up.

KITCHEN CAPERS

When summer's bounty comes in, make freezer "soup kits" to enjoy all winter. Combine corn, carrots, celery, onions, broccoli, tomatoes, and potatoes in containers or freezer bags, and put in the freezer. Then reach for one whenever the need arises.

A+ Ingredients

TOMATOES
Support heart health

POTATOES
Maintain strong bone structure

ONION
Fights inflammation

CULINARY Q & A

? Is there any difference between stock and broth? I see both terms used to describe the same product.

! There is a difference, but it's minor. In professional kitchens, broth is often seasoned (so that it can be consumed on its own), while stock is not (because it is designed to be seasoned later to suit a particular recipe). With commercial brands, the distinction essentially vanishes; both stock and broth are seasoned. Your best option when you're shopping for a stock is to look for a brand that contains the least amount of sodium. That gives you the most versatility when you're cooking.

THE DAY-AFTER TURKEY SOUP

This is the perfect go-to recipe anytime you have a partially eaten turkey in your fridge. The superstar ingredient is the vinegar. It makes the meat easier to remove from the bones and also draws out calcium and flavor.

YIELD: 6–8 servings   **PREP:** 10 minutes   **COOK:** 3 hours

1 leftover turkey carcass

Water

2 tbsp. of white vinegar

2 cups of barley

4 carrots, sliced

3 celery ribs, diced

2 large onions, diced

1 can (28 or 32 oz.) of
   diced tomatoes

1. Put the turkey carcass in a large stockpot, cover it with water, and add the vinegar.

2. Cover the pot, and simmer over low heat for 2 hours, adding more water as needed.

3. Remove the carcass, and let it cool. Pull the meat from the bones, and put it back in the pot, along with the rest of the ingredients, except the diced tomatoes.

4. Cook the soup for 50 minutes, then stir in the tomatoes, and cook for another 10 minutes.

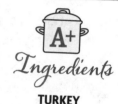

A+

Ingredients

TURKEY
Boosts immunity

BARLEY
Maintains healthy
blood pressure

CARROTS
Keep skin healthy

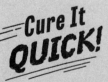

If you can, make soups and stews a day ahead and stash them in the refrigerator. Then warm them on the stove (not the microwave) before serving time. Spending quality time in the chiller and then being reheated slowly will let the flavors blend and intensify.

KITCHEN CAPERS

Cure It QUICK!

SUPERCHARGED CHICKEN SOUP We all know that chicken soup is a powerful weapon in the fight against cold and flu germs. But you can add even more oomph to your favorite recipe (or even instant chicken broth) with this simple trick: Heat 1 cup of soup or broth, then stir in 1 tablespoon of vinegar, 1 crushed garlic clove, and hot-pepper sauce to taste. Pour the mixture into a bowl or mug, and sip your way to good health. Repeat as necessary until you're back in the pink of health again.

GAZPACHO ITALIANO

Balsamic vinegar gives an Italian twist to this refreshing summertime classic. Serve it with a loaf of crusty Italian bread and a bottle of chilled white vino.

YIELD: 6–8 servings	PREP: 30 minutes	WAIT: 4–24 hours

3 large tomatoes, quartered

1 cucumber, peeled and sliced

1 red bell pepper, chopped

1 small red onion, chopped

1 large garlic clove, minced

1 ½ cups of tomato juice

⅓ cup of balsamic vinegar

½ tsp. of salt

¼ tsp. of red pepper flakes

⅓ cup of chopped fresh basil leaves (for garnish)

1. Put the first first five ingredients into a food processor, and pulse until coarsely chopped.

2. Add the tomato juice, vinegar, salt, and red pepper flakes, and process again. Make sure you don't overprocess—this soup should be chunky! If necessary, work in batches.

3. Transfer soup to a large bowl; cover it tightly. Refrigerate for 4 to 24 hours.

4. Serve in chilled soup bowls, with the basil sprinkled on top.

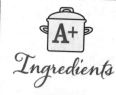

A+ Ingredients

CUCUMBER
Boosts hydration

BELL PEPPER
Supports a healthy immune system

GARLIC
Fights cold and flu germs

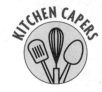

KITCHEN CAPERS

When you cook vegetables, freeze the cooking liquid. It makes a flavorful and nutritious base for soups and stews. The same goes for either pan juices or cooking liquid from meat and fish.

CULINARY Q & A

? I've read that commercial balsamic vinegars are really wine vinegar with artificial flavorings added. But I can't begin to afford the real thing! Is there any alternative?

! Nothing compares to traditional balsamic vinegar, which by law is made in small quantities and aged for at least 12 years in wooden barrels. However, balsamic vinegar that's labeled *condimento* is very good and cheaper than the "real deal." Another option is to use a commercial version that's labeled "balsamic vinegar of Modena" and add one large pinch of brown sugar for every cup of vinegar.

KALE & KIELBASA SOUP

Nothing warms up a cold winter evening like a bowl of hearty, stick-to-your ribs soup. And you'll never find a recipe that lives up to that description more than this one does.

YIELD: 4 servings	PREP: 15 minutes	COOK: 25 minutes

1 tbsp. of extra virgin olive oil

8 oz. of kielbasa or fresh Italian sausage, thinly sliced crosswise

1 large leek (white and light green parts), sliced

1 bunch of kale, rinsed, de-stemmed, and chopped

3 cups of chicken broth

1 can (15 oz.) of white beans, rinsed and drained

1 tbsp. of red wine vinegar

½ tsp. of kosher or sea salt

Freshly ground black pepper to taste

Parmigiano-Reggiano cheese, freshly grated

1. Heat the oil in a large, heavy saucepan over medium heat. Add the sausage, and cook until browned.

2. Add the leek and cook for about 3 minutes, then add the kale and cook until it's wilted (about 3 minutes).

3. Stir in the chicken broth and beans, and bring to a boil. Then reduce the heat and simmer until the kale is tender (10 to 15 minutes).

4. Stir in the vinegar, and season with salt and pepper. Sprinkle cheese on top to taste.

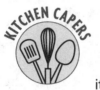

KITCHEN CAPERS Remove fat from a meat-based soup by freezing it for 30 minutes. The fat will congeal on top. Skim it off using a spatula or spoon, and toss the stuff in the trash. Don't use the garbage disposal, or you'll get a major clog!

A+
Ingredients

KIELBASA
Helps maintain muscle mass

KALE
Boosts your immune system

WHITE BEANS
Help balance blood sugar

INSTANT GRATIFICATION

Hot & Sour Soup—Fast!

This recipe will go head-to-head with anything you'll find at the best Chinese restaurant in town. Heat 2 cups of chicken broth, 2 tablespoons of rice vinegar, 1 tablespoon of chili-garlic sauce, and ½ tablespoon of grated fresh ginger over medium heat. When it reaches a slow boil, mix in a beaten egg, and continue cooking for one or two minutes. This recipe makes two to four servings.

HAMBURGER VEGETABLE SOUP

While this hearty, old-timey soup is still tasty when made with frozen or canned vegetables and dried herbs, it is especially delectable and even more healthy at the height of summer when made with fresh-from-the-garden crops.

YIELD: 6–8 servings   **PREP:** 15 minutes   **COOK:** 30 minutes

1 tbsp. of extra virgin olive oil

1 lb. of ground beef

1 cup of diced onions

2 cups of beef broth

3 cups of corn kernels (fresh or frozen)

3 cups of diced tomatoes (fresh or frozen)

3–4 tbsp. of minced fresh parsley

2 tbsp. of minced fresh basil (or 2 tsp. dried)

1 ½ tsp. of crumbled fresh rosemary (or ½ tsp. dried)

1 tbsp. of red wine vinegar

1 garlic clove, minced

¼ cup of chopped nasturtium stems

Salt and freshly ground black pepper to taste

1. Heat the olive oil in a large stockpot, and brown the ground beef, breaking it up with a spoon as it cooks.

2. Drain off the fat at the bottom of the pot. Then add the diced onions, and cook, stirring frequently, until they're transparent.

3. Add the beef broth, corn, tomatoes, parsley, basil, rosemary, vinegar, and garlic, and simmer the mixture for 30 minutes, stirring to combine.

4. While the soup is cooking, blanch the nasturtium stems in a separate pot, and toss them into the soup pot at the end of the cooking time, stirring well.

5. Season your finished soup with salt and pepper to taste, and serve it hot.

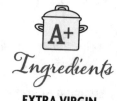

A+ Ingredients

EXTRA VIRGIN OLIVE OIL
Promotes cardiovascular health

GROUND BEEF
Helps build strong bones and teeth

CORN
Helps maintain vision

KITCHEN CAPERS Always make sure you have more cooking oil (or butter) on hand than a recipe calls for. Very often, when you're browning meat or sautéing veggies, the pan will need more than you'd expect.

LOVELY LENTIL SOUP

Lentil soup ranks high on the roster of cold-weather comfort foods, and this version can be on your table within an hour after you prep the ingredients.

YIELD: 6 servings	PREP: 10 minutes	COOK: 50–60 minutes

1 qt. of chicken stock

2 cups of water

1 cup of brown or green lentils*

1 can (15 oz.) of diced tomatoes

3 carrots, peeled and diced

2 celery ribs, diced

1 large onion, diced

2 tsp. of red wine vinegar

Salt and black pepper to taste

* Don't use red lentils, which get mushy in soup.

1. Combine the chicken stock and water in a large stockpot. Bring to a simmer, and add the lentils.

2. Cover and simmer until the lentils are mostly cooked through (about 20 minutes for the brown version; 30 for green).

3. Add the tomatoes. Cover and return to a simmer, then add the carrots, celery, and onion. Simmer for another 15 minutes, or until the veggies are tender.

4. Stir in the vinegar, and season with salt and pepper.

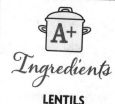

A+ Ingredients

LENTILS
Enhance digestion

CARROTS
Promote oral health

CELERY
Helps fight
free radicals

KITCHEN CAPERS
When you're making any tomato-based soup or sauce, and the recipe doesn't already call for vinegar, stir in 2 tablespoons of it before completing the cooking process. You'll be astounded by how much it enhances the flavor!

CULINARY Q & A

? I've heard that onion skins are actually good for you. Is that true?

! Yes! Onion skins contain quercetin, a compound with the power to help lower blood pressure and LDL (bad) cholesterol, reduce inflammation, fight allergies, relieve depression, and more. Tap into this medicinal gold mine by tossing a whole, unpeeled onion or two into the pot the next time you're making soup. Then just fish it out before serving time.

BLACK BEAN SOUP

This Tex-Mex-style soup is quick to make and full of healthy protein. It's no wonder that it's the perfect recipe to keep on hand for impromptu get-togethers!

YIELD: 2–4 servings	PREP: 10 minutes	COOK: 15 minutes

1 can (15 oz.) of black beans

½ red onion, chopped

2 tbsp. of extra virgin olive oil (more if needed)

3 cups of chicken stock

1 cup of fresh or frozen corn kernels

½ cup of tomato-based salsa

1 garlic clove, minced

1 small jalapeño pepper, seeded and chopped

2 tbsp. of adobo sauce

1 tbsp. of red wine vinegar

1. Drain and rinse the black beans, and set aside.

2. In a medium saucepan, sauté the onion in the olive oil until the onion begins to soften (about 2 minutes).

3. Add the remaining ingredients, and simmer over medium heat for 10 to 15 minutes.

4. Serve along with bowls of various toppings (see Kitchen Capers, below).

KITCHEN CAPERS To round out the flavor of any black bean soup, top it with sour cream, chopped tomatoes, tortilla chips, fresh cilantro, shredded cheese, or any combination thereof.

A+ Ingredients

BLACK BEANS
Promote a healthy digestive tract

CORN
Supports the nervous system

JALAPEÑO PEPPER
Boosts weight loss

INSTANT GRATIFICATION

Bare-Slate Chicken Stock

Homemade chicken stock doesn't come any easier than this: Mix 3 pounds of uncooked chicken wings, 3 quarts of water, 1 large chopped onion, and 1 minced garlic clove in a slow cooker. Cook on low for 8 to 10 hours or high for 4 to 5 hours. Then strain out the solids. If you like, refrigerate the stock until the (very little) fat solidifies on top, and then skim it off. Either use your stock immediately, or freeze it to have on hand for future soups and stews. **Note:** *Don't use chicken legs, backs, or necks for this recipe. They tend to give a "liver-y" taste to the stock.*

BRACING BALSAMIC ROOT VEGETABLE SOUP

Root vegetables make some of the most satisfying soups of all, and the balsamic vinegar in this version brings out their natural sweetness and adds essential nutrients.

YIELD: 4 servings   **PREP:** 15 minutes   **COOK:** 25 minutes

4 medium potatoes

2 carrots

2 onions

2 red turnips

2 white turnips

2 tbsp. of extra virgin olive oil

2 tsp. of grated fresh ginger

2 tsp. of minced garlic

6 cups of water

4 tsp. of balsamic vinegar

Salt and black pepper to taste

½ cup of torn mustard greens

1. Chop the potatoes, carrots, onions, and turnips into bite-size pieces, and set them aside.

2. Pour the olive oil into a large pot, add the ginger and garlic, and sauté until fragrant.

3. Pour in the veggies, and stir until heated. Add the water, cover, and bring to a boil. Lower the heat and simmer, covered, for 15 minutes, or until the vegetables are fork tender.

4. Stir in the vinegar. Taste the soup, and season with salt, pepper, and/or more vinegar as desired. Serve sprinkled with the mustard greens.

KITCHEN CAPERS To enhance the flavor of onions, sauté them for five minutes in olive oil or butter before adding them to soups, stews, or casseroles. For a caramelized flavor, stir 1 teaspoon of sugar in before adding the onions.

A+ Ingredients

POTATOES
Fight inflammation

TURNIPS
Enhance iron absorption

MUSTARD GREENS
Fight free-radical damage

CULINARY Q & A

? I find fresh ginger all but impossible to grate because of the stringy fibers. Is there any way to do it easily?

! There sure is! Store the root in a plastic bag in the freezer, where it will keep for about a year. Then, when you need some for a recipe, just slice off a piece, and let it cool before you grate it. This works because freezing causes the water in the ginger to expand, breaking down the tough fibers in the process.

CHILLED BERRY SOUP

This simple—and delicious—soup provides a boatload of berries' health-giving benefits for both your body and your mind. Healthy eating doesn't get any better than that!

YIELD: 4 servings	PREP: 10 minutes	CHILL: 4–24 hours

3 cups of fresh mixed berries

2 tbsp. of sugar

1 tbsp. of freshly squeezed orange juice

1 tsp. of finely grated lemon zest

1 tsp. of lemon vinegar

Small fresh mint leaves for garnish

Vanilla ice cream or frozen yogurt (optional)

1. Combine all of the ingredients except the mint leaves and optional topping in a medium-size heat-proof bowl, and toss to coat thoroughly.

2. Set the bowl over a large saucepan of simmering water and cook for 10 minutes, stirring occasionally.

3. Remove from the heat and let cool for 15 minutes. Then set the bowl, covered, in the refrigerator to chill for at least 4 and no more than 24 hours.

4. To serve, divide the soup among four bowls and garnish each one with mint leaves. Top each serving with a scoop of vanilla ice cream or frozen yogurt, if you like.

A+ Ingredients

BERRIES
Support brain function

LEMON ZEST
Helps ease asthma symptoms

MINT
Promotes good digestion

KITCHEN CAPERS

To freeze fresh berries, spritz a cookie sheet with nonstick cooking spray, spread the berries out in a single layer, and freeze until solid. Slide them from the tray into bags or containers to store in the freezer.

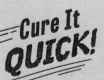
Cure It QUICK!

GIVE BRUISES THE BLUES When you've had a run-in with the corner of a coffee table, blueberries can aid the healing process. They'll also help strengthen your blood vessels so they're better able to fend off future damage. This simple soup is a dandy way to up your intake. To make four servings, combine 1 cup each of blueberries, plain yogurt, and heavy (a.k.a. whipping) cream in a blender. Puree for five seconds (no longer). Fold in another 1 cup each of blueberries and plain yogurt, 3 tablespoons of sugar, and 1 tablespoon of balsamic vinegar. Chill well, and enjoy! **Note:** *Blueberries also help reduce the swelling of varicose veins.*

SQUASH & LEEK SOUP

Thanks to its roster of heavy-hitting health boosters, this warm, sweet, and spicy soup is a handy weapon to have when the cold and flu season rolls around. It also just happens to be delicious and easy to make. What more could you ask for?

YIELD: 6 servings   **PREP:** 15 minutes   **COOK:** about 90 minutes

1 acorn squash

2 tbsp. of sunflower oil

3 celery ribs, chopped

2 leeks, chopped and rinsed well

1 tbsp. of apple cider vinegar

1 tsp. of chili flakes

1 tsp. of coriander

½ tsp. of ground cinnamon

½ tsp. of ground nutmeg

½ tsp. of turmeric

Salt and freshly ground black pepper to taste

4 cups of water

Chopped fresh parsley (optional)

Plain full-fat yogurt (optional)

1. Put the whole, unpeeled squash in a baking dish and bake it for 60 minutes at 375°F.

2. Remove from the oven, cut the squash open, and let it cool for 5 to 10 minutes. Then peel it, scoop out the seeds, and set aside.

3. In a stockpot, heat the oil on medium. Add the celery and leeks and cook, stirring frequently, until translucent (about 5 minutes).

4. Add the squash, vinegar, and spices to the pot, and mix well.

5. Add the water and bring to a boil. Reduce the heat and simmer for 15 to 20 minutes, leaving the lid slightly askew so that some of the steam escapes and the soup thickens slightly.

6. Serve hot, and garnish with parsley and/or yogurt, if desired.

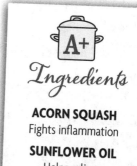

A+

Ingredients

ACORN SQUASH
Fights inflammation

SUNFLOWER OIL
Helps relieve arthritis pain

LEEKS
Boost immunity

KITCHEN CAPERS

When you accidentally oversalt a soup or stew, correct the damage by stirring in 1 teaspoon each of vinegar and brown sugar for every quart of liquid. Crisis averted!

BLOODY MARY SOUP

This more substantial version of the classic cocktail will wake up any meal. If you prefer the nonalcoholic version, simply leave out the vodka. You'll get the same spicy punch.

YIELD: 12 cups   **PREP:** 10 minutes   **CHILL:** 4–24 hours

4 medium ripe tomatoes, diced

4 scallions, thinly sliced

1 large cucumber, diced

1 orange or yellow bell pepper, diced

1 jalapeño pepper, minced

4 cups of tomato juice

3 ½ cups of chicken broth

½ cup of sherry vinegar

2 tbsp. of freshly squeezed lime juice

4 garlic cloves, minced

Hot-pepper sauce to taste

Salt and pepper to taste

Vodka (optional)

1. In a large bowl, combine the tomatoes, scallions, cucumber, bell pepper, and jalapeño pepper.

2. Stir in the tomato juice, chicken broth, vinegar, lime juice, and garlic.

3. Taste the blend and add hot-pepper sauce to suit your desired level of firepower. Season with salt and pepper. Cover and chill for 4 to 24 hours.

4. Serve with a jigger and a bottle of good-quality vodka, so guests can spike their soup, or not, as desired.

KITCHEN CAPERS Vinegar loses much of its punch when heated. For a milder flavor, add the vinegar to a soup or stew at or near the beginning of the cooking process. For more pungency, stir the vinegar into the dish after removing it from the heat source.

Ingredients

BELL PEPPER
Promotes healthy skin

LIME JUICE
Aids digestion

VODKA
Supports sound sleep

INSTANT GRATIFICATION

A Slow Road to Fast Results

Use roasted garlic instead of fresh to make a soup or stew taste like it's cooked all day. The roasting process can take up to an hour, but it's a snap to do. Use your fingers to peel away the outer layers of the garlic, but leave the head intact. Trim about ¼ inch off the top of the head to expose the tops of the cloves. Drizzle 2 teaspoons of extra virgin olive oil over the exposed surface. Wrap the bulb in aluminum foil, and bake at 400°F for 40 minutes. Check every 10 minutes and when a center clove feels soft when poked with a sharp knife, the garlic is done.

CROWD-PLEASING POTATO & BLUE CHEESE SOUP

If you and your family find traditional potato soups a little on the bland side, give this one a try. It'll impress even the pickiest eaters in your clan—guaranteed!

YIELD: 12 servings	**PREP:** 25 minutes	**COOK:** 35 minutes

2 tbsp. of extra virgin olive oil

1 cup of chopped onions

5 garlic cloves, minced

6 cups of vegetable broth

4 lbs. of red-skinned potatoes, diced

⅓ cup of crumbled blue cheese

1 tbsp. of balsamic vinegar

Salt and freshly ground black pepper to taste

½ cup of olive tapenade (for serving)

1. Heat the oil over medium heat in a 6-quart pot. Add the onions and garlic and cook, stirring, until tender.

2. Add the vegetable broth and potatoes, stir, and bring to a boil. Reduce the heat to low, cover, and cook until the potatoes are tender (about 30 minutes).

3. Pour one-third of the mixture into a blender, mix until smooth, and transfer to a large bowl. Repeat two more times with the remaining broth and potato mixture.

4. Return the blend to the pot, and add the cheese and vinegar. Increase the heat to medium, and cook until the soup is hot and bubbling. Season to taste.

5. Divide soup among 12 bowls. Serve the tapenade on the side.

Ingredients

ONIONS
Boost immunity

GARLIC
Supports bone health

BLUE CHEESE
Helps maintain a healthy nervous system

KITCHEN CAPERS

Crumbling blue cheese by hand tends to produce chunks of varying sizes. To ensure more evenly sized pieces, use a fork to do the job.

CULINARY Q & A

? What's the best way to store blue cheese?

! Wrap the original packaging tightly in aluminum foil, and put the wrapped wedge into a sealed glass storage container to keep the cheese from sharing its strong aroma with its fellow refrigerator residents. Keep it in the cheese drawer, where the humidity is higher than in the rest of the fridge. The cheese should keep for three to four weeks.

CHILLED GRAPE & ALMOND SOUP

This soup is a centuries-old favorite in Spain, known as *ajo blanco*. For an extra-silky texture, soak the blanched almonds in milk for 10 to 15 minutes or so before processing.

YIELD: 4–6 servings	**PREP:** 15 minutes	**CHILL:** 30–40 minutes

4 slices of French or Italian bread

1 cup of blanched almonds

3 garlic cloves, peeled and sliced

5 tbsp. of extra virgin olive oil

2 ½ cups of cold water

2 tbsp. of sherry vinegar

Salt to taste

½ cup of seedless green grapes

Chopped fresh parsley

Toasted slivered almonds

1. Soak the bread in cold water for 5 minutes. Then puree it with the blanched almonds and garlic in a food processor. (See page 139 for an easy way to blanch almonds.)

2. With the motor still running, slowly pour in the olive oil until you have a smooth paste.

3. Add the water and vinegar, and process until the mixture is thin and smooth. Season with salt.

4. Pour the mixture into a large bowl and float the grapes on top. Cover and refrigerate for 30 to 40 minutes. Serve in individual soup bowls, garnished with the parsley and slivered almonds.

When making cold soup, keep in mind that chilling food dulls its flavor. Always taste the soup before serving, and adjust the seasonings (including vinegar and any herbs) as needed.

KITCHEN CAPERS

A+
Ingredients

ALMONDS
Promote brain health

GARLIC
Fights bacterial infections

GRAPES
Fend off fatigue

Cure It **QUICK!**

A TASTY TRIPLE-THREAT TEAM Cranberries are renowned for their ability to help keep kidneys working efficiently. Apricots help guard against heart disease. And balsamic vinegar supports healthy blood pressure, cholesterol, and glucose levels. This recipe packs all that power into one soup. To make four to six servings, mix 2 ½ cups of pure apricot juice or nectar, 2 cups of whole-berry cranberry sauce, 1 cup of cold water or club soda, and 1 tablespoon of white balsamic vinegar. Chill well and garnish with fresh mint.

VEGETABLE SOUP OVER EASY

Soul-satisfying homemade soups don't come any faster or easier to whip up than this one. You and the gang can have it on the table in less than half an hour.

YIELD: 8 servings	**PREP:** 10 minutes	**COOK:** 15 minutes

4 cups of vegetable or chicken broth

1 bag (32 oz.) of frozen vegetable blend

1 can (15 oz.) of white beans, drained and rinsed

½ cup of sun-dried tomatoes

2 tbsp. of white wine vinegar

½ tsp. of dried basil

½ tsp. of dried oregano

Salt and freshly ground black pepper to taste

1. Bring the broth to a boil in a large pot, and add the frozen vegetables. Reduce to a simmer and cook until the vegetables have thawed (about 5 minutes).

2. Add the beans, tomatoes, vinegar, and herbs. Continue to simmer until the soup is hot (about 10 minutes).

3. Taste and season with salt, pepper, and additional herbs and vinegar as needed.

4. Serve with warm, crusty bread. Leftovers will keep in the refrigerator for up to a week and in the freezer for 3 months.

A+ Ingredients

FROZEN VEGETABLES
Help fight bacteria and viruses

SUN-DRIED TOMATOES
Help prevent anemia

WHITE WINE VINEGAR
Supports heart health

KITCHEN CAPERS

Before you refrigerate a just-cooked soup, bring it to room temperature. To do the job quickly, fill a large plastic beverage bottle with water almost to the top, cap the bottle, and freeze it. Then use the frozen bottle to stir the soup or stew in the pot. It'll be fridge-ready in no time.

CULINARY Q & A

? Is there any way to reduce the gassiness caused by canned beans?

! There is, and it couldn't be easier. Simply pour off the canning liquid and rinse the beans thoroughly before you add them to soups, stews, or other recipes. The water will wash away some of the complex sugars (oligosaccharides in scientific lingo) that contribute to gassiness. A good "shower" also removes up to 40 percent of the sodium found in canned beans, making them healthier.

LIGHTLY DOES IT ONION SOUP

When it comes to onion soup, most of the hoopla centers on the kind that's topped with toasted French bread and melted cheese. And it is delicious! But when you're in the mood for something lower in calories (still with bold onion flavor), try this version.

YIELD: 8 servings	PREP: 15 minutes	COOK: 45 minutes

4 tbsp. of unsalted butter

5 large onions, chopped

5 cups of beef broth

1 celery rib, chopped

1 large potato, peeled and chopped

1 cup of dry white wine

1 tbsp. of white wine vinegar

2 tsp. of sugar

1 cup of light cream

1 tsp. of minced fresh parsley

Freshly ground black pepper to taste

1. Melt the butter in a large nonreactive pan. Add the onions and sauté for about 10 minutes.

2. Add the beef broth, celery, and potato. Bring to a boil. Cover, reduce the heat, and simmer for 30 minutes.

3. Puree the mixture in a blender. Return to the pan and stir in the wine, vinegar, and sugar. Bring to a boil and cook for 5 minutes.

4. Reduce the heat, and mix in the cream and parsley. Taste, and add pepper. Do not let the soup boil at this stage, or the cream will curdle.

 KITCHEN CAPERS Light cream has a butter-fat content of about 20 percent, making it ideal for thin cream soups or light sauces. If you don't have any, make some by mixing ¾ cup of whole milk with 3 tablespoons of unsalted butter.

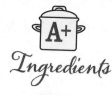

A+
Ingredients

ONIONS
Promote heart health

BEEF BROTH
Helps balance blood sugar

LIGHT CREAM
Helps build strong bones

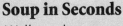 INSTANT GRATIFICATION

Soup in Seconds

Well, maybe not seconds—but within 10 minutes max. Just combine whatever leftover vegetables you have on hand with chicken or beef broth in a blender and process until smooth. Pour the mixture into a pan, and heat it up. Stir in 1 to 2 tablespoons of vinegar (whatever type you like). Season to taste with salt and freshly ground black pepper, and serve it up.

COLD & SPICY PLUM SOUP

This refreshing soup is full of antioxidants and tons of vitamins.
Plus, it will win rave reviews at any warm-weather lunch or dinner!

YIELD: 6 servings   **PREP:** 10 minutes   **CHILL:** 2–5 hours

2 lbs. of very ripe purple plums, halved

1 cup of freshly squeezed orange juice

2 long strips of orange zest

½ cup of raw honey

1 tsp. of sugar

4 whole cloves

2 cinnamon sticks

½ tsp. of cardamom

½ cup of plain or vanilla yogurt

1 tsp. of balsamic vinegar

1. Put the plums (with pits) in a pot with the orange juice, orange zest, honey, sugar, and spices. Bring to a boil, reduce the heat, and simmer, covered, until the fruit comes off the pits easily (about 30 minutes).

2. Using a slotted spoon, skim off and discard as many pits as possible. Transfer the fruit to a food mill placed over a large bowl. Remove any remaining pits, along with the cloves and cinnamon sticks.

3. Process the fruit, skins and all. Mix in the yogurt, cover the bowl, and chill for 2 to 5 hours.

4. Before serving, stir in the vinegar. Taste and add more juice, yogurt, vinegar, or sugar as needed.

Ingredients

PLUMS
Help build strong bones

ORANGE JUICE
Helps fend off free radicals

YOGURT
Fights colds and flu

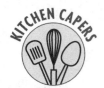

KITCHEN CAPERS

After grating the zest from an orange or citrus fruit, it will harden up within a day or two. To keep it soft, wrap it very tightly in plastic wrap and refrigerate.

CULINARY Q & A

? I always have a hard time zesting citrus fruit. It ends up tasting bitter no matter what I do. Do you have any advice?

! When zesting citrus fruits, always go gently so you remove only the thin, colored top coat of the skin. If you go any deeper, you'll pick up white pith, which has an unpleasantly bitter taste. To ensure the best flavor, you should also only zest just before you need it. That's when the flavors are at their strongest.

CREAMY ROASTED BEET & PARSNIP SOUP

It seems that parsnips don't get much "airplay" in most kitchens. But with their potent load of potassium and fiber, they truly should! Parsnips can even help reduce blood pressure and risk of heart disease. So do youself a favor, and give this flavorful soup a try.

YIELD: 6 servings	**PREP:** 20 minutes	**COOK:** 35 minutes

½ cup of sour cream

1 tbsp. of apple cider vinegar

1 tbsp. of orange juice

1 tbsp. of packed brown sugar

1 tsp. of grated orange zest, divided

5 beets, peeled and diced (about 4 cups)

1 lb. of parsnips, peeled and diced

1 small sweet onion, chopped (about 1 cup)

2 garlic cloves, peeled and sliced

2 tbsp. of extra virgin olive oil

Salt and freshly ground black pepper to taste

5 cups of vegetable broth

1. Stir the sour cream, vinegar, orange juice, brown sugar, and ½ teaspoon of the orange zest in a small bowl. Cover and set aside in the refrigerator.

2. Spread the beets, parsnips, onion, and garlic in a single layer in a 17- by 11-inch roasting pan. Toss with olive oil, and season with salt and pepper.

3. Bake at 425°F until the beets are tender (about 25 minutes).

4. Puree half of the vegetables, half of the broth, and the remaining ½ teaspoon of orange zest in a blender. Pour it into a 3-quart pot. Repeat the process with the remaining veggies and broth.

5. Bring to a boil. Reduce heat and cook for 10 minutes. Divide the soup among six serving bowls, and top each with 1 tablespoon of the sour cream mixture.

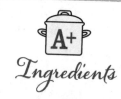

A+

Ingredients

SOUR CREAM
Promotes cardiovascular health

BEETS
Boost heart health

PARSNIPS
Help maintain strong bones

KITCHEN CAPERS Whenever you whip up a recipe using store-bought broth or soup base concentrate from a jar (like the Better Than Bouillon® brand), add a tablespoon or two of vinegar to it. It'll give any kind of soup or stew more old-fashioned, full-bodied flavor—and a bigger health kick, too!

TASTE-TEMPTING TORTELLINI SOUP

When you're hankering for a really substantial meal, but you lack the time—or the inclination—to fuss around in the kitchen for hours, this winner has your name written all over it. It can go from a wish to a finished dish in half an hour flat.

YIELD: 6 servings   **PREP:** 15 minutes   **COOK:** 15 minutes

3 tbsp. of extra virgin olive oil

½ cup of minced celery

½ cup of minced onions

4 cups of chicken broth

1 package (9 oz.) of refrigerated cheese tortellini

1 can (15 oz.) of cannellini beans, drained and rinsed

1 can (15 oz.) of diced tomatoes, drained

2 tbsp. of balsamic vinegar

½ tbsp. of dried basil

Salt and freshly ground black pepper to taste

Freshly grated Parmesan cheese

1. Heat the oil in a large pot, and sauté the celery and onions until translucent. Add the chicken broth and bring to a boil.

2. Add the tortellini and cook, uncovered, for about 9 minutes (or according to the timing guidelines on the package label).

3. Add the beans, tomatoes, vinegar, and basil, and simmer for 5 minutes, stirring occasionally.

4. Season with salt and pepper, and serve with a bowl of grated Parmesan cheese on the side.

KITCHEN CAPERS You can freeze chopped onions—either raw or sautéed—in an airtight container for up to 3 months. Then just add them directly to soups and stews without thawing. If you froze the onions raw, first let them thaw, and blot them dry with paper towels before sautéing.

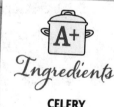

A+
Ingredients

CELERY
Promotes liver health

CHICKEN BROTH
Fights inflammation

CHEESE TORTELLINI
Boosts bone health

CULINARY Q & A

? When an onion has a green sprout in the center, should I throw it out?

! Not at all! That greenery is perfectly harmless—although not very tasty. If you'd like to remove it, slice the onion in half lengthwise and pluck out the sprout.

STUFFED-PEPPER SOUP

If you love stuffed peppers, you'll go crazy over this souped-up version (pun intended). Use whatever color pepper you like—green, red, orange, or yellow. If you're doubling the recipe, you might want to use two different colors for an extra-festive look.

YIELD: 6 servings   **PREP:** 20 minutes   **COOK:** 40 minutes

1 lb. of ground beef

1 large bell pepper, diced

1 small onion, diced

1 can (14 oz.) of beef broth

1 can (10 ¾ oz.) of condensed tomato soup

1 can (29 oz.) of diced tomatoes

2 cups of cooked rice

2 tbsp. of apple cider vinegar

1 tbsp. of brown sugar

Salt and freshly ground black pepper

Shredded cheddar cheese

1. In a large pot over medium-high heat, crumble and brown the ground beef. Add bell pepper and onion. Sauté until the meat is cooked (7 to 10 minutes).

2. Drain off the excess fat, and put the beef mixture back in the pot. Add the beef broth, tomato soup, and diced tomatoes, and mix well. Stir in the rice.

3. Add the vinegar and brown sugar. Taste and season with salt and pepper. Cover and simmer on low for about 30 minutes to let the flavors blend.

4. Serve topped with cheese.

When you're using very lean ground beef, heat 2 or 3 teaspoons of cooking oil in the pan before you add the meat. This will help keep it from sticking, especially if your pan is not the nonstick variety.

A+

Ingredients

GROUND BEEF
Boosts energy

BELL PEPPER
Helps eyesight

TOMATOES
Support cardiovascular health

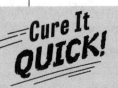

Cure It **QUICK!**

HERE'S TO YOUR HEART SOUP On nutritionist's list of the heart-healthiest foods, black beans rank near the top. They also happen to be one of the most flavorful legumes of all. To put 'em to work in a flash, process a can of them in a blender or food processor. Then pour the puree into a pan, add a can of drained whole beans, and mix in your favorite flavor enhancers—for example, a can of diced tomatoes with green chiles or a few spoonfuls of salsa. Heat the mixture, stir in a tablespoon or so of hot-pepper or red wine vinegar, and serve it up.

SWEET POTATO & CAULIFLOWER SOUP

The stars of this "show" are two of the healthiest foods on the planet: sweet potatoes and cauliflower. It's a snap to make and so delicious it'll become an instant family favorite.

YIELD: 8 servings	**PREP:** 15 minutes	**COOK:** 25 minutes

- 1 tbsp. of extra virgin olive oil
- 1 medium yellow onion, diced
- 1 garlic clove, crushed
- 3 cups of cauliflower florets (fresh or frozen)
- 1 large sweet potato, peeled and diced
- 5 cups of chicken or vegetable broth
- 2 tbsp. of apple cider vinegar
- Assorted toppings

1. Heat the oil in a medium-size pot, and sauté the onion until glossy. Add the garlic and continue cooking, stirring frequently, until fragrant.

2. Add the cauliflower and sweet potato and cook, stirring, for 2 minutes. Add the broth, reduce the heat to low, and simmer, uncovered, until the sweet potato is fork tender (15 to 20 minutes).

3. Puree with an immersion blender until smooth. Stir in the vinegar, bring to a quick boil, then reduce the heat and simmer for 3 minutes.

4. Serve hot, garnished with your favorite toppings, such as chives, pumpkin seeds, toasted pine nuts, croutons, sour cream, or yogurt.

A+
Ingredients

CAULIFLOWER
Helps your body detox

SWEET POTATO
Fights inflammation

APPLE CIDER VINEGAR
Enhances digestion

KITCHEN CAPERS

To prevent sour cream or yogurt from curdling in hot soup, bring it to room temperature before adding it to the pot. Then heat it gently and only until the mixture is warmed through. Don't let it boil!

CULINARY Q & A

? Is there any way to rescue soup in which yogurt or sour cream has curdled?

! Yes, there is! You can strain the soup through a sieve into a blender and process it until it's smooth. Just make sure you don't fill the blender jar any more than two-thirds full with liquid, and begin blending at low speed, gradually increasing to high. That's all there is to it!

EASY NEW ENGLAND CLAM CHOWDER

Creamy-white clam chowder has been pleasing palates since not long after Myles Standish and crew first set foot on Plymouth Rock. This is an updated version.

YIELD: 6 servings   **PREP:** 20 minutes   **COOK:** 35 minutes

1 package (12 oz.) of frozen chopped clams, thawed, drained, and liquid reserved

2 cups of diced potatoes

1 cup of chopped celery

1 cup of chopped onions

1 ½ tsp. of salt

Water

1 qt. of half-and-half

2 tbsp. of unsalted butter

¼ cup of whole milk

3 tbsp. of cornstarch

3 tbsp. of red wine vinegar

Black pepper to taste

1. Set aside drained clams. Then combine the clam liquid, potatoes, celery, onions, and salt in a pan. Add just enough water to cover the mixture. Simmer until the potatoes are fork tender (8 to 10 minutes).

2. Meanwhile, combine the half-and-half and butter in a large stockpot and bring to a boil, stirring constantly.

3. In a small bowl, mix the milk and cornstarch together and stir into the half-and-half mixture while it's still boiling. Remove from the heat.

4. Stir in the vegetable mixture. Add the vinegar, and the clams. Season with pepper.

KITCHEN CAPERS Use fresh or frozen clams for soups and stews; canned clams are too soft for this purpose. Always add clams to any hot mixture at the last minute. If they cook too long, they turn rubbery.

Ingredients

CLAMS
Promote strong bones

POTATOES
Fight inflammation

ONIONS
Boost immunity

INSTANT GRATIFICATION

Creamy Pumpkin Soup—Pronto

This satisfying soup can be on your table in 10 minutes flat. To make four servings, mix 6 cups of canned pumpkin, 4 cups of vegetable broth, 2 cups of sautéed onions, 1 cup of unsweetened coconut milk, 8 cloves of roasted garlic, 2 teaspoons each of ground nutmeg and paprika, and 1 teaspoon of cayenne pepper. Process until smooth. Pour the mixture into a pot and heat. Season to taste with salt and freshly ground black pepper, and stir in 2 tablespoons of balsamic vinegar.

CHEERY CHERRY SOUP

A bowl of this cold soup is perfect on a hot summer day! And cherries are full of health benefits that, among other things, can help relieve pain and inflammation.

YIELD: 4 servings	PREP: 20 minutes	CHILL: 30–60 minutes

½ cup of balsamic vinegar

1 lb. of cherries, pitted

1 cup of plain yogurt

1 cup of sour cream

2 tbsp. of chopped fresh mint

2 tsp. of raw honey

Salt and freshly ground black pepper to taste

2 tbsp. of heavy cream

4 fresh mint sprigs for garnish

1. Pour the vinegar into a small pan. Bring to a boil and reduce by half. Cool to room temperature and set aside.

2. Combine the cherries, yogurt, sour cream, mint, honey, and salt and pepper in a blender or food processor and puree until smooth.

3. Cover and chill for 30 to 60 minutes. Taste, and adjust the seasonings as desired.

4. Ladle into chilled soup bowls and drizzle each one with the reduced vinegar and heavy cream. Garnish with the mint and serve immediately.

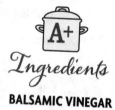

A+ Ingredients

BALSAMIC VINEGAR
Supports healthy blood pressure

CHERRIES
Boost immunity

MINT
Promotes good digestion

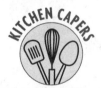

KITCHEN CAPERS When picking out cherries, remember the darker they are in color, the richer they are in antioxidants—and the more beneficial to your health.

CULINARY Q & A

? My local farmers' market has fabulous cherries that I'd love to buy in bulk and keep on hand. Can I freeze them?

! Yes! Pitted or not, they'll keep in fine condition for up to a year in ziplock freezer bags. But it's important to follow the right procedure: Rinse and dry the cherries thoroughly, and then put them into the bag and seal it closed. The less air that gets into the bag, the longer the cherries will keep. To use your stash, thaw it for eight hours or so in the refrigerator or for 30 minutes at room temperature.

GERMAN POTATO SALAD SOUP

If you're partial to German potato salad, do yourself a favor and give this soup a try. You can use a high-quality canned version, as called for in the recipe, or pick up some fresh potato salad at your local deli. Either way, you've got a real treat in store!

YIELD: 4 servings	**PREP:** 10 minutes	**COOK:** 20 minutes

1 tbsp. of extra virgin olive oil

1 cup of chopped onions

1 cup of chopped red bell peppers

2 cans (15 oz. each) of German potato salad

1 bottle (12 oz.) of light ale

1 cup of diced ham

¾ cup of chicken broth

2 tbsp. of red wine vinegar

1 tbsp. of chopped parsley

Salt and ground black pepper

Rye croutons (optional)

1. Heat the oil on medium in a Dutch oven or large saucepan. Sauté the onions and peppers until the onions just start to brown (5 to 7 minutes), stirring occasionally.

2. Add the potato salad, ale, ham, and chicken broth, and stir to combine.

3. Bring to a boil, reduce the heat to low, and simmer, uncovered, for 10 minutes, stirring occasionally.

4. Stir in the vinegar. Add the parsley, salt, and pepper. Serve topped with croutons, if desired.

KITCHEN CAPERS

A major key to success with this recipe—or any other soup or stew that contains ham—is to dice the meat into very small pieces. That way, the flavor will be evenly distributed!

A+ Ingredients

OLIVE OIL
Supports heart health

ALE
Enhances digestion

HAM
Promotes muscle health

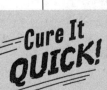

Cure It QUICK!

BEETS BEAT HIGH BLOOD PRESSURE Beets can help lower and prevent high blood pressure. This soup is a great way to put these robust roots to work. In a pan, combine 2 cups of chicken broth, 1 can (10 ¾ ounces) of condensed mushroom soup, 1 cup of diced canned beets, 2 tablespoons of unsalted butter, and 1 tablespoon of apple cider vinegar. Cook over medium heat for 30 to 40 minutes. Add 1 cup of diced potatoes, and cook until tender. Season to taste with salt and freshly ground black pepper, and serve with a dollop of sour cream and a sprinkling of chopped fresh dill on each bowl.

OKTOBERFEST STEW

This classic stew is made with apple cider vinegar, which boasts a variety of health benefits. These include boosting weight-loss abilities, helping to maintain healthy cholesterol and blood sugar levels, promoting skin health, and more!

YIELD: 4 servings   **PREP:** 20 minutes   **COOK:** 1 hour

1 tbsp. of extra virgin olive oil

1 large sweet onion, chopped

1 tsp. of minced garlic

1 (10 oz.) smoked sausage, cut into bite-size pieces

2 cups of shredded green cabbage

½ tsp. of freshly ground black pepper

¼ tsp. of ground caraway seeds

1 cup of dark beer*

2 cups of chicken broth

2 medium potatoes, peeled and cut into bite-size pieces

2 tbsp. of apple cider vinegar

2 tbsp. of chopped fresh parsley

* Preferably a German Oktoberfest lager.

1. Pour the olive oil into a large pot over medium-high heat. Add the onion and garlic and sauté until translucent (about 3 minutes).

2. Add the sausage and sauté until lightly browned (about 4 minutes).

3. Stir in the cabbage, pepper, and caraway seeds. Sauté until the cabbage is soft (about 4 minutes).

4. Add the beer and simmer until the liquid is reduced by half (about 5 minutes).

5. Stir in the chicken broth and potatoes. Return to a simmer. Reduce the heat to low, and cook until the potatoes are tender and the liquid is reduced by a little over half (about 40 minutes). Stir in the vinegar.

6. Serve hot, topped with the parsley.

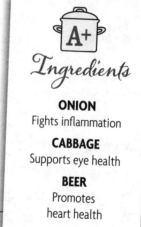

A+ Ingredients

ONION
Fights inflammation

CABBAGE
Supports eye health

BEER
Promotes heart health

KITCHEN CAPERS
To save stirring and pot-watching time, you can cook just about any stew, covered, in a 350°F oven. The heat surrounds the pan and cooks the contents evenly—freeing you up to get on with other activities.

GRAND & GLORIOUS BEEF STEW

Why "grand and glorious"? Because when you serve it up to your guests (or even your picky kids), this recipe will earn oohs and aahs all around. And it's easy to make, too!

YIELD: 6 servings	**PREP:** 15 minutes	**COOK:** 1 ½ hours

2 lbs. of stew beef

3 large carrots, peeled and cut into 1-inch chunks

2 cups of sliced fresh mushrooms

2 sweet onions, chopped

1 cup of beef broth

¼ cup of apple cider vinegar

2 tbsp. of brown sugar

1 cup of sour cream

Chopped fresh parsley for garnish

1. Trim the excess fat from the beef and cut it into bite-size pieces.

2. Combine the beef, carrots, mushrooms, onions, beef broth, vinegar, and brown sugar in a Dutch oven or casserole dish.

3. Cover and bake at 300°F for 1 ½ hours, or until the beef is fork tender. Remove the dish from the oven, and stir in the sour cream. Sprinkle the parsley on top, if desired, and serve immediately.

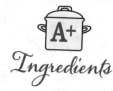

A+ Ingredients

BEEF
Helps maintain muscle mass

CARROTS
Keep skin healthy

MUSHROOMS
Help prevent anemia

KITCHEN CAPERS Packaged "stew meat" sold in supermarkets often contains gristly, misshapen scraps of various sizes from different parts of the animal. Instead, opt for boneless chuck roast, and cut it into 1 ½-inch cubes at home. It will cook more evenly and be more tender, too!

CULINARY Q & A

? I've always lined the floor and racks of my oven with aluminum foil to reduce cleanup. But recently a friend told me that's not a good idea. Is she right?

! Unfortunately, yes. While a foil lining will make for fast, easy oven cleaning, it will also hinder the flow of air that food needs to cook efficiently and effectively. Plus, the heat reflected by the foil can throw off your thermostat, and lining the floor of your oven can damage both the heating element and the oven lining. The bottom line: Spending a little time and elbow grease to clean up is the way to go!

PULLED PORK STEW

When you get a gang of pulled pork lovers together, you'll hear all kinds of recipe variations. But the proof of the puddin' is in the tasting. So give this winner a try!

YIELD: 8 servings	**PREP:** 10 minutes	**COOK:** 3 hours

5 lbs. of boneless pork picnic shoulder

2 cups of dark beer or stout (like Guinness®)

½ cup of barbecue sauce*

½ cup of dark brown sugar

¼ cup of apple cider vinegar

2 tbsp. of chili powder

2 tbsp. of instant coffee

* *Either a commercial brand or a DIY version (see Chapter Two for some recipes).*

1. Put the meat in a large ovenproof pot or Dutch oven. Whisk the remaining ingredients together and pour over the pork. Cover and bring to a simmer on the stove top.

2. Move the pot to the oven and bake at 325°F until the pork is fork tender (about 3 hours), basting frequently and turning the meat over at the 90-minute mark.

3. Remove and discard the skin and any excess fat. Skim the top layer of fat from the juices in the pot.

4. Using two forks, shred the pork and toss with the juices in the pot. Reheat on the stove and serve.

KITCHEN CAPERS Quickly remove excess fat from a brothy soup with a gravy separator. For chunky stew, set a large lettuce leaf or two on the surface of the stew to absorb the fat. Then toss the greenery in the trash.

A+ Ingredients

PORK
Boosts skin health

BEER
Encourages healthy sleep

COFFEE
Promotes brain function

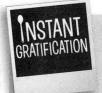

INSTANT GRATIFICATION

Dump-and-Go Beef Goulash

Pop this dish into a slow cooker, and you can walk away and forget it until it's time to dig in. To make four servings, combine 1 can (6 ounces) of tomato paste, ½ cup of water, 2 tablespoons of apple cider vinegar, and 1 envelope of sloppy joe seasoning in a 3-quart slow cooker. Stir in 2 to 2 ¼ pounds of cubed stew beef, 1 chopped green pepper, and 1 sliced celery rib. Cover and cook on high for 4 to 5 hours or low for 8 to 10 hours. Serve over hot cooked noodles.

SLOW COOKER BALSAMIC CHICKEN STEW

Cooking dinner doesn't get much easier than this simple, delicious stew. Start it just before you leave for work in the morning, and it'll be all ready to enjoy by the time you get home!

YIELD: 6–8 servings	**PREP:** 15 minutes	**COOK:** 4–10 hours

3 ½ lbs. of skinned chicken pieces

½ cup of dry white wine

3 tbsp. of tomato paste

6 garlic cloves, chopped

1 tsp. of dried basil

1 tsp. of dried oregano

½ tsp. of salt

1 ¾ cups of chicken broth, divided

3 tbsp. of balsamic vinegar

2 tbsp. of all-purpose flour

4 medium tomatoes, chopped

3 ¼ cups of frozen green beans

Egg noodles or rice

1. Put the chicken pieces in a 5- or 6-quart slow cooker. Mix the wine, tomato paste, garlic, basil, oregano, and salt in a small bowl, and pour the mixture over the chicken. Add ¼ cup of chicken broth; cover and refrigerate the rest of the broth.

2. Cover and cook until the chicken is tender (4 to 5 hours on high or 8 to 10 hours on low).

3. Forty minutes before the cooking time is up, whisk the vinegar, flour, and reserved chicken broth in a bowl until smooth. Gradually stir the vinegar mixture into the slow cooker liquid without disturbing the chicken. Layer the tomatoes and green beans on top. Cover and cook on high until the mixture simmers. Serve over egg noodles or rice.

Don't remove the lid of your slow cooker (except when specified in a recipe). If you do, you may need to add 15 to 20 minutes to the cooking time.

KITCHEN CAPERS

A+

Ingredients

CHICKEN
Helps weight loss

TOMATOES
Promote brain health

GREEN BEANS
Boost immunity

Cure It QUICK!

"EAT YOUR VEGETABLES!" STEW You should be eating at least five servings of veggies per day. Here's an easy way to do so: Put 1 tablespoon of extra virgin olive oil, 4 small diced zucchini, and 1 small diced eggplant in a skillet, and cook for three minutes, stirring often. Mix in 1 cup of halved grape tomatoes and cook for another two minutes. Remove from the heat, season with freshly ground black pepper to taste, and stir in 2 to 3 teaspoons of balsamic vinegar.

QUICK & EASY CHILI CON CARNE

When you have a hankerin' for chili, this is the recipe to reach for. It freezes well, so make a double batch, and next time you can put it on the table even faster!

YIELD: 6 servings	**PREP:** 10 minutes	**COOK:** 20 minutes

1 lb. of ground beef

2 cups of finely chopped onions

2 tbsp. of chili powder

1 garlic clove, finely chopped

1 can (10 ¾ oz.) of condensed tomato soup

1 can (15 oz.) of kidney beans

1 tbsp. of malt vinegar

Salt and freshly ground black pepper to taste

Assorted toppings

1. Brown the beef on medium-high in a heavy pot. Stir in the onions, chili powder, and garlic. Cook, stirring frequently, until the onions are tender.

2. Add the tomato soup, kidney beans, and vinegar. Bring to a boil.

3. Reduce the heat and simmer, uncovered, stirring occasionally, for about 15 minutes. Taste and season with salt and pepper.

4. Serve with shredded cheddar cheese on the side and—for those who might like additional firepower— a dish of chopped jalapeño or habanero peppers.

KITCHEN CAPERS

Leftover chili is delicious over a split baked potato and topped with shredded cheese. It also makes a mighty fine filling for tacos, burritos, or omelets.

CULINARY &

? Are "chili" powder and "chile" powder the same thing? I see both spellings in the supermarket.

! No, they aren't. Commercial chili powders contain spices such as cumin and paprika, along with salt and preservatives. Chile powder is made from ground whole dried chili peppers with no additives. In recipes that call for chili powder, you can substitute a pure chile powder until it's as hot as you'd like. If you prefer a more complex flavor with no preservatives, you can make your own (see DIY Chili Powder on page 179).

A+

Ingredients

ONIONS
Boost immunity

TOMATO SOUP
Supports weight loss

KIDNEY BEANS
Help balance blood sugar

CRESCENT CITY GUMBO

There are as many gumbo recipes as there are strings of beads flying at a Mardi Gras parade! But this one delivers true New Orleans flavor with very little effort.

YIELD: 8 servings	PREP: 15 minutes	COOK: 35 minutes

½ cup of peanut oil

½ cup of all-purpose flour

1 cup of chopped celery

1 cup of chopped green bell peppers

1 cup of chopped sweet onions

2 tsp. of Creole seasoning

2 tsp. of chopped garlic

5 ¼ cups of chicken broth

4 cups of shredded cooked chicken

½ lb. of andouille sausage, cut into ¼-inch slices

1 ½ cups of frozen black-eyed peas, thawed

1 lb. of extra-large shrimp, peeled and deveined

1. Heat the oil in a 4- to 6-quart Dutch oven over medium-high heat. Gradually whisk in the flour and cook, stirring constantly, until the flour is chocolate colored (5 to 7 minutes). Be careful the mixture doesn't burn!

2. Reduce the heat and stir in the celery, bell peppers, onions, Creole seasoning, and garlic. Gradually stir in the chicken broth. Cook for 3 minutes, stirring.

3. Add the cooked chicken, sausage, and black-eyed peas. Heat to boiling, then reduce to low. Simmer for 20 minutes, stirring occasionally. Then stir in the shrimp and cook for 5 minutes, or until the shrimp are just pink.

KITCHEN CAPERS When you peel shrimp, don't throw the shells away—turn them into broth! Just wash and cover them with water in a pan, boil, reduce to a simmer, and then cover and cook for 30 minutes. Let the shells cool, strain, and then toss them in the trash.

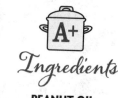

A+

Ingredients

PEANUT OIL
Boosts immunity

BLACK-EYED PEAS
Help prevent anemia

SHRIMP
Aids weight loss

INSTANT GRATIFICATION

DIY Creole Seasoning

When you need Creole seasoning, make your own. It's better than any commercial brand, and chances are you've already got everything you need. Combine 2 ½ tablespoons of paprika; 2 tablespoons each of salt and garlic powder; and 1 tablespoon each of black pepper, cayenne pepper, dried oregano, dried thyme, and onion powder. Store in an airtight container, and use as needed.

MANGO CHICKEN CHILI

The sweet-hot combination of mangoes and jalapeño peppers gives this chili an out-of-the-ordinary flavor that'll have you and your family clambering for seconds.

YIELD: 4 servings	**PREP:** 15 minutes	**COOK:** 15 minutes

1 tbsp. of extra virgin olive oil

1 medium white onion, chopped

4 garlic cloves, minced

4 cups of chicken broth

2 ½ cups of frozen mango chunks

¼ cup of tomato paste

3 tbsp. of sugar

2 tbsp. of red wine vinegar

2 jalapeño peppers, chopped

1 cup of shredded cooked chicken

1 medium tomato, chopped

1. In a medium-size pan, heat the oil on medium and sauté the onion until it begins to soften (1 to 2 minutes). Add the garlic and heat for about 20 seconds. Pour in the chicken broth and bring to a simmer.

2. As the broth simmers, put the mango, tomato paste, sugar, vinegar, and peppers in a food processor, and puree. Add water if necessary.

3. Pour the mango mixture into the broth mixture. Add the chicken and tomato, and stir. Bring to a simmer and cook, stirring, for about 10 minutes. Then serve.

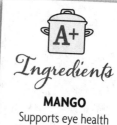

A+

Ingredients

MANGO
Supports eye health

JALAPEÑO PEPPERS
Promote weight loss

CHICKEN
Boosts nervous system

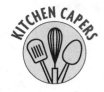

KITCHEN CAPERS

When you need to puree ingredients for soups and stews, either a blender or a food processor will do. If the quantity of your ingredients totals more than 3 to 4 cups, use a food processor to avoid a mess.

CULINARY Q & A

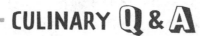

? Do I really have to preheat the oven? Isn't that a waste of time and energy?

! Getting your oven to the temperature specified in a recipe is anything but wasteful! It could spell the difference between a great dish and one that's barely edible. When food starts out in a cold oven, it cooks unevenly. You can easily wind up with one part of your dish overcooked and rubbery and another part not cooked at all. Food also cooks faster in a preheated oven. When it has the right temperature environment from the get-go, it can start cooking immediately and carry on right to the finish line.

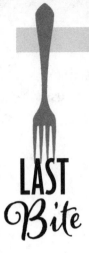

SECRETS FOR SUPER SOUPS AND STEWS

CONSIDER YOUR SOUP'S COMPANIONS

You can make soup out of just about any edible ingredients under the sun. But when you're making it as a first course for a special meal, choose a soup that will complement the dishes that will follow it. For example, a rich, creamy corn chowder might be a perfect prelude to a simple grilled steak and sautéed vegetables, but it would be major overload served with a rich entrée like beef stroganoff.

KEEP SOUP ON ICE

Almost any soup will keep fine in your freezer for up to three months. Stocks can last for as long as six months. To ensure success, follow these guidelines:

- Let the soup or stock cool completely, then freeze it in the quantities you use most often—whether that's individual or family-size servings. When in doubt, remember that smaller is better. The bigger the batch you have to thaw before reheating, the longer it will take.

- Use either freezer-proof containers or sealable plastic bags. Leave room for the liquid to expand a little as it freezes (½ inch should be plenty).

- Stocks can be spooned into ice cube trays or silicone muffin liners. Once frozen, transfer them to a bag or larger container for storage.

- Do not freeze any soup (or stew) that contains cream (sweet or sour), yogurt, cream cheese, or egg yolks. These will separate or become watery. If you're making a dish specifically for freezing purposes, omit these ingredients and add them later.

- To defrost frozen soup or stock, thaw it overnight in the refrigerator, then reheat the liquid in a pan until it's piping hot. Or, put it in the microwave and cook on high for a few minutes.

While ziplock freezer bags work well for stocks and thin soups, rigid plastic or glass containers are better for stews and heartier soups that contain lots of solid ingredients along with the liquid. Sturdy aluminum foil trays work especially well for stews because they can go from freezer to fridge for thawing and then into the oven for the final baking.

ICY STEW SECRETS

Stews can fare just as well in the deep freeze as soups and stocks do. To ensure success, follow the same general soup routine outlined at left, but take these additional precautions:

Choose lean cuts when you're making stews to freeze. Fatty meats can turn rancid after a long time in the freezer, so if you do choose to freeze 'em, try to eat them within a few weeks.

Cover the meat fully with the liquid before freezing. Otherwise, the meat will dry out and be subject to taste-destroying freezer burn.

Cook thawed meat until it's piping hot all the way through before serving. And don't refreeze any leftover meat a second time after it's been thawed. Otherwise, it could be at risk for bacteria.

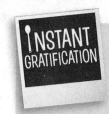

INSTANT GRATIFICATION

DIY Chili Powder

When you're fresh out of chili powder that you need for a recipe—or if you'd prefer a custom-made version with no salt or other preservatives added—give this simple recipe a try. Mix 2 teaspoons each of cumin and garlic powder with 1 teaspoon each of cayenne pepper, dried oregano, and paprika. Multiply the ingredients as desired, and store the blend in an airtight container away from light and heat sources to keep it potent.

KEEP IT CREAMY

While it is possible to salvage a soup in which dairy products have curdled (see the Culinary Q & A box on page 167), it's a whole lot easier to prevent trouble to begin with. Here's a trio of ways to do just that:

1. Opt for full-fat dairy delights like whole milk, full-fat sour cream or yogurt, and heavy (a.k.a. whipping) cream. Low-fat or nonfat versions tend to separate in the blink of an eye.

2. Buffer the meeting by first stirring ½ cup or so of soup into your dairy product. Then remove the hot soup from the heat, add the dairy-soup mixture, and reheat the finished soup on a very low burner.

3. Always add any acidic ingredients, like vinegar, tomatoes, or citrus juice, to a milk-based soup, rather than the other way around.

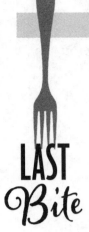

COOL IT!

If you serve a soup that is much too spicy, it can be downright embarrassing! Fortunately, there are some simple ways to lower the heat without having to sacrifice flavor or nutrition. Any one or a combination of these ploys will do the trick:

Add more ingredients. Simply stirring in more stock, juice, or plain tomato sauce will reduce the spiciness considerably. So will adding neutral solids that complement your recipe—for example, meat, tomatoes, potatoes, rice, or sweet bell peppers.

Sweeten it up. Mixing a little honey or sugar—either brown or white— will produce a welcome cool front.

Act with vim and vinegar. Stirring in ¼ cup or so of balsamic, wine, or apple cider vinegar will temper the inferno on its own. To double the cooling effect, use vinegar and sweetener.

Give it a dairy delight. The casein protein contained in milk bonds to and washes away the capsaicin molecules that make peppers hot. So top the dish with a generous sprinkling of shredded cheese or a hefty dollop of sour cream. To cover your bases, also adorn the table with individual dishes of these fire fighters so guests can add more as needed.

CULINARY Q & A

? Whenever I use pasta in my homemade soups, it turns mushy, even though I follow the recipe to the letter. What am I doing wrong?

! Most likely, you're simply using the wrong kind of pasta. The best kinds to use are those made from 100 percent semolina flour. Also, small, compact shapes like orzo, macaroni, and rotini fare far better in soups than the larger, ribbon-style versions like spaghetti and linguine.

HOW HOT IS HOT?

When it comes to spicy food, what one person considers steamy may taste mild to others. But in 1912, a pharmacist named Wilbur Scoville came up with a scale that objectively measures the heat in peppers and hot sauces. He called it the Scoville Organoleptic Test, and it's still used today. The scale begins at 0 Scoville Heat Units (SHUs) and goes up…and up. Here's a sampling of heat ratings:

Scoville Heat Units	Peppers
0–100	Bell pepper, pimento
100–1,000	Banana pepper, Cubanelle
1,000–10,000	Guajillo pepper, 'Fresno Chili' pepper, jalapeño
10,000–100,000	Malagueta pepper, chiltepin pepper, cayenne pepper
0.1–0.6 million	Habanero chili pepper, Red Savina habanero
0.6–3.2 million	Carolina Reaper, Dragon's Breath, Naga Morich, Pepper X

BE A BREAD WINNER

A luscious soup or stew and warm homemade bread go together like Hope and Crosby, Abbott and Costello, or gin and tonic. And since bread freezes beautifully, it's easy to keep it at your beck and call. Here's a trio of ways white vinegar can help you when you're fixin' to make a loaf or two:

Make it rise faster and give it a yummy texture to boot. Just add 1 tablespoon of vinegar for every 2½ cups of flour called for. (But remember to reduce the other liquid ingredients by the amount of vinegar you use!)

Give it a shine. To add luster to the crust, put your bread in the oven as usual. Then two minutes before the baking time is up, remove the loaf, brush the top with vinegar, and put it back in the oven to finish baking.

Keep the crust soft. If you prefer a soft crust, simply brush vinegar on the top of the loaf just before you pop it into the oven.

Note: *As you might expect, these tricks work just as well with home-baked rolls as they do with loaves of bread.*

Chapter Six

Vibrant Vegetables

As nutritionists and medical pros are constantly reminding us, one of the crucial keys to good health is to eat a wide variety of vegetables—and plenty of them. In these pages, you will discover scads of vinegar-enhanced recipes for old favorites, like spuds and green beans. You'll also have a chance to sample some ultra-healthy produce that's probably never appeared on your radar, like celeriac and broadleaf plantain (yes, that pesky "weed").

HEART-HEALTHY VEGGIE CASSEROLE

This hearty and healthy blend never fails to win raves even from folks who are not big-time vegetable fans. It makes a scrumptious side dish for any kind of poultry or meat but it's also substantial enough to enjoy with a salad for lunch or a light supper.

YIELD: 6 servings	PREP: 15 minutes	COOK: 2 hours

1 can (28 oz.) of diced tomatoes

1 green bell pepper, diced

1 medium onion, diced

2 carrots, sliced

2 cups of broccoli florets

2 cups of cauliflower florets

1 cup of uncooked brown rice

¾ cup of water

2 tbsp. of white wine or mixed-vegetable vinegar*

1 tsp. of chicken or vegetable soup base

Hot-pepper sauce to taste

Salt and freshly ground black pepper to taste

2 cups of shredded cheese

For a DIY version, see the Garden Harvest Vinegar recipe on page 23.

1. Cover the bottom of a 13- by 9-inch baking pan with a single layer of tomatoes.

2. Mix the pepper, onion, carrots, broccoli, and cauliflower in a large bowl. Spread a layer of the veggie blend over the tomatoes. Follow up with a layer of rice.

3. Continue layering tomatoes and mixed vegetables until you've run out, finishing with a layer of tomatoes.

4. Mix the water, vinegar, soup base, hot-pepper sauce, salt, and pepper in a small bowl, and sprinkle the mixture over the vegetables.

5. Cover, and bake at 350°F for 1 ½ hours. Remove the cover, top with the cheese, and bake for an additional 15 to 30 minutes.

A+

Ingredients

TOMATOES
Support heart health

CARROTS
Keep skin healthy

CAULIFLOWER
Promotes proper heart function

KITCHEN CAPERS

When you're substituting fresh tomatoes for canned (or vice versa), keep this guideline in mind: A 28-ounce can of diced tomatoes equals 2 to 2 ½ cups of fresh diced ones.

BLACK-EYED PEAS WITH GARLIC & KALE

Kale, garlic, apple cider vinegar, and black-eyed peas rank high on every dietitian's list of nutritional superpowers. Put this team together for a dietary wonder worker!

YIELD: 6 servings	**PREP:** 10 minutes	**COOK:** 20–25 minutes

1 ½ lbs. of kale leaves, rinsed and dried

1 tbsp. of chopped fresh garlic

1 tbsp. of extra virgin olive oil

2 cups of black-eyed peas (dried and cooked, or canned), drained

Pinch of dried red pepper

1 tbsp. of apple cider vinegar

1. Chop the kale leaves (stems discarded) into 1-inch pieces. Bring about 2 inches of water to a boil in a large pot, and add the kale. Cover and cook, stirring occasionally, until tender (15 to 20 minutes).

2. Drain the kale. Then combine the garlic and olive oil in a large skillet. Cook the garlic over low heat, stirring, until it starts to sizzle. Add the peas and red pepper, and cook, stirring constantly, until blended. Stir in the kale.

3. Add the vinegar just before serving, either hot or at room temperature.

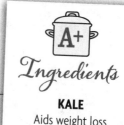

A+ Ingredients

KALE
Aids weight loss

GARLIC
Supports bone health

BLACK-EYED PEAS
Promote skin and eye health

KITCHEN CAPERS

To soften up kale, wash and dry the leaves, then freeze them in a bag for a few hours or up to a month. This will break down the rigid fibers better than cooking can.

CULINARY Q & A

? Every time I remove a few cloves of garlic from a head, the remaining ones go bad quickly. Is there any way to keep them fresh longer?

! Garlic has a ton of antioxidants, making it a powerful tool against colds and flu. And if you freeze it, it'll stay fresh for at least 6 to 12 months. First, peel the cloves and chop them in a food processor. Then, in a small bowl, mix the fragments with extra virgin olive oil at about a 1:1 ratio by volume. Spoon the mixture into ice cube trays, and pop them into the freezer. Transfer the frozen cubes to freezer bags or containers.

BROCCOLI WITH WALNUTS & BALSAMIC VINEGAR

This simple recipe belongs in every cook's repertoire. Not only does it pair well with just about any entrée you can think of, but it's also quick and easy to prepare.

YIELD: 6 servings	**PREP:** 10 minutes	**COOK:** 6 minutes

1 ½ tbsp. of extra virgin olive oil

1 ½ tbsp. of minced garlic

3 cups of fresh broccoli florets or 1 bag (20 oz.) of frozen

½ cup of toasted chopped walnuts

2 tsp. of balsamic vinegar

Kosher or sea salt to taste

1. Heat the oil in a small skillet over medium heat. Add the garlic, and cook, stirring continuously, until the garlic is just beginning to turn brown (30 to 90 seconds). Immediately pour into a large mixing bowl to stop cooking.

2. Insert a steamer into a large pot, add 1 to 2 inches of water, and bring to a boil over high heat. Add the broccoli to the steamer, and cook, covered, until the broccoli is tender-crisp (4 to 5 minutes).

3. Transfer the broccoli to the bowl, and mix with the garlic and residual oil. Add the walnuts and vinegar. Taste and season with the salt.

A⁺ Ingredients

EXTRA VIRGIN OLIVE OIL
Promotes cardiovascular health

BROCCOLI
Supports brain function

WALNUTS
Help maintain heart health

KITCHEN CAPERS

The high fat content of walnuts makes them prone to turning rancid. So to ensure the best flavor, buy them in small quantities from a supplier with a rapid turnover. Refrigerate shelled nuts in an airtight container; they should keep well for about four months.

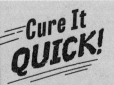

Cure It QUICK!

BOOST YOUR IMMUNE SYSTEM And lower your risk for colds and flu—with Brussels sprouts! Thanks to their potent load of vitamin C, they are one of the most powerful sources of antioxidants. Here's a quick and delicious way to enjoy them. In a large bowl, toss 1 ½ pounds of Brussels sprouts with 2 tablespoons of extra virgin olive oil. Season with kosher salt and freshly ground black pepper to taste. Spread the sprouts on a rimmed baking sheet and roast at 425°F, stirring occasionally, until tender and caramelized. Toss them with another tablespoon of olive oil, 1 tablespoon of balsamic vinegar, and 1 teaspoon of raw honey. Toss to coat evenly, and serve 'em up! (This recipe makes six servings.)

TURNIP GREENS FOR STRONG BONES

Unless you hail from Dixie, there's a good chance you've never even thought of cooking turnip greens. If that's the case, try this simple down-home casserole!

YIELD: 6 servings   **PREP:** 10 minutes   **COOK:** 35–40 minutes

1 package (14 oz.) of frozen turnip greens

1 can (10½ oz.) of cream of mushroom soup

½ cup of mayonnaise

2 tbsp. of white wine vinegar

2 tsp. of prepared horseradish

2 eggs, beaten

Salt and ground black pepper to taste

1 cup of saltine cracker crumbs

1 cup of shredded sharp cheddar cheese

1. Combine the turnip greens, soup, mayo, vinegar, horseradish, and eggs in a bowl, and mix well. Season with salt and pepper.

2. Spoon the mix into a greased 9- by 13-inch baking dish. Bake at 350°F for 30 minutes.

3. Sprinkle the cracker crumbs and shredded cheese over the top, and bake for an extra 5 to 10 minutes, or until the cheese melts.

4. Serve piping hot to accompany baked ham, pork chops, or roasted chicken.

A+

Ingredients

TURNIP GREENS
Help maintain healthy bones

MAYONNAISE
Promotes cardiovascular health

EGGS
Support memory and cognition

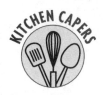

KITCHEN CAPERS When buying fresh turnip greens, remove the leaves from the mid-rib, wash, and pat them dry. Wrap the leaves loosely in paper towels and refrigerate them in a tightly sealed plastic bag for up to three days.

CULINARY Q & A

? Is it really true that you can stay healthier and live longer simply by packing your diet with certain "superfoods"?

! Many foods, such as the ones singled out in this chapter, do contain large concentrations of powerful nutrients. But no single type of edible can do anything on its own. Rather, the key to staying in (or getting into) the pink of health is to eat a varied, well-balanced diet that provides all the essential nutrients you need for good health. And couple wholesome eating habits with plenty of sleep and regular exercise.

HEALTH-BOOSTIN' HONEY & HORSERADISH BEETS

When you combine beets with honey, horseradish, and vinegar, the result is a beautiful harmony of earthy, sweet, and tangy. This dish makes a perfect complement to pork or fish cakes. Even if you don't think you care much for beets, give it a try—you'll love it!

YIELD: 4 servings   **PREP:** 15 minutes   **COOK:** 30 minutes

1 lb. of whole baby beets

1 tbsp. of white vinegar

⅔ cup of beet cooking liquid

2 tbsp. of raw honey

2 tbsp. of red wine vinegar

1 tbsp. of cornstarch

2 tbsp. of grated fresh horseradish

1 tbsp. of unsalted butter

Salt and freshly ground black pepper to taste

1. Put the beets in a pan and cover with water. Add white vinegar and boil until tender (about 30 minutes). Drain and reserve the liquid. Rinse the beets with cold water. Using your fingers, slip off the skins and root ends.

2. In a nonreactive pan, combine the reserved beet cooking liquid and honey. Bring to a boil over medium heat.

3. Combine the red wine vinegar and cornstarch. Add the mixture to the hot liquid, and stir until thickened.

4. Add the beets, and stir to coat well. Mix in the horseradish and butter, and heat until the butter melts. Season with salt and pepper.

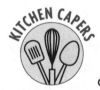 **KITCHEN CAPERS** To keep your hands from turning red when touching beets, wear disposable latex gloves. Don't have any? Just dampen your palms with white vinegar instead!

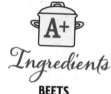 **A+ Ingredients**

BEETS
Support healthy liver function

RAW HONEY
Alleviates allergies

HORSERADISH
Enhances digestion

 INSTANT GRATIFICATION

Get to Harvard in a Hurry

Harvard beets, that is. Thanks to the magic of slow cookers, this sweet-and-tangy treat is easy to whip up quick. Just mix ½ cup of sugar, 2 tablespoons of flour, and ¼ cup each of water and white vinegar in a bowl. Dump two 16-ounce cans of whole beets (drained) into your slow cooker. Pour the vinegar-sugar mixture over the beets, and stir. Cover and cook on high for three to four hours or six to eight hours on low. (This recipe makes four to six servings.)

COLOR UP YOUR PLATE!

One of the simplest ways to ensure that you're getting all the nutrients you need for good health is to examine your plate at each meal. If the food on it is mostly white or pale shades, your food is probably overprocessed and lacking in essential nutrients. On the other hand, a plate that's filled with a colorful cast of characters will deliver health benefits galore. Here's the rainbow rundown:

Food Color	Key Phytonutrient	Some Foods That Contain It
Red	**Lycopene** helps to fend off infections, colds, and flu. **Betacyanin** battles bad bacteria.	Tomatoes, radishes, strawberries, cherries, raspberries, grapes, peppers, beans, watermelon, cranberries, beets, apples
Orange	**Beta carotene** strengthens your immune system and lowers your risk for contracting illnesses.	Oranges, squash, carrots, sweet potatoes, cantaloupe, papayas, apricots
Yellow	**Lutein** helps preserve your eyesight. **Quercetin** fights inflammation throughout your body.	Raspberries, cherries, peppers, grapefruit, squash, lemons, corn, beans, bananas, pineapple, apples
Green	**Indoles** have potent antioxidant and immunity-boosting properties.	Broccoli, Brussels sprouts, kiwis, grapes, peppers, dark leafy greens, beans, apples, asparagus, celery, okra, cucumbers
Blue and purple	**Anthocyanin** fights free radicals that can lead to premature aging and boosts cardiovascular health.	Eggplant, red cabbage, blue and purple potatoes, blackberries, raspberries, grapes, blueberries, cherries, plums

Note: *This is only a partial list of the potful of treasure at the end of the edible rainbow!*

BALSAMIC ONIONS, PEPPERS, & TOMATOES

If you can, make this Italian classic ahead of time, and stash it in the fridge. All the flavors will have a chance to blend, and the finished result is one amazing combo!

YIELD: 4 servings	PREP: 10 minutes	COOK: about 20 minutes

5 tbsp. of extra virgin olive oil

5 tbsp. of unsalted butter

2 large sweet onions, sliced

5 fresh tomatoes coarsely chopped

3 bell peppers (green, yellow, and red), cut into strips

1 tbsp. of balsamic vinegar

Salt to taste

1 tbsp. of water

1. Heat the olive oil and butter in a large, heavy pan. Add the onions and cook over medium heat, stirring frequently, until the onions are golden brown. Follow up with the tomatoes and peppers, and cook until the water they release has evaporated.

2. Stir in the vinegar and salt, and cook, stirring, for about 3 to 4 minutes.

3. Add the water, cover, and cook until heated through. Serve immediately, or refrigerate for up to 48 hours.

A+

Ingredients

BUTTER
Fends off food cravings

ONIONS
Fight inflammation

TOMATOES
Support cardiovascular health

KITCHEN CAPERS Peppers or other veggies on the limp side will still work in recipes. Dunk them briefly in hot tap water, then into a bowl of ice water with 1 tablespoon of vinegar mixed into it. Soon, they'll perk right up!

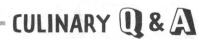

CULINARY Q & A

? Is fresh produce really better for you than frozen or canned versions?

! Yes—but *only* when you pick fully ripe produce fresh from your own garden or from a local organic farmer and eat it the same day. Even the organic produce that you see in supermarkets and "natural" food chains has traveled a *long* way to get there. Those fruits and vegetables have been harvested before they've ripened completely, which depletes nutrients and flavor. On the other hand, frozen and canned produce is processed quickly and close to the source—before vitamins and other essential nutrients have had a chance to go AWOL. So it's sometimes a better choice than fresh!

FRUITY RED CABBAGE

Red cabbage works very well in this sweet-and-sour treatment. This version incorporates carrots, pears, and currants, providing an out-of-the-ordinary taste treat—and an extra boost of nutrients. Another bonus: It's even better when it is prepared one to three days ahead of time, so the flavors can fully blend.

YIELD: 4 servings **PREP:** 25 minutes **COOK:** about 1 ¼ hours

2 tbsp. of unsalted butter

1 medium onion, diced

2 medium carrots, diced

2 fresh pears, peeled, cored, and diced

1 head (about 2 lbs.) of red cabbage, cored and thinly sliced

1 cup of pear juice or nectar

⅓ cup of dried currants or golden raisins

⅓ cup of dry red wine

¼ cup of balsamic vinegar

¼ cup of packed light brown sugar

½ tsp. of dried thyme

Salt and freshly ground black pepper to taste

1. Melt the butter over medium heat in a large pan. Add the onion and carrots. Cover and cook until the vegetables are soft (about 5 minutes).

2. Remove the cover, and stir in the pears. Cook, uncovered, until the onion is golden brown (about 3 minutes).

3. Add all of the remaining ingredients and bring the mixture to a boil. Reduce the heat to medium-low. Then cover and cook, stirring frequently, until the cabbage is tender (50 to 60 minutes).

4. Raise the heat to medium-high and cook uncovered, stirring frequently, until the liquid is evaporated (5 to 7 minutes). Serve the dish immediately while hot, or cover and refrigerate it for up to 3 days. Reheat gently before serving.

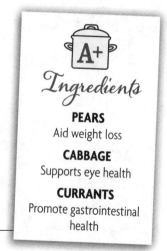

A+

Ingredients

PEARS
Aid weight loss

CABBAGE
Supports eye health

CURRANTS
Promote gastrointestinal health

KITCHEN CAPERS When a recipe calls for unsalted butter, and you only have the salted kind, just reduce the amount of additional salt you add. As a rule of thumb, there is about ¼ teaspoon of salt in every stick of salted butter.

MAPLE-ROASTED SWEET POTATOES

Sweet potatoes, pure maple syrup, and balsamic vinegar are a trio beyond compare—in terms of both scrumptious flavor and powerful health benefits. If that statement sounds extreme, just wait until you get a taste of this recipe.

YIELD: 4 servings	PREP: 10 minutes	COOK: 35 minutes

4 small sweet potatoes, peeled and cut into 1-inch cubes

¼ cup of extra virgin olive oil, divided

¼ cup of pure maple syrup, divided

2 tsp. of kosher salt

1 tsp. of freshly ground black pepper

4 large shallots, peeled and thinly sliced

2 tbsp. of balsamic vinegar

1. In a large bowl, combine the sweet potatoes, half of the olive oil and maple syrup, and the salt and pepper. Spread the potatoes in a single layer on a baking sheet.

2. Roast at 400°F for 30 minutes until golden brown. Check after 15 minutes, and stir if necessary.

3. While the potatoes are cooking, put the remaining olive oil in a large skillet. Add the shallots, and sauté until they start to caramelize. Stir in the remaining maple syrup and the vinegar. Season with salt and pepper to taste.

4. Add the roasted sweet potatoes to the shallot mixture, and transfer to a warm serving dish.

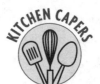 **KITCHEN CAPERS** Whenever a recipe calls for shallots, bear in mind that in most cases, "1 shallot" means one clove—not the whole, garlic-like head.

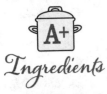 **A+** *Ingredients*

SWEET POTATOES
Help regulate blood pressure

MAPLE SYRUP
Boosts immune system

SHALLOTS
Help calm anxiety

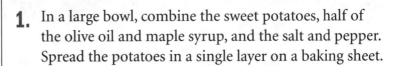 ## CULINARY Q & A

? Why do so many cooking recipes that call for maple syrup specify Grade B? What is this grade business all about?

! Pure maple syrup is full of antioxidants and comes in four different strengths: Light, Medium, and Dark Amber, and Grade B. While you can use whatever type you prefer, each one has its own ideal niche. Light Amber is best for delicate sweets. Medium is the type sold as a table syrup for pancakes and waffles. Dark Amber lends itself well to baking. The most robust of them all, Grade B, is generally used for cooking and baking.

SWEET VINEGAR CABBAGE WITH APPLES

The intense flavors of this super side dish make it a perfect partner for pork chops or steak. Try it with some of the hearty meat casseroles coming up in Chapter Seven.

YIELD: 4 servings	PREP: 15 minutes	COOK: 50 minutes

1 small red cabbage, thinly sliced

2 tbsp. of unsalted butter

1 sweet-tart apple, peeled, cored, and thinly sliced

1 small onion, diced

½ tsp. of ground nutmeg

Salt and cayenne pepper to taste

3 tsp. of dark brown sugar

½ tsp. of ground cinnamon

½ tsp. of ground cloves

2 tbsp. of apple cider vinegar

1. Soak the cabbage in cold water for about 15 minutes. Drain in a colander and transfer to a large pan.

2. Combine the butter, apple, onion, and nutmeg with the cabbage, and mix. Season with salt and cayenne pepper. Cover and cook over low heat for 45 minutes, stirring occasionally.

3. Stir in the brown sugar, cinnamon, cloves, and vinegar. Cook for another 5 minutes, then spoon the mixture into a warm serving dish.

KITCHEN CAPERS To retain the color of red cabbage, add vinegar to the cooking water—whether a recipe calls for it or not. Also, avoid cutting red cabbage with a carbon-steel knife or cooking it in an aluminum pan. Both will cause discoloration.

A+ Ingredients

CABBAGE
Fights inflammation

APPLE
Helps ease joint pain

ONION
Promotes cardiovascular health

INSTANT GRATIFICATION

Made-in-a-Snap Squash

You couldn't ask for an easier way to cook butternut squash than this winner: Just cut the squash in half lengthwise, scoop out the seeds, and cut the flesh into 4-inch squares with the skin intact. Score the flesh with crosshatch cuts about ½ inch deep, and rub it all over with extra virgin olive oil. Arrange the pieces, skin side down, on a baking sheet. Sprinkle with salt and black pepper to taste, and bake at 400°F until tender and lightly browned (about 45 minutes). Serve hot or at room temperature, doused with balsamic vinegar to taste. (This recipe makes six to eight servings.)

GARLICKY ROASTED POTATOES

These simple gems are great with a grilled steak or roasted chicken.
Or all on their own. Sprinkle your favorite grated cheese on top and dig in!

YIELD: 6–8 servings	PREP: 40 minutes	COOK: 55 minutes

½ cup of extra virgin
olive oil

4 garlic cloves, crushed

3 tbsp. of fresh rosemary
leaves or 1 ½ tsp. of dried

9 medium-size Yukon Gold
potatoes (about 2 ½ lbs.),
cut into 1-inch chunks

Salt and freshly ground
black pepper to taste

2 tbsp. of balsamic vinegar

1. In a small pan, cook the oil and garlic until the garlic just starts to turn color. Don't let it brown! Remove from the heat and stir in the rosemary. Cover and let stand for 30 minutes.

2. Strain the oil into a roasting pan, and add the potatoes. Season with salt and pepper, and then toss well to thoroughly coat the potatoes.

3. Bake at 400°F in the top third of the oven, turning the potatoes occasionally with a spatula, until they're crispy outside and tender inside (about 50 minutes). Sprinkle with the vinegar, toss, and bake another 5 minutes. Serve immediately.

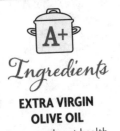

Ingredients

**EXTRA VIRGIN
OLIVE OIL**
Promotes heart health

ROSEMARY
Boosts memory

**YUKON GOLD
POTATOES**
Fight free radicals

To remove grease splatters from your oven and stove top, mix 2 cups of white vinegar and ½ cup of lemon juice in a spray bottle. When a spill occurs, let the surface cool, then spritz it and wipe it with a paper towel.

KITCHEN CAPERS

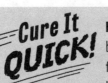

Cure It QUICK!

HOORAY FOR ONIONS! These bulbs are one of the best sources of quercetin, a bioflavonoid that helps fight free radicals that can cause premature aging, higher risk of disease, and more. And here's a sweet-and-tangy onion recipe for you to try: Peel and quarter three large red or sweet onions, and toss them in a bowl with ¼ cup of balsamic vinegar, 3 tablespoons of extra virgin olive oil, ½ teaspoon of sugar, and sea salt and black pepper to taste. Spread them in an even layer in a large, ovenproof skillet. Cover with aluminum foil, and roast at 350°F for 20 minutes. Remove the foil, toss the onions to coat them with the sauce, and return the skillet to the oven, uncovered, for another 20 minutes.

WHITE BEANS WITH TOMATOES & THYME

This blend makes a dandy side dish for pork or poultry. But it's filling enough to serve on its own for a winter lunch, accompanied by a green salad and warm, crusty bread.

YIELD: 4 servings	PREP: 15 minutes	COOK: 70 minutes

1 cup of dried cannellini beans

2 celery ribs, chopped

1 medium onion, chopped

Salt and freshly ground black pepper to taste

4 tbsp. of white wine vinegar

2 tbsp. of extra virgin olive oil

3 sprigs of fresh thyme

2 garlic cloves, crushed

2 fresh, ripe tomatoes, chopped

½ medium cucumber, peeled and sliced

Torn fresh flat-leaf parsley

1. Cover the beans with cold water, and soak for at least 2 but no more than 24 hours.

2. Drain the beans, and combine them in a pan with the celery and onion. Cover with water, and bring to a boil. Reduce heat, and cook for 30 minutes.

3. Season with salt and pepper, and continue cooking until beans are just tender (30 minutes). Then drain.

4. Combine the vinegar, olive oil, thyme, and garlic in a large pan, and heat gently. Add the beans and simmer for 10 minutes. Stir in the tomatoes and cucumber, and heat until warmed through. Serve immediately, sprinkled with the parsley.

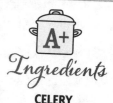

A+ Ingredients

CELERY
Promotes heart health

ONION
Supports oral health

CUCUMBER
Boosts hydration

KITCHEN CAPERS

Tiny pantry bugs love dried beans. To foil them, store your legumes in airtight containers. For extra protection, tuck a couple of dried chili peppers inside.

CULINARY Q & A

? I've never had any pantry bugs, but ants and fruit flies drive me crazy when I'm cooking in the summertime. What's a good, safe way to get rid of them?

! Your best anti-ant defense is to wash your kitchen surfaces with equal parts of white vinegar and water. As for the fruit flies, pour apple cider vinegar into a small bowl. Add a few drops of dishwashing liquid, mix, and set it on a kitchen counter. The bugs will be tempted by the vinegar, fall into the drink, and drown!

HONEY-VINEGAR BEETS WITH MUSHROOMS

Here, the magical duo of honey and red wine vinegar combines with the sweetness of beets, the earthy flavor of mushrooms, and the mild tang of shallots to produce a tasty treat that'll have your family asking for seconds—or thirds.

YIELD: 6 servings   **PREP:** 30 minutes   **COOK:** 25 minutes

- 1 lb. of beets (about 6 medium)
- 1 tbsp. of white vinegar
- 8 tbsp. (1 stick) of unsalted butter, divided
- 3 tbsp. of minced shallots
- 1 lb. of mushrooms, thinly sliced
- 2 tbsp. of raw honey
- 2 tbsp. of red wine vinegar
- 1 cup of chicken stock
- 1 ½ tbsp. of green peppercorns, packed in brine or water, drained

1. Put the beets in a saucepan of water and add the white vinegar. Bring to a boil, and cook until the beets are just tender (about 15 minutes). Drain, peel, and cut the beets into thin slices. Set aside.

2. Melt 6 tablespoons of the butter in a skillet over moderate heat. Add the shallots and sauté until soft (about 2 minutes). Raise the heat to high, and add the beets and mushrooms. Sauté, stirring often, for 2 minutes.

3. Stir in the honey, vinegar, and chicken stock. Reduce the heat, and simmer, uncovered, until the beets are more tender (about 2 minutes). Using a slotted spoon, transfer the veggies to a warm serving bowl.

4. Boil the remaining liquid over high heat until it's reduced to roughly ⅓ cup (about 2 minutes). Stir in the remaining 2 tablespoons of butter. Mix in the peppercorns, pour the sauce over the beet-mushroom mixture, and serve immediately.

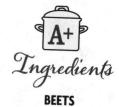

A+ Ingredients

BEETS
Promote heart health

SHALLOTS
Boost metabolism

MUSHROOMS
Help relieve anemia

KITCHEN CAPERS

To wash mushrooms quickly—and keep them from darkening—plunge them into a solution made from 2 quarts of water, ½ cup of vinegar, and ¼ cup of salt. Swirl the mushrooms in the liquid to dislodge any dirt, and then lift them out of the bath and dry them gently with paper towels.

BUILD-UP-YOUR-BONES BEET GREENS

Every time you turn around, it seems, you hear another nutritional guru touting the importance of eating plenty of dark leafy greens. If you're looking for a way to pack more of these wonder workers into your diet, you can't beat this recipe.

YIELD: 4 servings   **PREP:** 10 minutes   **COOK:** 20–35 minutes

1 tbsp. of extra virgin olive oil

2 medium yellow onions, chopped

1 tsp. of dried rosemary

1 tsp. of dried thyme (or more to taste)

1 garlic clove, minced

¼ cup of balsamic vinegar

Salt and freshly ground black pepper to taste

4 cups of chopped beet greens

1. In a large skillet, heat the oil on medium. Add the onions, and reduce the heat to medium-low. Cook, stirring frequently, until the onions are golden brown and caramelized (15 to 20 minutes).

2. Add the rosemary, thyme, garlic, and vinegar. Stir well to combine. Taste, and add more herbs if you'd like. Season with the salt and pepper.

3. Cook, stirring frequently, for 5 to 15 more minutes. Mix in the beet greens, cook until they're just wilted, and serve immediately.

KITCHEN CAPERS When a burner on your gas stove won't light, chances are the problem is a dirt-clogged igniter head. The solution: Turn off the gas and remove the burner head. Dip the head of a retired toothbrush in white vinegar and scrub until the crud washes away.

A+

Ingredients

ONIONS
Fight inflammation

BALSAMIC VINEGAR
Supports healthy blood pressure

BEET GREENS
Help build strong bones

INSTANT GRATIFICATION

Quick and Easy Beet Greens
In the mood for greens and got no time to waste?
If so, then heat 2 tablespoons of extra virgin olive oil in a large pan. Add three thinly sliced shallots, and sauté for two minutes. Add two bunches of chopped beet greens and stir until tender. Season with salt and pepper. Then stir in 1 to 2 teaspoons of apple cider vinegar, and serve. (This recipe makes two servings.)

BAKED PROVENÇAL VEGETABLES

Vegetables baked in shallow earthenware dishes are major favorites in the south of France. Roasting the veggies separately brings out even more of their rich flavor.

YIELD: 4 servings   **PREP:** 20 minutes   **COOK:** 50 minutes

6 medium tomatoes, sliced

4 Japanese eggplants, unpeeled and halved lengthwise

4 small zucchini, sliced lengthwise

1 red onion, sliced

5 tbsp. of extra virgin olive oil, divided

4 tbsp. of thyme vinegar

2 garlic cloves, crushed

2 tsp. of chopped fresh thyme

Salt and black pepper to taste

1. Brush the vegetables with 1 to 2 tablespoons of the olive oil, spread them out on a baking sheet, and roast at 400°F for 10 minutes, turning them over at about the midpoint.

2. Put the vinegar, garlic, thyme, salt, and pepper in a bowl, and whisk in the remaining olive oil. Add the roasted veggies, and toss until coated.

3. Transfer to a baking dish, and cover with foil. Bake at 400°F for about 25 minutes. Uncover, and cook for another 15 minutes.

4. Serve immediately with warm bread and a wedge of Parmesan cheese (with hand grater) on the side.

A+

Ingredients

TOMATOES
Support bladder health

EGGPLANT
Promotes heart health

ZUCCHINI
Aids digestion

KITCHEN CAPERS
To clean the window on your oven door, saturate it with full-strength vinegar. Let it sit, open, for 15 minutes. Then wipe the grease away with a damp sponge.

CULINARY 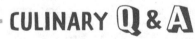 Q & A

? I love to use Pyrex® baking dishes, but I've found that glass ovenware collects brown food stains like there's no tomorrow. Is there a way to remove the marks?

! Yes! Fill the afflicted dish with 1 part vinegar and 4 parts water, and heat the mixture to a slow boil in the oven. Let it boil on low for five minutes, then carefully pull the pan out of the oven. Wait until it's cooled down and then scrub the surface lightly with a plastic scouring pad. Those unsightly splotches will be splitsville!

ROASTIN' THE BLUES

Blue- and purple-fleshed potatoes are chock-full of anthocyanins—the same phytonutrients that give many berries their potent antioxidant kick. They also have more flavor than any white tater can ever hope to deliver—as one taste of this dish will prove.

YIELD: 10–12 servings   **PREP:** 15 minutes   **WAIT:** 45–60 minutes

1 ½ lbs. of baby carrots

1 ½ lbs. of pearl onions, peeled

1 ½ lbs. of small blue potatoes (2 inches across), halved

1 tbsp. of extra virgin olive oil

2 tsp. of chopped fresh thyme

2 tsp. of fresh rosemary

½ tsp. of freshly ground black pepper

⅓ cup of balsamic vinegar

⅓ cup of chicken broth

⅓ cup of dry red wine

1. In a 12- by 15-inch roasting pan (not a ceramic baking dish!), combine the carrots, onions, potatoes, olive oil, thyme, rosemary, and pepper. Roast at 450°F, stirring occasionally, until tender (40 to 50 minutes).

2. Move the pan to the stove top over medium heat. Add the vinegar, broth, and wine. Stir until the brown drippings have been scraped free of the pan and the veggies are coated (2 to 4 minutes).

3. Spoon the mixture into a bowl, and serve it garnished with rosemary sprigs or roasted garlic, if desired.

KITCHEN CAPERS

To peel pearl onions quickly, immerse them in boiling water for one to two minutes (depending on their size). Drain and drop them into a bowl of ice water. Then just pinch each little bulb at its root end.

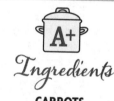

A+

Ingredients

CARROTS
Promote oral health

BLUE POTATOES
Fight free radicals

RED WINE
Helps balance blood sugar

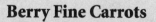

INSTANT GRATIFICATION

Berry Fine Carrots

Don't be surprised if Bugs Bunny himself comes knockin' when you whip up this treat. Sauté 1 cup of chopped onions in 4 tablespoons of unsalted butter until the onions are transparent. Add 2 pounds of baby carrots, cover, and cook over low heat until tender. Stir in ⅓ cup of raspberry or blackberry vinegar and ¼ cup of chicken stock. Increase the heat and stir until the liquid evaporates. Serve immediately.

SLOW & EASY GREEN BEANS

Green beans rank high on just about everybody's list of favorite vegetables. Here's one of the most people-pleasing ways to prepare them.

YIELD: 6–8 servings	PREP: 15 minutes	COOK: 8–10 hours

2 packages (10 oz. each) of frozen French-style green beans, partially thawed

4 slices of bacon, diced

1 small onion, diced

1 tbsp. of all-purpose flour

¼ cup of water

¼ cup of apple cider vinegar

2 tbsp. of sugar

1 tbsp. of jarred diced pimento

Salt and black pepper

1. Put frozen beans in a slow cooker. Then fry the diced bacon until crisp, and drain, keeping 2 tablespoons of the drippings. Sauté the onion in the remaining drippings until soft but not brown.

2. Dissolve the flour in the water, stir into the onion mixture, and cook until slightly thickened. Combine the bacon with the vinegar, sugar, and pimento. Add salt and pepper, and stir into onion mixture.

3. Pour the mixture over the beans in the cooker, and stir well. Cover, and cook on high for 1 hour. Reduce the heat to low, and cook for another 7 to 9 hours.

Ingredients

GREEN BEANS
Boost mood

APPLE CIDER VINEGAR
Helps balance blood sugar

PIMENTO
Aids weight loss

KITCHEN CAPERS

For the above recipe, store the bacon slices in the freezer ahead of time. When you're ready, dice them with kitchen shears directly over the pan. It's a lot neater than chopping them on a cutting board!

CULINARY 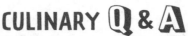 Q & A

? How can you use a slow cooker when you need to be gone longer than the specified cook time in a recipe?

! Simply plug your cooker into an automatic timer, and set it to start the action while you're gone. But keep these two guidelines in mind: Always make sure the food is well chilled when you put it into a cooker that has a delayed starting time. And never let the food stand for more than two hours before it starts cooking.

FENNEL & SWISS CHARD WITH PASTA

The delicate bitterness in Swiss chard makes it a perfect partner to sweet fennel and balsamic vinegar. You've got a real winner on your table with this trio!

YIELD: 4 servings	**PREP:** 15 minutes	**COOK:** 20 minutes

¼ cup plus 2 tbsp. of extra virgin olive oil

1 medium onion, diced

1 fennel bulb, stalks removed and thinly sliced

2 garlic cloves, minced

¾ cup of water

4 tbsp. of balsamic vinegar

Pinch of hot-pepper flakes

8 cups of cooked pasta

1 lb. of Swiss chard leaves, roughly chopped

½ cup of freshly grated Parmesan cheese

1. Heat ¼ cup of oil in a large skillet, and sauté the onion for about 5 minutes. Add the fennel and garlic, and cook, stirring, until the garlic begins to brown. Add the water and vinegar, cover with the lid partway, and let the liquid evaporate. Add the hot-pepper flakes.

2. While the liquid is reducing, cook pasta according to the package directions. Add the chard 2 minutes before the end of the cooking time.

3. Drain the pasta and chard, reserving about 1½ cups of the cooking water. Add 1 cup of the water to the fennel mixture, and stir. Add the grated cheese and 1 to 2 tablespoons of the remaining oil. Toss to coat. Garnish with raw fennel slices and shredded Parmesan, if desired.

To slice a fennel bulb, chop off the stems and fronds. Cut the bulb in half lengthwise. Remove the bottom and cut each side crosswise into crescent-shaped pieces.

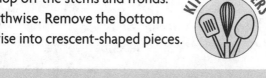

KITCHEN CAPERS

A+ Ingredients

FENNEL
Promotes brain health

PASTA
Helps balance blood sugar

SWISS CHARD
Helps build strong bones

Cure It QUICK!

PUT POTATO POWER TO WORK Colorful spuds are full of health-boosting nutrients. To make four servings of this battle-worthy winner, warm ¼ cup of extra virgin olive oil in a nonreactive skillet. Add 1 pound of small new potatoes (any color), and sauté, until they're tender and lightly browned. Add 3 tablespoons of dill-peppercorn vinegar, and cook for another three minutes. Sprinkle with about 3 tablespoons of fresh minced dill, season to taste with salt and pepper, and dig in!

RAINBOW MIXED PEPPERS

This colorful medley is tailor-made for serving buffet style. And, it'll virtually fly off the table, so multiply the ingredients as needed to suit the size of your gathering.

YIELD: 6–8 servings   **PREP:** 25 minutes   **COOK:** 40 minutes

6 bell peppers (a mix of green, red, orange, and yellow)

4 small jalapeño peppers

8 ripe tomatoes, quartered

4 medium onions, quartered

2 tbsp. plus ¼ cup of extra virgin olive oil

2 tbsp. of lemon vinegar

½ tsp. of oregano

Salt and black pepper

3 scallions (including tops), finely snipped

1. Cut the bell peppers and jalapeños in half, put them on a broiler pan, and flatten them with the back of a spoon. Broil until charred. Pop the peppers into a paper bag, close the top, and let them steam for 10 minutes. Remove them from the bag, slip off the skins, and scrape away the seeds. Set aside.

2. Put the tomatoes and onions on a baking sheet, and brush them with 2 tablespoons of the olive oil. Bake at 350°F until tender-crisp. Remove from the oven and cool.

3. Mix the vinegar and oregano. Slowly whisk in the remaining ¼ cup of olive oil. Add salt and pepper to taste.

4. To serve, arrange the vegetables on a large platter, drizzle with the dressing, and sprinkle the scallions on top.

A+

Ingredients

BELL PEPPERS
Support healthy eyesight

JALAPEÑO PEPPERS
Boost weight loss

ONIONS
Promote heart health

KITCHEN CAPERS When roasting one or two peppers, don't use the broiler. Instead, grip each pepper with tongs and hold it over an open flame until the skin blackens. Put it in a bag to remove the skin, as described above.

CULINARY Q & A

? Is there a secret to making sweet onions last longer? Mine go downhill much faster than other types do.

! Onions are amazing to boost your skin health and mood and fight off colds and flu! Keep them firm longer by putting them in a brown paper bag and storing them in the crisper drawer inside your refrigerator.

VEGGIE BAKE CASSEROLE

This colorful and substantial casserole is intended to be served directly from the dish you cook it in. So choose a pot, like an enameled Dutch oven, that can go safely from the stove top to the oven—and that looks attractive enough to adorn your table.

YIELD: 8 servings   **PREP:** 25 minutes   **COOK:** 70–90 minutes

4 tbsp. of extra virgin olive oil

1 large red onion, chopped

1 small butternut squash (about 1 lb.), peeled and cut into ½-inch pieces

4 celery ribs, cut into ¼-inch slices

4 small zucchini, cut into ½-inch slices

1 small eggplant (about 1 lb.), cut into ½-inch pieces

1 cup of water

1 can (16 oz.) of crushed tomatoes with juice

2 tbsp. of chopped fresh basil

2 tbsp. of chopped fresh parsley

1 tbsp. of balsamic vinegar

1 tbsp. of sugar

2 cups of fresh white bread crumbs

1 cup of grated sharp cheddar cheese

Salt and black pepper to taste

1. Heat the oil in an oven-safe pot over medium heat on the stove top. Add the onion and squash, and sauté until they're lightly browned.

2. Mix in the celery, zucchini, and eggplant, and cook, stirring occasionally, for about 5 minutes.

3. Add the water, tomatoes, basil, parsley, vinegar, and sugar. Cover, and simmer until the vegetables are tender (60 to 90 minutes). Remove from the heat.

4. Combine the bread crumbs, cheese, salt, and pepper, and spread the mixture in an even layer over the top of the vegetables.

5. Slide the pot under a hot broiler for a few minutes to crisp and brown the topping. Serve the dish right away.

A+ Ingredients

BUTTERNUT SQUASH
Helps ease
joint pain

ZUCCHINI
Enhances digestion

EGGPLANT
Helps maintain
gastrointestinal health

KITCHEN CAPERS
If you have stainless steel appliances, keep them spotless and gleaming by wiping the surfaces periodically with a sponge or soft cloth dampened with a little white vinegar.

ANTI-AGING ITALIAN-STYLE ONIONS

Onions pack a potent load of compounds that can help to boost the health of your skin (and other body parts) over time. This simple side dish is a classic favorite in Rome, where women are renowned for their beautiful skin.

YIELD: 4–6 servings   **PREP:** 40 minutes   **COOK:** 10–15 minutes

½ cup of raisins

Hot water

3 tbsp. of extra virgin olive oil

1 ½ lbs. of cipolline onions, peeled*

¼ cup of balsamic vinegar

1 ½ tbsp. of sugar

Kosher or sea salt to taste

* *Available in many large supermarkets, or substitute pearl onions, either fresh or frozen.*

1. Put the raisins in a bowl, cover them with hot water, and let them soften for 30 minutes.

2. Heat the oil in a skillet over medium-high heat. Add the onions, and cook until they're golden brown (about 10 minutes).

3. Pour off the oil. Drain the raisins, and add them, along with the vinegar, sugar, and salt, to the skillet. Stir until the sauce thickens (2 to 3 minutes).

4. Serve with any kind of meat or poultry or as a topping for pasta or baked potatoes.

KITCHEN CAPERS You can store any leftover raisins (or even newly purchased ones) in a tightly sealed container at room temperature for several months. In the freezer or fridge, they should stay in fine shape for up to a year.

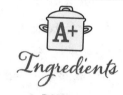

A+

Ingredients

RAISINS
Fight tooth decay

EXTRA VIRGIN OLIVE OIL
Supports weight loss

BALSAMIC VINEGAR
Maintains healthy glucose levels

INSTANT GRATIFICATION

Marinated Stuffed Peppers

This old-time delish dish entails some waiting time before eating, but it couldn't be quicker to prepare—and as quirky as it sounds, it's truly delicious! Simply stuff large green peppers with vinegar-based coleslaw, but don't use anything that contains mayonnaise (it'll affect the aging process). Then stack the peppers in a stone crock, and cover them with white vinegar. Let 'em age for four weeks, then dig in!

APPLES & GREENS WITH GARLIC & BEER

Sautéed greens and vinegar go together like the Fourth of July and fireworks. If you don't have the collard greens, substitute spinach, kale, beet greens, or turnip greens.

YIELD: 6 servings	PREP: 20 minutes	COOK: 35–40 minutes

¼ lb. of bacon, chopped

1 red onion, chopped

2 cups of lager beer

⅓ cup of malt vinegar

2 tbsp. of pure maple syrup

1 tbsp. of molasses

1 tart, crisp apple, cored and chopped

½ tsp. of crushed red pepper flakes

2 lbs. of collard greens, stemmed and chopped

8 garlic cloves, minced

1. Cook the bacon but don't let the it get brown and crispy. Transfer it to paper towels. Pour off and discard half of the drippings—or save them for another use.

2. Sauté the onion in the drippings over medium-high heat until slightly browned. Add the next six ingredients. Simmer over medium heat, and stir in the greens and bacon. Cover and simmer for 20 minutes.

3. Add the garlic and simmer, covered, for 5 more minutes. Season with salt and pepper, and adjust the sweetness with more maple syrup or molasses as desired.

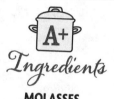

A+ Ingredients

MOLASSES
Promotes skin health

APPLE
Supports heart health

GREENS
Enhance digestion

KITCHEN CAPERS

To store leftover bacon drippings, let them cool in the pan until solidified. Spoon them into a tightly lidded glass container. Store for about three months in the fridge or nine months in the freezer.

CULINARY Q & A

? My backyard is full of plantain! I was going to blast it with weed killer, but a neighbor told me this obnoxious weed is actually edible. Is that true?

! Yes. Not only is broadleaf plantain edible, but it packs a bigger nutritional punch than any other kind of leafy greens. What's more, it's even higher in beta-carotene than carrots. The young leaves are delicious in salads or sautéed. While older leaves are also edible and healthy, they tend to have a bitter taste.

OUT-OF-THIS-WORLD ONION RINGS

If you like onion rings, you'll go bananas over this vinegar-enhanced version.
They're crispy on the outside but tender and sweet on the inside. Enjoy
them on sandwiches, drizzled with sauce or simply unadorned.

YIELD: 4–6 servings **PREP:** 40 minutes **COOK:** 10–15 minutes

Oil for frying

1 cup of milk

1 tbsp. of white vinegar

½ cup of sour cream

1 cup of all-purpose flour

1 tsp. of garlic powder

Salt and freshly
ground black
pepper to taste

1 large sweet onion,
thickly sliced (¼ to
½ inch) and separated
into rings

1. Add about 1 inch of oil (or enough to cover onion rings) to a cold Dutch oven or deep fryer, and heat it to 365°F.

2. In a medium-size bowl, mix the milk and vinegar. Let sit for 5 minutes, then whisk in the sour cream.

3. In a separate bowl, combine the flour, garlic powder, salt, and pepper.

4. Using a fork, dip each onion ring in the milk blend, then dredge it in the flour mixture. Repeat both steps of the dipping process and set the rings on a plate.

5. Working in batches, insert the batter-covered rings into the hot oil and cook until the outsides are crisp and light golden brown (3 to 4 minutes).

A+ Ingredients

MILK
Helps build healthy bones

SOUR CREAM
Helps boost red
blood cell counts

ONION
Fights coughs and colds

KITCHEN CAPERS

For this recipe or any other frying job, use an oil that has a high smoke point. Grapeseed, peanut, safflower, and sunflower oils are all good options.

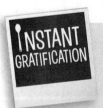

INSTANT GRATIFICATION

Dandy Dipping Sauce

To make a quick, delicious, and out-of-the-ordinary sauce for your Out-of-This-World Onion Rings (above), mix 2 parts mayonnaise with 1 part salsa. You can use whatever kind you fancy, but a fruity type, like peach or mango, produces a sweet-spicy flavor that's a perfect complement to onion rings or sweet potato fries.

CELERIAC IN VINEGAR-MUSTARD SAUCE

Is your family getting a little tired of the same old vegetables? If so, then perk up their appetites by delivering a brand-new taste treat in the form of celeriac!

YIELD: 2–4 servings	**PREP:** 15 minutes	**WAIT:** 2–3 hours

1 ½ tsp. of lemon juice

1 large celeriac (about 1 lb.)

3 tbsp. of hot water

3 tbsp. of prepared mustard*

2 tbsp. of apple cider vinegar

6 tbsp. of extra virgin olive oil

½ tsp. of dried tarragon

Salt and freshly ground black pepper to taste

4 tbsp. of chopped fresh parsley

* Use a favorite commercial mustard or one of the DIY versions in Chapter Four.

1. Boil water, and add the lemon juice. Scrub the celeriac root, peel it, and cut it into matchstick strips. Blanch the strips for 2 minutes. Drain, and set aside.

2. Combine the hot water, mustard, and vinegar in a blender. With the motor still running, slowly drizzle in the olive oil. Blend until thick, then add the tarragon, salt, and pepper.

3. Pour the dressing over the celeriac, cover, and marinate for 2 to 3 hours at room temperature. Garnish with parsley.

Ingredients

CELERIAC
Promotes brain function

MUSTARD
Helps build strong bones

PARSLEY
Fights fatigue

KITCHEN CAPERS Celeriac turns brown quickly after it's peeled. So if you aren't using it right away, put it—either whole or sliced—into a bowl of water with a tablespoon of white vinegar added.

CULINARY Q & A

? I'd love to use celeriac more, but its thick skin is impossible to remove with a vegetable peeler. Is there a simple way to peel this stuff?

! Celeriac is great to use in recipes because of its high vitamin count! Here's how to peel it easily: Cut off about ³/₈ inch from the root and stalk ends, and rest the root flat on a cutting board. Then, use a sharp knife to cut from top to bottom, rotating the root as you slice off wide strips of skin.

BOOST-YOUR-BRAINPOWER BABY PEAS

When you're assigned a side dish for a potluck gathering, reach for this recipe.
It's a snap to make, it multiplies well to suit the size of your crowd, and it's delicious!

YIELD: 8 servings	PREP: 15–20 minutes	COOK: 5 minutes (optional)

½ lb. of bacon

2 packages (16 oz. each) of frozen baby peas, thawed

1 red onion, chopped

1 cup of chopped toasted walnuts

¼ cup of white wine vinegar

2 tbsp. of water

1 tbsp. of chopped chives

1 tbsp. of Dijon mustard

1 tbsp. of sugar

½ cup of walnut oil

1. Cook the bacon until crisp. Drain on paper towels, then crumble. Combine the peas, onion, walnuts, and bacon in a bowl.

2. Mix the vinegar, water, chives, mustard, and sugar in another bowl. Slowly whisk in the walnut oil. Taste and season with freshly ground black pepper.

3. Pour the dressing over the pea mixture, and toss to coat thoroughly. Cover, and chill until serving time. To serve hot, transfer the contents to a pan, heat on low, and pour into a warmed serving dish.

KITCHEN CAPERS

To save time, toast large batches of nuts, and store them in the freezer. They'll keep for up to three months. Just measure out what you need for a recipe, and let the nuts come to room temperature before you use them.

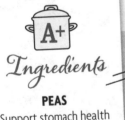

A+

Ingredients

PEAS
Support stomach health

WALNUTS
Help boost metabolism

CHIVES
Promote healthy sleep

Cure It QUICK!

HAVE A (HEALTHY) HEART SWEET POTATO FRIES
Sweet potatoes rank among the top heart-healthiest foods. These oven-baked fries give you a simple way to shore up your cardiac defenses. Cut two large sweet potatoes (peeled or not, as you prefer) into wedges or wide strips. Toss them with enough extra virgin olive oil to coat them thoroughly, and stir in 2 teaspoons of apple cider vinegar. Season with salt and pepper if desired, and spread the taters in a slight layer on a lightly oiled, rimmed baking sheet. Bake for 20 minutes at 400°F, then turn and bake for another 20 minutes, until the potatoes are soft on the inside and crisp on the outside. (This recipe makes four servings.)

GREAT NORTHERN BAKED BEANS

If you find baked beans a tad too sweet to suit you, give this version a try. They are less sweet than most of their counterparts but still have the zip that makes them delicious!

YIELD: 8–10 servings	**PREP:** 15 minutes	**COOK:** 1 hour

½ lb. of bacon

1 small onion, diced

4 cans (15 oz. each) of white beans, undrained

1 cup of ketchup

½ cup of molasses

2 tbsp. of apple cider vinegar

1 tbsp. of brown mustard*

Try the Mighty Marvelous Mustard recipe on page 133.

1. Cook (do not crisp) the bacon in a Dutch oven or small stockpot. Transfer to paper towels and set aside. When cool, chop it into ½-inch pieces.

2. Pour off all but about 2 tablespoons of the bacon drippings. Sauté the onion until transparent. Add the beans, ketchup, molasses, vinegar, mustard, and bacon. Stir to combine.

3. Cover and bake in the oven at 350°F for 1 hour. Or, if you prefer, simmer on the stove top for 1 hour, stirring occasionally to prevent sticking. Serve, or cool to room temperature and refrigerate for up to 3 days.

KITCHEN CAPERS

To keep bacon strips flat, rather than cooking curly or ruffled, arrange them in a single layer on a baking sheet with sides and bake at 400°F for 10 to 15 minutes (no turning needed). Blot thoroughly with paper towels before serving or using in a recipe.

A+

Ingredients

BACON
Helps maintain muscle mass

KETCHUP
Supports eye health

MOLASSES
Boosts sexual health

CULINARY Q & A

? Is there any way to salvage overcooked dried beans?

! Dried beans are a great source of protein and nutrients! And you can easily save overcooked ones with vinegar (any kind will work). Simply remove the pot from the heat, and stir in 2 teaspoons per quart of beans. If that doesn't do the trick, gradually add more vinegar until the beans perk up. Having said all that, if the beans are seriously overcooked, try mashing them to make bean dip instead. (You'll find some recipes for bean dip coming up in Chapter Eight.)

BRUSSELS SPROUTS & GOOD COMPANY

If you don't usually care for Brussels sprouts, do yourself a favor and give this tasty oven-roasted recipe a try. You'll change your tune in a hurry!

YIELD: 4 servings   **PREP:** 15 minutes   **COOK:** 30 minutes

½ lb. of carrots, sliced

½ lb. of fresh Brussels sprouts, halved

½ lb. of small new blue or purple potatoes, halved

2 large shallots, quartered

3 tbsp. of extra virgin olive oil, divided

Freshly ground black pepper to taste

2 tbsp. of balsamic vinegar

1 tbsp. of raw honey

1. In a large bowl, combine the carrots, Brussels sprouts, potatoes, and shallots with 2 tablespoons of the olive oil and pepper. Toss to coat thoroughly.

2. Transfer the vegetables to a baking sheet and roast at 425°F until tender and caramelized (about 30 minutes). Turn at the halfway point, so they cook evenly.

3. Return the roasted veggies to the bowl. Add the remaining 1 tablespoon of olive oil (more if necessary), along with the vinegar and honey.
Toss to coat evenly, and serve.

KITCHEN CAPERS When buying fresh brussels sprouts, pick small, firm, and bright green ones. If they're dull, loose-leaved, or larger than 1 ½ inches in diameter, they're not good.

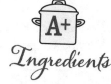

A+

Ingredients

BRUSSELS SPROUTS
Fight inflammation

BLUE POTATOES
Help build strong bones

SHALLOTS
Help calm anxiety

INSTANT GRATIFICATION

Balsamic Roasted Asparagus

Anything as delectable as spring's first tender asparagus spears deserves ultra-simple treatment. To make six servings, blanch 1 pound of trimmed spears in boiling salted water for 30 seconds. Immediately dip them in ice water to stop the cooking. Drain, and spread the spears on a lightly oiled rimmed baking sheet. Then drizzle the asparagus with ¼ cup of extra virgin olive oil, and roast at 400°F until tender and lightly browned. Arrange on a serving platter, and top with 1 tablespoon of balsamic vinegar, and season to taste with salt and freshly ground black pepper.

SPICY GRILLED SWEET POTATOES

When summer grilling time rolls around, pull out this unconventional treat. It makes an especially tasty companion for grilled chicken, pork, and other grilled veggies.

YIELD: 6–8 servings	PREP: 10 minutes	COOK: about 20 minutes

4 medium sweet potatoes (about 3 lbs.)

2 tbsp. of apple cider vinegar

1 tsp. of coarse sea salt

1 tsp. of cumin

1 tsp. of paprika

½ tsp. of chipotle powder*

½ tsp. of ground cinnamon

¼ cup of extra virgin olive oil

* *If you like a less smoky flavor, substitute chili powder or ground cayenne pepper.*

1. Cover the potatoes with cold, salted water in a large pot, and boil. Reduce the heat, and simmer until slightly tender (about 7 minutes). Drain well.

2. Let the potatoes cool, then cut them lengthwise into ¼-inch slices.

3. Mix the vinegar, salt, and spices in a small bowl. Then slowly whisk in the olive oil. Brush the mixture onto the sweet potato slices.

4. Arrange the slices on a lightly oiled rack, and grill until grill marks appear and the potatoes are cooked through (about 15 minutes). Serve immediately.

A+ Ingredients

SWEET POTATOES
Fight inflammation

APPLE CIDER VINEGAR
Enhances digestion

EXTRA VIRGIN OLIVE OIL
Promotes heart health

KITCHEN CAPERS

To loosen up food residue inside of your refrigerator, heat ½ cup of vinegar. Pour it into a heat-proof bowl, and set it in the fridge for five minutes. It'll unstick the gunk, so you can just wipe it away.

CULINARY Q & A

? What's the least messy way to clean a grill rack?

! This method works like a charm—for both barbecue grill and oven racks. Put each rack in a large, heavy-duty plastic trash bag. Add 1 cup of white vinegar, ⅓ cup of dishwashing liquid, and enough hot water to almost fill the sack. Seal the bag tightly and put it in a bathtub full of warm water for 60 minutes. Remove the rack from its bag and scrub it with a brush. Then rinse the rack with water and let it air-dry. Bingo—clean grill and oven racks with no greasy cleanup!

OVEN-ROASTED BABY CARROTS

If children or teenagers join you for dinner even occasionally, this recipe belongs in your repertoire. It's a blockbuster hit with kids of all ages!

YIELD: 8 servings	PREP: 10 minutes	COOK: 40 minutes

2 lbs. of fresh baby carrots

6 garlic cloves, peeled

4 small onions, quartered

2 tbsp. of extra virgin olive oil

2 tsp. of white balsamic or white wine vinegar

1–2 tsp. of dried thyme

Salt and black pepper to taste

1. Combine the carrots, garlic, and onions in a large bowl. Drizzle with the oil and vinegar. Sprinkle with the thyme, and season with salt and pepper.

2. Divide the mixture between two greased 15- by 10- by 1-inch baking pans. Cover with foil, and bake at 450°F for 20 minutes.

3. Remove the foil, stir, and bake uncovered for 10 minutes. Stir again, and continue baking until the carrots are tender-crisp (about 10 minutes).

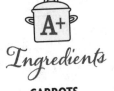

Ingredients

CARROTS
Promote healthy skin

GARLIC
Fights cold and flu germs

ONIONS
Boost immunity

Aerosol cooking sprays are convenient, but here's a healthier option: Get an olive oil mist sprayer. Then, just add your favorite oil and spray away! You can refill your mister at a much lower cost, plus you won't be adding unnecessary chemicals or propellants to food.

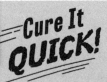

THE EYES HAVE IT! Carrots are famous for their high levels of beta-carotene, which is essential for preventing oxidative stress in your eyes, thereby helping fend off cataracts and supporting eye health. Well, guess what? Acorn squash also packs this powerful antioxidant. Tap into its ultra-rich gold mine this way: Grab an acorn squash that weighs about 2 pounds. Cut it in half, scoop out the seeds, and cut the flesh into ½- to ¾-inch-thick crescents. In a nonreactive pan fitted with a steamer insert, heat 1 cup of red wine vinegar on medium-high until it boils. Add the squash, cover the pot, and steam until tender. Serve, sprinkled with sea salt to taste, or transfer to a tightly sealed container and refrigerate for up to five days.

CHEESY SPAGHETTI SQUASH

There's no getting around it: Spaghetti squash tends to be on the bland side. But not when you mix it with a flavorful bunch of partners like the ones in this simple recipe!

YIELD: 4–6 servings	PREP: 15 minutes	COOK: 30 minutes

1 medium spaghetti squash, halved and seeded

4 tbsp. of extra virgin olive oil

Kosher or sea salt

2 garlic cloves, minced

3 tsp. of white wine vinegar

¼ cup of minced fresh parsley

2 tbsp. of minced fresh basil

¾ cup of shredded Gruyère cheese

Salt and black pepper to taste

½ cup of toasted pine nuts

1. Rub the squash with 1 tablespoon of oil, and sprinkle with salt. Put it, cut side down, on a rimmed baking sheet, and roast at 375°F until fork tender (about 25 minutes). Let it cool until comfortable to handle, then use a fork to pull strands away from the skin.

2. Put the strands in a colander, cover with paper towels, and press down to expel excess moisture. Set aside.

3. In a Dutch oven or large skillet, heat 3 tablespoons of olive oil over medium heat. Add the garlic, and cook until fragrant. Stir in the squash, vinegar, and herbs. Cook until heated through.

4. Remove from heat, and stir in cheese. Top with the pine nuts, salt, and pepper.

KITCHEN CAPERS

The most versatile Dutch oven models are round with straight sides that are at least 4 inches deep. Oval versions are fine for ovens, but on the stove top, the ends extend over the burners, cooking unevenly.

A+

Ingredients

SPAGHETTI SQUASH
Promotes cardiovascular health

GRUYÈRE CHEESE
Supports bone health

PINE NUTS
Boost immunity

CULINARY Q & A

? What's the best substitute for Gruyère cheese in a recipe?

! An ounce of Gruyère cheese has a whopping 8.5 grams of protein! But if you don't have any on hand, American Swiss cheese and Norwegian Jarlsberg have a similar flavor. Both can also work well in casseroles. If you can find Emmentaler (which, like Gruyère, is made in Switzerland), that's even better because it melts to a very smooth, even consistency.

SWEET POTATOES & WINTER SQUASH

Here's a hearty blend that's tailor-made to pair with your favorite pork or poultry recipe on a cold winter evening. You couldn't ask for a more satisfying warmer-upper!

YIELD: 8 servings	PREP: 15 minutes	COOK: 50 minutes

2 lbs. of carrots, cut into ½-inch diagonal slices

2 lbs. of sweet potatoes, peeled and chopped into ½-inch cubes

1 lb. of acorn or butternut squash, peeled and cut into 2-inch wedges

2 orange bell peppers

1 red onion, chopped

2 tbsp. of extra virgin olive oil

2 tbsp. of balsamic vinegar

2 tbsp. of red wine vinegar

2 tbsp. of brown sugar

2 tbsp. of pure maple syrup

2 tbsp. of chopped thyme

2 tbsp. of fresh parsley

1. Combine the carrots, sweet potatoes, squash, peppers, and onion in a large bowl. Toss with the olive oil to coat thoroughly. Spread the vegetables out on a large rimmed, lightly oiled baking sheet.

2. Roast at 375°F, stirring twice, until they're browned and tender (50 minutes). Transfer to a serving bowl.

3. Mix the vinegars, brown sugar, maple syrup, and thyme in a small bowl. Taste, and season with salt and pepper. Toss the mixture with the vegetables, sprinkle parsley on top, and serve it up.

 KITCHEN CAPERS Want the easiest way to peel an onion? Cut the bulb in half lengthwise. Grip the skin along the cut edge of one half and pull down. It'll slide right off. Repeat with the other half. Bingo—a naked onion!

 **A+**

Ingredients

CARROTS
Promote oral health

SWEET POTATOES
Help prevent constipation

SQUASH
Helps maintain vision

 INSTANT GRATIFICATION

Baby Zucchini in Red Wine Vinegar

This is a scrumptious and unexpected way to prepare zucchini. To make four servings, heat 1 tablespoon of crushed mustard seeds in ⅔ cup of red wine vinegar in a small pan. Remove from the heat. Bring another pan of salted water to a boil, and add 1 pound of baby zucchini. Blanch for one minute, then drain and transfer to a large bowl, and mix in one sliced red onion. Pour the mustard-vinegar blend on top, and serve as a side for any kind of meat.

SUFFERIN' SUCCOTASH!

Sylvester the Cat himself would give two thumbs up to this version of the classic southern side dish. Unlike many succotash recipes, this healthier version contains no bacon.

YIELD: 6 servings	PREP: 10 minutes	COOK: 15 minutes

2 tbsp. of unsalted butter

1 cup of chopped yellow onions

1 garlic clove, minced

2 cups of frozen corn kernels

1 package (10 oz.) of frozen baby lima beans

½ cup of chopped red bell peppers

1 tsp. of dried basil

½ cup of chicken broth

½ tsp. of sugar

1 tbsp. of balsamic vinegar

1. Melt the butter in a Dutch oven or large skillet over medium heat.

2. Add the onions and garlic. Cook, stirring occasionally, until the onions soften but do not brown (about 3 minutes).

3. Mix in the corn, lima beans, red peppers, and basil. Cook for 4 minutes, stirring occasionally.

4. Add the broth and sugar. Season with salt and pepper, and cook until the liquid has almost evaporated (7 minutes). Remove from the heat, stir in the vinegar, and serve.

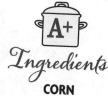

Ingredients

CORN
Helps maintain vision

LIMA BEANS
Help boost energy levels

RED BELL PEPPERS
Promote youthful skin

KITCHEN CAPERS Remove blackened, cooked-on grease from any pan with this trick: Mix 1 cup of apple cider vinegar with 2 tablespoons of sugar. While pan is still hot, cover its surface with the mixture. Let the pan sit for an hour or so. Then scrub lightly. The grime'll slide right off!

CULINARY Q & A

? My new house came with a pristine smooth-top stove too delicate for commercial cleansers. What's the best alternative?

! Mix ¼ cup of white vinegar and 3 drops of lemon essential oil in a small handheld spray bottle. Sprinkle baking soda over the dirty areas of the stove top, and spray the vinegar and oil over the soda. (It'll fizz.) Wait for 5 to 10 minutes until the mixture becomes pasty, and wipe it away with a damp, soft cloth.

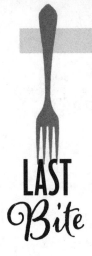

COOKING IN THE SLOW LANE

While there are scads of cookbooks dedicated to slow cooking, you don't really need 'em. Most stove-top or oven recipes can be adapted to work in this time- and labor-saving device. But make sure to keep these basic guidelines in mind:

Check the cooking time. Recipes that work best in a slow cooker are those that take at least 45 minutes to cook in a traditional oven.

Reduce the liquid. Remember: Liquid does not evaporate in a slow cooker. So use about half the amount called for in the original recipe.

Cut the seasonings. Reduce the quantities of herbs and spices in proportion to the amount of liquid you're adding. Whenever possible, use fresh herbs and whole spices rather than crushed or ground. This is because some flavor tends to dissipate during slow cooking. Always taste just before serving.

Delay the dairy. Milk, cream, and sour cream tend to break down during long cooking times. Add to the slow cooker during the last 30 minutes. Or, you can substitute condensed soup or evaporated milk, which will hold up for hours.

Procrastinate with pasta and rice. When cooked for long periods of time, they become starchy and pasty. So, instead, cook them on the stove top, and stir them into the slow cooker a few minutes before serving.

Mind the meat. Less tender (and cheaper) cuts are better suited to slow cooking than leaner versions are. Browning isn't necessary, but do trim away excess fat, which can cause overcooking. Always wipe meat thoroughly before adding.

Ensure vegetable victories. Cut all vegetables into pieces that are similar in size and shape. And always add tender, quick-cooking vegetables like peas and leafy greens during the last 20 to 30 minutes of cook time.

To speed up cleaning time after using a food processor, spritz the work bowl and the blade or shredding disk with aerosol cooking spray before adding any food. When you've finished your processing job, squirt a few drops of dishwashing liquid and a little warm water in the bowl, and blend briefly. In most cases, you can just rinse and dry.

TIMELY TOMATO TRANSLATIONS

More than almost any other vegetable, fresh tomatoes vary like night and day in flavor and nutrient content. So do yourself and your family a favor: Whenever a recipe calls for fresh tomatoes and they're out of season—or you can't find fresh-picked, vine-ripened (preferably heirloom) versions, just used canned tomatoes. Besides packing more true tomato flavor, they'll contain a full load of health-giving nutrients. Here's how to make the correct substitution:

- One 28-ounce can of tomatoes equals 10 to 12 whole tomatoes, or about 2 pounds.

- One 14 ½-ounce can equals 5 or 6 whole tomatoes, or about 1 pound.

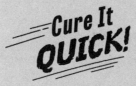

Cure It QUICK!

LYCOPENE ON CALL

We all know that cooked tomatoes offer up even more immunity-boosting lycopene than their fresh-from-the-vine counterparts do. The addition of health-enhancing balsamic vinegar gives you double-barreled firepower. To make four servings' worth of protection, toss 2 pounds of halved plum or Campari tomatoes with 2 tablespoons each of extra virgin olive oil and balsamic vinegar, and 1 teaspoon of dried thyme (or more to taste). Arrange the coated tomatoes, cut side up, on a rimmed baking sheet, and roast at 350°F for one hour. Reduce the heat to 250°F and continue roasting until the tomatoes are tender and fairly dry (about 90 minutes). Drizzle with more olive oil and serve hot, cold, or at room temperature. For more potent tomato protection, see the Heart-Healthy Veggie Casserole on page 184.

FULL STEAM AHEAD

Steaming vegetables ensures that they retain more nutrients, more color, and a texture that's just right. There's only one catch: Unless you keep an eagle eye on the water level under the steamer unit, it can evaporate—burning the pot and its contents at the same time. The simple solution: Put four or five glass marbles on the bottom of the pot before you add the water. When the level gets low, the marbles will start rolling and bouncing around, making a racket that will remind you to add more H_2O.

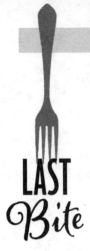

VEGETABLE PREP 101

Preparing fresh vegetables for cooking can be either a relaxing, almost meditative process or a royal pain in the neck. A food processor can go a long way toward speeding up the process, but sometimes you need to take a hands-on approach. In either case, it helps to know the basic vocabulary:

Chopping, dicing, and mincing describe the same basic technique. The only difference is the size and shape of the results. Chopping produces small, irregularly shaped pieces. Dicing creates small cubes that are uniform in size. Mincing reduces diced vegetables to fine, tiny pieces just short of a puree.

Slices are flat and uniform in size. To slice round veggies, like potatoes, cut a thin strip from one side and hold the cut side flat on the board to keep it steady. Then make downward cuts.

Roll cutting is a technique used for cylindrical vegetables like asparagus, carrots, and zucchini. Start by making a diagonal cut at a 45-degree angle an inch or so from the end. Then roll the vegetable and slice again at the same angle about an inch from the first cut, and so on. Diagonal slices expose more of the veggie's insides, so they'll cook faster and absorb more flavor.

Julienne, a.k.a. matchstick, cuts produce thin strips of uniform size. To julienne (let's say) a zucchini, first cut it into 2-inch lengths. Stand each one on its end, holding it firmly with your fingertips, and cut straight down to create thin slices. Stack up a few slices, and cut them into fine strips.

CULINARY Q & A

? Is it true that organic veggies have more flavor than conventionally grown ones?

! Yes and no. Some kinds of vegetables (and fruits) are naturally more flavorful than others. In particular, heirloom varieties have the kind of sweet, full-bodied taste that you'll almost never find in modern hybrids. Using organic growing methods brings out more of the natural flavor. But if there wasn't much to begin with, nothing you can do will put it there.

SLOW COOKER CONVERSION TIMES

Here's how to translate conventional cooking times to slow cooking times:

Oven or Stove Top Time	Slow Cooker on Low	Slow Cooker on High
15–30 minutes	4–6 hours	1 ½–2 ½ hours
35–45 minutes	6–8 hours	3–4 hours
50 minutes–3 hours	8–12 hours	4–6 hours

ADD LIFE TO YOUR VEGGIES

When it comes to storage life, all vegetables are not created equal. Some, such as carrots, have real staying power, while others—for example, corn and peas—start losing flavor and nutrients the minute they're plucked from the plant. Here's how to prolong the lives of the most popular veggies:

Broccoli: Store unwashed in the refrigerator crisper for up to five days.

Cabbage: Store unwashed heads in the fridge crisper for up to two weeks.

Carrots: Wash well, place in a plastic bag, and refrigerate for up to five weeks.

Celery: Wrap tightly in aluminum foil, and store in the crisper for up to one month.

Corn: Best if eaten immediately. Can store for a few days in a sealed plastic bag in the refrigerator crisper.

Leaf lettuce: Wash and gently pat dry. Store in a sealed plastic bag in the refrigerator crisper for up to four days.

Onions: Wrap individually in newspaper and store in a cool, dry, dark place for up to one month. Do not refrigerate.

Peas: Best if eaten upon purchase. Store in a sealed plastic bag in the refrigerator crisper for up to three days.

Peppers: Store, unwrapped, in the refrigerator crisper for up to two weeks.

Potatoes: Keep in a cool, dark place. Do not refrigerate.

Tomatoes: Keep at room temperature, away from sunlight.

Winter squash: Store in a warm, dry place with good air circulation for up to 3 months.

Chapter Seven

Marvelous Meat, Poultry, & Fish

It's probably safe to say that in most households, meat, poultry, or fish forms the centerpiece of most meals. No matter which variety your clan favors, or whether you prefer your protein fried, baked, broiled, or grilled over charcoal in the backyard, this chapter is for you. You'll discover how vinegar can turn your favorite steaks, chops, fillets, or roasts from pretty darn good to simply spectacular.

HERE'S TO YOUR HEART HAM LOAF

In addition to the essential protein provided by the ham and eggs, this recipe serves up plenty of heart-healthy quercetin in the onion and lycopene in the ketchup.

YIELD: 4–6 servings	PREP: 15 minutes	COOK: 40–50 minutes

1 ½ lbs. of ground cooked ham

½ onion, minced

2 eggs, beaten

½ cup of bread crumbs

½ cup of milk

½ tsp. of dry mustard

½ tsp. of Worcestershire sauce

1 ½ cups of brown sugar

½ cup of apple cider vinegar

½ cup of ketchup

1 tbsp. of Dijon or spicy brown mustard

1. Mix the ham, onion, eggs, crumbs, milk, dry mustard, and Worcestershire sauce in a bowl. Shape it into a loaf, and put it in a lightly oiled loaf pan. Bake it at 350°F until the center is no longer pink (40 to 50 minutes).

2. Combine the brown sugar, vinegar, ketchup, and prepared mustard in a pan over medium heat. Bring it to a boil, stirring well to dissolve the sugar. Reduce the heat, and simmer for 5 minutes. Remove the pan from the stove, and let it cool.

3. When the loaf is done, remove it from the oven, let it sit for about 10 minutes, and transfer it to a serving platter. Cut the loaf into thick slices, and serve them drizzled with the sauce.

As soon as you bring home an uncooked ham, rub vinegar on the cut end to prevent mold from forming.

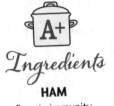

A+
Ingredients

HAM
Boosts immunity

EGGS
Promote brain function

KETCHUP
Supports eye health

Cure It QUICK!

PRACTICE SAFE CELLS How? By upping your intake of pickle juice. It's packed with antioxidants that help prevent damage to all the cells in your body, helping reduce your risk for illness and cardio-vascular disease—and keep your skin healthy and young-looking. So what's this tip doing in a chapter about meat? Just this: One easy and tasty way to enjoy pickle juice is to use it in a basting sauce for ham. Stir cloves and mustard into the juice, and dribble some of the mixture over the ham every 30 minutes until the meat's done.

CHICKEN THIGHS WITH RED WINE VINEGAR

This recipe delivers a full load of nutrients that your ticker needs to stay healthy—thanks to the olive oil, garlic, and red wine vinegar. What's more, it's a great venue for your homemade vinegar (it'll also work just as well with a store-bought version).

YIELD: 8 servings   **PREP:** 5 minutes   **COOK:** 30 minutes

4 tbsp. of extra virgin olive oil

4 garlic cloves, chopped

8 boneless, skinless chicken thighs

1 tbsp. of fresh rosemary

1 ½ cups of red wine vinegar

1. Pour the olive oil into a large skillet, add the garlic, and sauté for about 2 minutes.

2. Add the chicken thighs, and sprinkle the rosemary over them. Brown the chicken on both sides, then pour the vinegar over it.

3. Cover, and cook for about 20 minutes, turning the chicken at the halfway mark. Then serve it up. (It's great over wild rice with a side of broccoli!)

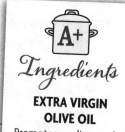

A+

Ingredients

EXTRA VIRGIN OLIVE OIL
Promotes cardiovascular health

CHICKEN
Helps weight loss

ROSEMARY
Boosts memory

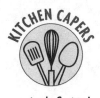

KITCHEN CAPERS

When you bring an uncooked chicken or turkey home, pour ¼ cup of white vinegar into the cavity, and swish it around. It'll slow down the growth of harmful bacteria. Nothing can halt bacterial growth indefinitely, though, so cook that bird within about 48 hours.

CULINARY Q & A

? What's the hoopla about extra virgin olive oil? What's wrong with the other types?

! When you want to coat your stomach against the effects of hot beverages, spicy food, or liquor, swallowing a tablespoon of any kind of olive oil works fine. But for health (and beauty) purposes, only one grade cuts the mustard: extra virgin. To qualify for that distinction, the oil must be extracted from the fruit by a method known as "cold pressing," which ensures that the oil retains all of its health-giving benefits. And it contains no additives, and no chemicals are used in processing the oil.

LEMON ROASTED CHICKEN

Lemon vinegar gives a moist, tender oomph to the classic baked bird. If you have any leftovers, the vinegar also imparts a subtle but tasty tang to cold chicken sandwiches.

YIELD: 4 servings	**PREP:** 10 minutes	**COOK:** 1 hour

2 tbsp. of lemon vinegar*

2 tbsp. of extra virgin olive oil

1 whole chicken (about 4 lbs.)

½ tbsp. of sea salt

2 onions, quartered

1 bunch of fresh tarragon, washed and shaken dry

* Try the Fruity Vinegar on page 16 (see the Culinary Q & A).

1. Brush the vinegar and olive oil onto the interior and exterior of the chicken. Sprinkle with the salt.

2. Stuff the onions and tarragon into the cavity, tie the legs together, and set the bird breast side down on a rack in a shallow roasting pan.

3. Roast, breast side down, at 400°F for 30 minutes. Then turn it breast side up and continue roasting until the skin is dark brown and crisp and the juices run clear when you pierce the thigh with a fork (about another 30 minutes).

4. Move the chicken to a platter, and wait for about 10 minutes before carving.

A+ Ingredients

CHICKEN
Maintains healthy blood pressure

ONIONS
Fight inflammation

TARRAGON
Helps fight free radicals

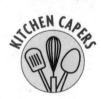

KITCHEN CAPERS

When shopping, always purchase meat or fish last. That way, it won't be sitting at room temperature in your cart while you check out the magazines, peruse the dog toys, compare nutrition labels on cracker boxes, and do other time-consuming stuff.

Cure It QUICK!

POWER UP YOUR IMMUNE SYSTEM Red bell peppers, capers, and protein-rich beef all give your immune system a healthy boost—thereby helping fend off colds, flu, and other illnesses. So the next time you toss some steaks on the grill, serve them topped with a hard-hitting, and great-tasting, pepper-caper relish. Here's how to make enough for four steaks: In a small bowl, mix 1 cup of grilled red pepper strips, ¼ cup of red wine vinegar, 2 tablespoons of chopped capers, and a teaspoon or so of oil from the caper jar. When the steaks are done, spoon the relish over each one.

UNSTUFFED CABBAGE

Medical science tells us that chronic inflammation lies at the root cause of just about every health condition, from asthma to muscle pain, high blood pressure, and diabetes. And cabbage ranks high on the list of anti-inflammatory foods.

YIELD: 4–6 servings   **PREP:** 15 minutes   **COOK:** 25 minutes

1 lb. of ground beef

1 cup of chopped onions

1 small head (about 1 lb.) of cabbage, shredded

1 can (28 oz.) of Mexican-style tomatoes, undrained

1 tbsp. of apple cider vinegar

1 tbsp. of brown sugar

Salt and freshly ground black pepper to taste

Hot cooked rice

1. In a Dutch oven, cook the ground beef and onions over medium heat until the meat is brown, with no pinkish patches, about 7 to 10 minutes.

2. Stir in the cabbage. Cover and cook until tender-crisp (about 5 minutes).

3. Add the tomatoes and juice, vinegar, and brown sugar. Taste and season with salt and pepper. Cook 10 minutes, stirring occasionally. Serve over the rice.

A+
Ingredients

GROUND BEEF
Boosts energy

CABBAGE
Fights inflammation

TOMATOES
Support cardiovascular health

KITCHEN CAPERS For any recipe that calls for shredded cabbage, you can prep it a day ahead. Simply blanch the shreds, then plunge them into cold water to stop the cooking. Drain, blot the cabbage dry, and refrigerate it in a plastic bag. The next day, add it at the last minute of cooking time.

CULINARY Q & A

? Is there an effective alternative to chemical cleansers to clean a porcelain stove?

! Natural cleansers are safer and healthier than chemical ones. Here's a version you can make at home: Fill a spray bottle with 2 cups of water, 2 teaspoons of white vinegar, 1 teaspoon of borax, ½ teaspoon of baking soda, and a squirt of dishwashing liquid. Shake well and spray your porcelain stove top, drip pans, gas burner grates, oven, and even the windows in your oven door. Wait 15 minutes before wiping it off. **Note:** *Do not use this formula on stainless steel appliances or smooth-surface cooktops.*

MAPLE-APRICOT PORK CHOPS

Balsamic vinegar, maple syrup, and apricot preserves give these chops an intense flavor that pairs well with rice, baked potatoes, or egg noodles. Add steamed broccoli or Brussels sprouts, and you've got dinner that'll bring your family running to the table.

YIELD: 4 servings	PREP: 12 minutes	COOK: 45 minutes

2 tbsp. of unsalted butter

1 large sweet onion, chopped

½ cup of balsamic vinegar

3 tbsp. of apricot preserves

2 tbsp. of pure maple syrup (preferably Grade B)

1 tsp. of dried thyme

1 tbsp. of extra virgin olive oil

4 pork chops, ½–¾ inch thick

Sea salt and freshly ground black pepper to taste

3–4 tablespoons of all-purpose flour

½ cup of chicken broth

1. Melt the butter in a medium saucepan, and cook the onion until golden brown and tender (15 to 20 minutes).

2. Stir in the vinegar, apricot preserves, maple syrup, and thyme. Bring to a boil over high heat, reduce to low, and simmer, stirring occasionally, for 5 minutes.

3. Heat the olive oil in a large skillet over medium heat. Sprinkle the chops with the salt and pepper, then dust them with the flour. Brown them on both sides.

4. Add the broth, reduce the heat to low, and simmer, covered, for 10 minutes. Uncover, and continue cooking for another 5 minutes.

5. Add the vinegar mixture to the skillet, and turn the chops to coat well. Cover, and simmer for 10 minutes longer.

A+ Ingredients

ONION
Supports heart health

MAPLE SYRUP
Helps fight free radicals

PORK CHOPS
Promote healthy brain function

KITCHEN CAPERS

When you're shopping for unsalted butter, always make sure those exact words appear on the label. The term *sweet cream butter* refers to any butter that's made from fresh cream—and these products *do* contain salt.

DYNAMIC DIETARY DUOS

We all know it takes teamwork to win a baseball game. Well, guess what? Putting that same strategy to work can also help to improve your health in a big way. Each one of these foods by itself is a health-giving all-star. But when you team them up in a recipe—or even eat them in the same meal or snack—they'll light up your scoreboard!

Dynamic Duo	Savvy Strategy	The Winning Result
Almonds + red wine	Vitamin E in the almonds works with resveratrol in the wine to boost the health of your blood vessel linings.	A happier, healthier heart!
Bananas + yogurt	A fiber called inulin in the bananas revs up the growth of yogurt's healthy bacteria.	Improved digestion and a healthier immune system
Blueberries + walnuts	Antioxidants in the berries help protect your brain cells from free radical damage, and the omega-3 fatty acids in walnuts boost your brainpower.	Improved memory and mental function, and possibly a lowered risk for Parkinson's disease
Chicken + carrots	The zinc in chicken enables your body to convert the carrots' beta-carotene into vitamin A.	A rugged immune system, stronger eyes, and healthier skin
Dark chocolate + raspberries	The catechins in chocolate and quercetin in raspberries intensify each other's disease-fighting prowess.	Thinner blood and a healthier heart
Eggs + cheese	The vitamin D in the egg yolks makes the calcium in the cheese more readily available to your body.	Stronger bones, clearer thinking, and a healthier heart
Onions + garlic	Working together increases the potency of their artery-clearing compounds.	Cleaner blood vessels and reduced arteriosclerosis risk
Vinegar + dark leafy greens	The acetic acid in vinegar unlocks the iron and calcium in spinach, kale, and other greens and allows your body to absorb them more easily.	Richer blood and stronger bones

NEW ENGLAND BOILED DINNER

To say that this single-pot dish has deep historic roots is putting it mildly. It's been comforting Yankee families and their guests for more than three centuries. As with any traditional recipe, it has countless variations, but this is one of the easiest and tastiest.

YIELD: 6–8 servings   **PREP:** 15 minutes   **COOK:** 3 ½ hours

4 lbs. of corned beef brisket

Water to cover

2 tbsp. of apple cider vinegar

16 baby carrots, sliced

16 pearl onions, peeled

16 small new potatoes

2 medium turnips, chopped

1 medium cabbage, cut into 8 wedges

Dark, spicy mustard

Prepared horseradish

1. Put the meat in a Dutch oven or large kettle, and cover with cold water, to which you've added the vinegar. Cover and simmer until the meat is tender (about 3 hours).

2. Skim off the excess fat, and add the carrots, onions, potatoes, and turnips. Boil, uncovered, for 20 minutes. Add the cabbage, and continue cooking until it's soft (15 minutes).

3. Transfer the meat to a large, warmed platter. Drain the vegetables and arrange them around the meat. Serve bowls of mustard and horseradish on the side.

KITCHEN CAPERS Whenever you boil corned beef to use in a recipe, add 2 tablespoons or so of apple cider vinegar to the water. This will keep the meat from shrinking.

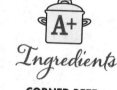

A+

Ingredients

CORNED BEEF
Helps maintain healthy cognitive function

CARROTS
Support oral health

CABBAGE
Promotes good digestion

INSTANT GRATIFICATION

Chicken Alfredo Pasta

This version of a cozy classic can be on your table in only 20 minutes. To make four servings, cook ½ pound of penne pasta in boiling water for 6 minutes. Add 1½ cups of frozen sugar snap peas, return to a boil, and cook until the pasta is al dente. Drain and return the mixture to the pan. Stir in a 15-ounce jar of Alfredo sauce, 1 tablespoon of white balsamic or white wine vinegar, and 2 cups of chopped cooked chicken. Cook over medium heat, stirring constantly, just until the chicken is heated through (3 to 4 minutes max).

PACK-IN-THE-PROTEIN QUICHE

Quiche is a highly versatile and almost-universally pleasing dish that works equally well for brunch, lunch, or a light supper. With a supply of refrigerated or frozen piecrusts on hand, it's as easy as, well, pie to whip up a tasty gem like this one at a moment's notice.

YIELD: 6–8 servings   **PREP:** 20 minutes   **COOK:** 55 minutes

1 deep-dish refrigerated piecrust

1 tbsp. of extra virgin olive oil

2 large onions, diced

2 tbsp. of balsamic vinegar

2 tbsp. of brown sugar

3 large eggs

1 cup of half-and-half

¾ cup of grated cheese

2 tsp. of dried thyme

Salt and black pepper to taste

1 package (8 oz.) of sausage

1. Prepare the pie crust according to package directions; set aside. Heat the oil in a skillet over medium heat. Sauté the onions until very soft (about 10 minutes). Add the vinegar and brown sugar, and cook, stirring, until caramelized (about 5 minutes).

2. In a bowl, beat the eggs. Mix in the half-and-half, cheese, and thyme. Season with salt and pepper.

3. Spread the onion mixture over the pie crust, and top with the crumbled sausage. Pour in the egg mixture, and bake at 350°F until just set (about 40 minutes). Cool on a wire rack for 15 minutes before serving.

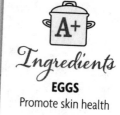

Ingredients

EGGS
Promote skin health

CHEESE
Supports bone health

SAUSAGE
Helps maintain oral health

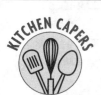

KITCHEN CAPERS

Here's a trick for reheating quiche so that the crust gets crisp and the filling stays moist: Heat it in a nonstick skillet—with no oil added—over low heat. This ploy works great with leftover pizza, too!

CULINARY Q & A

? When I make quiche, it comes out watery. Am I doing something wrong?

! Because it is full of eggs and veggies, a quiche is a delicious way to add protein and vitamins to your diet. But it can be tricky to make. Your problem likely lies with any vegetables you're using. Veggies release water as they cook, and this destroys the creaminess of the egg custard mixture. So precook the veggies and drain. If your quiche seems tough as well as watery, then you've simply overcooked it.

SLOW COOKER BALSAMIC CHICKEN & VEGETABLES

This is the kind of recipe that makes you wonder how you ever got along without a slow cooker. It proves beyond a shadow of a doubt that you can put a healthy, family-pleasing dinner on the table with a bare minimum of prep time.

YIELD: 8 servings   **PREP:** 10 minutes   **COOK:** 3–8 hours

4 boneless, skinless chicken breasts

1 lb. of baby carrots

1 lb. of red potatoes, halved

¼ cup of balsamic vinegar

¼ cup of raw honey

2 garlic cloves, minced

1 tsp. of dried basil

½ tsp. of dried oregano

Salt and black pepper

1 lb. of fresh green beans, trimmed

1. Put the chicken breasts, carrots, and potatoes in a 6- to 7-quart slow cooker. In a bowl, whisk together the vinegar, honey, garlic, basil, and oregano. Taste and add salt and pepper as desired.

2. Pour the vinegar mixture over the chicken and veggies. Cook on high for 3 to 4 hours or low for 6 to 8 hours.

3. Add the green beans during the last 30 minutes of cooking time.

KITCHEN CAPERS When your recipe tastes flat, don't automatically reach for the salt shaker. Instead, stir in a teaspoon or two of balsamic or full-bodied red wine vinegar. That'll provide the lacking pizzazz in a tastier—and healthier—way.

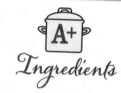

A+

Ingredients

CHICKEN
Boosts nervous system

CARROTS
Promote healthy skin

GREEN BEANS
Enhance sound sleep

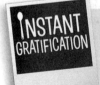

INSTANT GRATIFICATION

Doggone Delicious DIY Steak Seasoning

There are scads of steak seasonings at the grocery store, but it's a snap to make your own blend instead! Better yet—provided you buy your spices in bulk from a top-notch herb dealer, rather than the supermarket—you can make sure the spices you use are as fresh as possible. Here's a delicious basic recipe: In a small bowl, mix 2 tablespoons of sea salt, 2 teaspoons of brown sugar, 1 teaspoon of freshly ground black pepper, ½ teaspoon each of chili powder and paprika, and ¼ teaspoon each of garlic powder, garlic salt, onion powder, and turmeric. Pour the blend into an airtight glass container, and store it in a cool, dark place.

SIRLOIN TIPS WITH PEPPERS & ONIONS

When you want to serve up a simple but super-satisfying weeknight dinner, you can't go wrong with this humdinger. Pair it with baked potatoes and a green salad.

YIELD: 6 servings **PREP:** 20 minutes **COOK:** 10–15 minutes

¼ cup of balsamic vinegar

3 garlic cloves, minced

3 tbsp. of extra virgin olive oil

3 lbs. of sirloin steak, cut into 1-inch pieces

3 bell peppers (red, yellow, and green), sliced

1 large sweet onion, cut into thin wedges

2 tsp. of steak seasoning

1. Mix the vinegar and garlic in a bowl, then slowly whisk in the olive oil. Put the steak pieces in a shallow glass dish, and pour the marinade on top. Cover, and refrigerate for 3 to 24 hours. Then remove the pieces from the marinade, and discard the liquid.

2. Heat a drizzle of olive oil in a skillet. Transfer to a platter. Add the sirloin, and cook until browned.

3. Add the peppers, onions, and additional olive oil to the pan. Stir in the seasoning. Cook, scraping the brown bits from the skillet, until the veggies are browned and tender-crisp.

4. Return the meat to the pan. Stir until heated through, and serve.

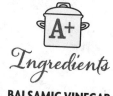

Ingredients

BALSAMIC VINEGAR
Supports healthy blood pressure

SIRLOIN STEAK
Helps prevent anemia

BELL PEPPERS
Promote skin health

KITCHEN CAPERS

Commercial steak seasonings vary in sodium content. So adjust the amount to suit your taste for saltiness. Or make your own seasoning. For an easy recipe, see Doggone Delicious DIY Steak Seasoning on page 230.

CULINARY Q & A

? I thought beef was one of the most fattening foods on the planet, but recently I heard that it can actually increase weight loss. Is this true?

! Yes, with two big "buts": First, the meat must come from cattle that graze only on untreated grass. This beef contains potent amounts of conjugated linoleic acid (CLA), which increases your body's ability to burn fat, fends off food cravings, and has been proven to help fight illnesses. Second, you need to eat beef in moderation. Otherwise, it'll pack on pounds, just as an overload of any other food will.

SWEET-AND-SOUR PORK FOR A CROWD

When you're making an entrée for any other big potluck gathering, don't panic. Just reach for this old-time recipe. It's been pleasing hungry event goers for decades!

YIELD: 24 servings	PREP: 15 minutes	COOK: 1 hour 45 minutes

5 lbs. of pork, cut into 1-inch cubes

Garlic salt

1 cup of vegetable shortening

2 cans (20 oz. each) of pineapple chunks

1 cup of cornstarch

2 qts. of chicken stock

3 cups of sugar

3 cups of apple cider vinegar

½ cup of soy sauce

4 large green bell peppers, cut in strips

Hot cooked rice

1. Season the pork with the garlic salt. Divide the pieces between two 9- by 13-inch pans, and add ½ cup of shortening to each one. Bake at 400°F for 1 hour, stirring often. Remove the pans from the oven, and pour off the fat.

2. Drain the pineapple, reserving the juice. Mix 1 cup of the juice with the cornstarch in a bowl. Stir in the stock, sugar, vinegar, and soy sauce. Mix in the peppers and pineapple.

3. Divide the mixture evenly between the two pans of cooked pork. Return to the oven, and bake at 400°F for 45 minutes, stirring frequently. Serve over the rice.

You can freeze this or just about any other casserole. Move it to the refrigerator up to two days before you want to use it. When serving time arrives, cover the dish with foil, and bake at 350°F for one hour. Remove the foil, and bake 30 minutes more, or until heated through.

KITCHEN CAPERS

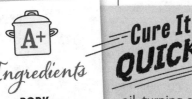

Ingredients

PORK
Boosts skin health

PINEAPPLE
Supports digestion

APPLE CIDER VINEGAR
Helps balance blood sugar

Cure It QUICK!

SPEEDY STROKE RECOVERY As little as 20 milligrams of zinc a day can greatly improve your brain function. Reach your quota with this recipe. Brown four lean pork chops in 2½ tablespoons of extra virgin olive oil, turning once. Remove the chops, and stir in ¾ cup of chicken broth and 6 tablespoons of raspberry vinegar. Add in the chops, and simmer, turning once, until thoroughly cooked. Transfer the meat to a serving platter. Raise the heat, and boil the sauce until slightly thickened (about 5 minutes). Add ½ cup of heavy (a.k.a. whipping) cream, and stir until thick. Pour the sauce over the chops, and serve.

OPEN-FACE GRUYÈRE CHICKEN MELT

Dark chicken meat with the addition of herbs, yogurt, and avocado makes this chicken melt a five-star fine-dining experience. You'll never settle for the standard version again!

YIELD: 4 servings	PREP: 10 minutes	COOK: 5 minutes

1 cup of plain full-fat yogurt

3 tbsp. of hearty dark mustard

¼ red onion, diced

2 tbsp. of chopped fresh chives

½ tsp. of dried thyme

2 cups of chopped cooked
   dark-meat chicken

1 cup of shredded Gruyère cheese

Salt and black pepper to taste

4 slices of sourdough bread

1 avocado, sliced

Balsamic syrup

1. Whisk the yogurt, mustard, onion, chives, and thyme in a medium-size bowl. Mix in the chopped chicken and grated cheese. Season with salt and pepper.

2. Divide the mixture evenly among the slices of bread. Broil until golden brown and bubbly (4 to 5 minutes).

3. Remove from the oven, and top with avocado slices. Drizzle with balsamic syrup (see the Kitchen Capers box, below), and serve immediately.

A+

Ingredients

YOGURT
Fends off colds
and allergies

GRUYÈRE CHEESE
Promotes
cardiovascular health

AVOCADO
Encourages deep,
restful sleep

KITCHEN CAPERS

To make balsamic syrup for this or any other recipe, simply boil ½ cup of balsamic vinegar in a small pan until reduced by half (three to four minutes). Let cool, and drizzle over the food at hand.

CULINARY Q & A

? I enjoy cooking with semi-firm cheeses like Gruyère, fontina, and cheddar, but they're so messy to grate. Are there any tricks to make the job neater?

! These cheeses are an excellent way to add more protein to your diet! Here is a method to easily grate them: First, freeze the cheese for 15 minutes. This will make it firmer. Then, rub a little oil on your hand grater or spritz it with cooking spray. This will prevent the cheese from sticking when you're ready to grate.

PORK CHOPS WITH APPLES & RAISINS

In this recipe, a fruity balsamic vinegar sauce adds a flavorful punch to standard pork chops. Serve it with potatoes and a green salad for an easy, nutritious weeknight dinner.

YIELD: 4 servings	PREP: 10 minutes	COOK: 20 minutes

⅓ cup of raisins

2 tbsp. of all-purpose flour

Salt and pepper to taste

1 tbsp. of olive oil

4 pork loin chops (about 1 inch thick)

3 large garlic cloves, minced

1 large tart apple, thinly sliced

1 cup of chicken or vegetable broth

¼ cup of balsamic vinegar

1 bay leaf

¼ tsp. of dried sage

1. Put the raisins in a bowl with enough boiling water to cover them. Let them sit for 20 minutes. Combine the flour, salt, and pepper, and dredge the chops in the mixture.

2. Heat the oil on medium-high. Add the chops, and brown lightly on one side. Toss in the garlic, and flip meat. Drain the raisins, and add with the apples to the chops. Cook until the second side is brown, stirring to mix the fruit.

3. Add the broth, vinegar, bay leaf, and sage. Cover, cook on low heat, turning the meat once, until it's juicy but firm (about 10 minutes). Move the chops to a platter. Cook the apples and raisins for 5 minutes and pour over the chops.

KITCHEN CAPERS Add vinegar to the water when parboiling meat for casseroles or stews. The toughest cuts will turn tender! Just ¼ cup of vinegar per 2 cups of water will do the trick.

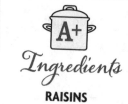

A+

Ingredients

RAISINS
Relieve congestion

PORK
Boosts the immune system

APPLES
Help prevent colds

INSTANT GRATIFICATION

Grilled Scallops with Prosciutto

Serve these up at your next party! For six servings, wash 18 large scallops and discard the small, tough side muscle. Cut nine paper-thin prosciutto slices in half lengthwise, and wrap a strip around the width of each scallop, trimming off any excess so that the strip overlaps by no more than an inch. Brush each scallop with extra virgin olive oil and season with freshly ground black pepper. Grill the scallops, exposed side down, over direct high heat until opaque in the center, turning once. Serve the scallops with a drizzle of balsamic syrup (see the Kitchen Capers box on page 233).

BEEF TENDERLOIN WITH WINE SAUCE

Beef tenderloin doesn't come cheap, to put it mildly. But when you've got a special occasion to celebrate, or you're planning a dinner for some of your favorite beef lovers, it's worth a splurge. And this is one fine way to cook it. As a bonus, the balsamic cranberry wine sauce delivers a triple-threat punch to your risk for cardiovascular disease.

YIELD: 8 servings	PREP: 10 minutes	COOK: about 45 minutes

3 tbsp. of unsalted butter, divided

1 center-cut beef tenderloin (2 lbs.)

Salt and ground black pepper to taste

⅓ cup of minced shallots

1 garlic clove, minced

1 cup of dry red wine

1 cup of 100 percent cranberry juice

¾ cup of beef broth

½ cup of balsamic vinegar

1 tbsp. of chopped fresh thyme

1 tbsp. of extra virgin olive oil

1. In a large, heavy skillet over medium-high heat, melt 2 tablespoons of the butter and brown the beef on all sides (about 2 minutes per side). Transfer the meat to a greased shallow roasting pan, and set the skillet and drippings aside. Season the beef with salt and pepper, and roast at 425°F until it reaches your desired degree of doneness (20 to 25 minutes).

2. In the skillet, melt the remaining 1 tablespoon of butter over medium heat. Add the shallots, and cook, stirring, for 1 minute. Mix in the garlic, and continue to cook, stirring, for 20 seconds.

3. Stir in the wine. Add the juice, broth, vinegar, and thyme. Boil, and cook, stirring occasionally, until slightly thickened (about 15 minutes). Reduce the heat to medium, and whisk in the olive oil. Strain the sauce into an attractive serving bowl.

4. Slice the beef, and serve with the sauce on the side.

A+ Ingredients

BEEF
Helps build muscle mass

SHALLOTS
Boost metabolism

CRANBERRY JUICE
Helps prevent urinary tract infections

KITCHEN CAPERS Never pour residual meat fat—or any other greasy substance—down the drain or into a garbage disposal. Instead, depending on the quantity, wipe it out with paper towels or pour it into a disposable container, and toss it into the trash can.

GRILLED TEQUILA TURKEY

The next time you host a barbecue, make sure the menu includes this tantalizing turkey tenderloin treat. It'll be a hit with any Margarita lovers, too!

YIELD: 4 servings	PREP: 20 minutes	COOK: 25 minutes

1 cup of chopped tomatoes

½ cup of chopped yellow bell peppers

1 jalapeño pepper, seeded and finely chopped

2 tbsp. of chopped fresh cilantro

2 tbsp. of red wine vinegar

1 package (20 oz.) of boneless turkey breast tenderloin

⅓ cup of fresh lime juice

¼ cup of tequila

2 tsp. of extra virgin olive oil

Black pepper to taste

1. Combine the first five ingredients in a bowl. Cover, and refrigerate for 2 hours so the flavors can blend.

2. While the veggies are marinating, put the turkey in a shallow dish. Stir the lime juice, tequila, olive oil, and black pepper until blended, and pour over the turkey. Cover, and refrigerate for 15 minutes to 2 hours. Drain, and discard the marinade.

3. Put a sprayed grill rack about 5 inches from the heat source. Grill the turkey on medium heat until it is no longer pink in the center and the juices run clear. An instant-read thermometer should read 165°F.

4. Cut the turkey into thin slices, and serve, topped with the tomato-pepper mixture.

You can ease your grill cleanup in a major way with this simple trick: Before you heat up the grill, spray the cleaning surface with a half-and-half solution of water and vinegar. Any residual grime will slide right off!

KITCHEN CAPERS

A+ Ingredients

TOMATOES
Support heart health

TURKEY
Promotes thyroid health

TEQUILA
Aids digestion

Cure It QUICK!

TAKE A HOT HEALTH TONIC The hot-pepper vinegar in this steak marinade helps increase your body's cortisone level, thereby helping to fend off illnesses. Mix ½ cup of extra virgin olive oil, ¼ cup of hot-pepper vinegar, ¼ cup of soy sauce, 2 tablespoons of chopped onions, 1 tablespoon of minced ginger, and 1 minced garlic clove. Pour over 2 pounds of flank steak. Cover and refrigerate for three hours. Grill the steak until done, slice into thin strips, and serve.

GRILLED TURKEY TENDERLOIN WITH PEACHES

Great grilling starts with turkey breast tenderloin. And here's one super-simple, super-healthy—and super-scrumptious—recipe to keep close at hand.

YIELD: 4 servings   **PREP:** 15 minutes   **COOK:** 35 minutes

2 tbsp. of extra virgin olive oil, divided

2 medium red onions, sliced ½-inch thick

1 package (24 oz.) of turkey breast tenderloin

3 fresh, ripe peaches, cut into wedges

2 cups of baby arugula

2 tbsp. of balsamic vinegar

2 oz. of blue cheese, crumbled

1. Drizzle 1 tablespoon of the olive oil over the onions; set aside. Grill the turkey, covered, over medium coals until the juices run clear and the internal temperature measures 165°F (about 8 minutes per side).

2. Grill the onions just until grill marks appear (about 5 minutes per side). Separate into rings. Follow suit with the peach wedges (about 2 minutes per side).

3. Toss the arugula with the onions, peaches, vinegar, and remaining olive oil. Arrange the turkey slices and arugula mixture on plates, and sprinkle with the cheese.

A+ Ingredients

TURKEY
Helps strengthen the immune system

PEACHES
Help calm anxiety

ARUGULA
Boosts immunity

KITCHEN CAPERS   Tip for frequent grillers: Buy a plastic or wicker tool tote, and stock it with your grilling staples—like salt, pepper, tongs, aluminum foil, paper towels, and a basting brush. Reserve a section for the basting sauce of the evening, and you'll be good to go!

CULINARY Q & A

? When I grill vegetables, brushed with an olive oil and vinegar mixture, they dry out. How can I prevent this problem?

! Grilled vegetables are scrumptious—and full of vitamins and nutrients to help boost your immune system and more! To keep them from drying out during the grilling process, simply use mayonnaise instead of oil. This will create a protective barrier on the surface of the veggies.

BEEF FILLETS WITH NECTARINE SAUCE

This protein-rich recipe is easy enough for weeknight dinners but also impressive enough for special occasions. And it'll please even the most finicky eaters!

YIELD: 4 servings	PREP: 10 minutes	COOK: 8–26 minutes

4 (4 oz. each) beef tenderloin fillets

2 tbsp. of unsalted butter

Salt and freshly ground black pepper to taste

3 scallions, sliced

2 medium nectarines, pitted and sliced*

¼ cup of orange marmalade

2 tbsp. of balsamic vinegar

* Or substitute fresh plums.

1. In a large, heavy skillet, cook the fillets in the butter over medium-high heat until the meat reaches your desired degree of doneness. Season with salt and pepper. Transfer to a serving platter, and keep warm.

2. In the same skillet, cook the scallions and nectarines until the fruit is tender (2 to 3 minutes).

3. Add the marmalade and vinegar. Cook, stirring constantly, until heated through. Pour the sauce over the warm fillets, and serve immediately.

KITCHEN CAPERS Before you cook hot dogs, give each one a few pokes with a fork. Then boil them for several minutes in water that has a tablespoon of vinegar added to it. Try it—you'll be amazed at the delicious difference it makes!

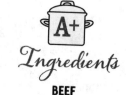

Ingredients

BEEF
Enhances the immune system

NECTARINES
Fight free radicals

BALSAMIC VINEGAR
Maintains healthy glucose levels

Tropical Shrimp Ceviche

This chilled shrimp dish makes a refreshing, nutritious appetizer for a barbecue. First, boil 1 pound of medium-size peeled, deveined shrimp in salted water for 2 minutes. Drain, cut each shrimp in half, and mix them with ½ cup each of coconut and white balsamic vinegar. Cover, and chill for 30 minutes. Mix in 1 cup of finely chopped red onion and 1 minced serrano chili pepper, and chill for another 30 minutes. Just before serving, stir in 1 cup of chopped fresh cilantro, 1 cup of diced cucumber, and 1 diced avocado.

SLOW COOKER POLYNESIAN SPARERIBS

Enjoy a taste of the islands—and get a jolt of ginger's anti-inflammatory kick—with these tantalizing ribs. Just pop 'em into a slow cooker and they'll fly on autopilot all day!

YIELD: 4 servings   **PREP:** 30 minutes   **COOK:** 4–10 hours

2 lbs. of boneless pork spareribs

⅓ cup of soy sauce

¼ cup of cornstarch

1 tbsp. of ground ginger

1 cup of sugar

½ cup of apple cider vinegar

¼ cup of water

1 tsp. of salt

½ tsp. of dry mustard

1-inch piece of fresh or crystallized ginger

1. Cut the meat into 3-inch pieces. Mix the soy sauce, cornstarch, and ground ginger until smooth, and brush the mixture over the ribs.

2. Arrange the ribs on the rack of a broiler pan, and bake at 425°F for 20 minutes to remove the fat. Drain on paper towels, and set aside.

3. Combine the sugar, vinegar, water, salt, mustard, and fresh or crystallized ginger in the slow cooker. Stir well.

4. Add the ribs, cover, and cook on low for 8 to 10 hours or on high for 4 to 5 hours. Serve immediately, or if you prefer your ribs to be brown and crispy, broil them for about 10 minutes before dishing them up.

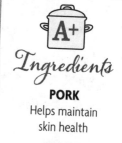

Ingredients

PORK
Helps maintain skin health

GINGER
Soothes acid reflux

APPLE CIDER VINEGAR
Enhances weight loss

KITCHEN CAPERS Prep your food for the slow cooker the night before, and refrigerate. Take it out when you wake up, so it'll come to room temp while you get dressed.

CULINARY Q & A

? Is it true that trichinosis is no longer a major concern in pork?

! Yes! And pork is a vital part of your diet because it benefits your skin, muscles, heart, and more. Studies show it even helps to prevent anemia. But still take basic precautions, so never taste raw pork and thoroughly wash in hot, soapy water any utensils or cutting boards that have come into contact with it. Also, always cook the meat to a temperature of 150° to 165°F before consuming it.

DUCK BREASTS WITH PICKLED PLUMS & CHERRIES

Duck lends itself beautifully to strong accompaniments like pickled fruits and tangy vinegars. And this version features white button mushrooms, which are the most potent vegetarian source of the fat-burning superstar conjugated linoleic acid (CLA).

YIELD: 4–6 servings	**PREP:** 10 minutes	**COOK:** 10–15 minutes

4 small (6 oz. each) boneless duck breasts

Salt and ground black pepper to taste

⅓ cup of unsalted butter

1 shallot, finely chopped

16 small white button mushrooms, stems removed

Pickled Plums & Cherries, drained*

2 tbsp. of orange vinegar

3 tbsp. of rich chicken stock

* See recipe on page 124.

1. Sprinkle the duck with salt and pepper. Heat the butter in a skillet, and brown the breasts. Sauté until the meat is tender but still pink inside. Remove, and keep warm.

2. In the same pan, sauté the shallot and mushrooms in the retained butter. Add the plums and cherries, and deglaze the pan with the orange vinegar. Stir in the chicken stock, and cook over high heat for 2 minutes.

3. To serve, slice the duck breasts diagonally and place them on a warmed serving platter. Top with the sauce and spiced fruit.

KITCHEN CAPERS Duck's strong flavor demands a rich, robust sauce. Wine, tomatoes, ginger, vinegar, and plenty of herbs can help camouflage the gamey taste.

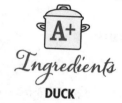

Ingredients

DUCK
Helps balance blood sugar

MUSHROOMS
Promote weight loss

CHERRIES
Help strengthen the nervous system

INSTANT GRATIFICATION

Chicken Wings on the Fly

Chicken fixes don't come much easier than this one.
First, mix 2 chopped garlic cloves with 2 ½ tablespoons of balsamic vinegar, 2 tablespoons of extra virgin olive oil, 2 tablespoons of honey, and 1 tablespoon of chopped fresh thyme. Season with salt and black pepper. Add 2 pounds of chicken wings, toss until coated, and sauté in olive oil until golden brown. Cook the marinade, partially covered with a lid, until it has thickened and the chicken is cooked through. Sprinkle with ½ tablespoon of fresh thyme, and serve.

PORK WITH FIG & PORT WINE SAUCE

If you *do* care a feather *and* a fig about serving healthy, tasty meals to your family—but you lack the time to spend hours preparing them—then this recipe is for you. The hands-on time is less than an hour, and the results are well worth it.

YIELD: 6 servings   **PREP:** 15 minutes   **COOK:** 50 minutes

8 dried figs, stemmed and chopped

¼ cup of port wine

¼ cup of water

6 tbsp. of unsalted butter, divided

2 ½ lbs. of pork tenderloin, trimmed and halved

2 tbsp. of red wine vinegar

1 ½ cups of light cream

2 tbsp. of finely minced shallots

1. Combine the chopped figs and wine in a pan, and soak for 1 hour. Add the water and 1 tablespoon of butter. Simmer until soft (about 20 minutes). Then puree in a blender.

2. In a skillet, heat the remaining butter, and brown the pork (about 5 minutes per side). Reduce the heat to low, cover, and cook until the meat is just pink (about 15 minutes). Remove, cut into roughly ½-inch slices, and keep warm.

3. Deglaze the pan with the vinegar. Add the cream and shallots. Cook, stirring, until thickened (about 3 minutes). Remove from the heat, stir in the fig mix, and reheat.

4. To serve, pour the sauce onto a warmed, rimmed platter, and arrange the pork slices on top.

A+

Ingredients

FIGS
Help maintain blood pressure

PORT WINE
Helps speed wound healing

PORK
Boosts skin health

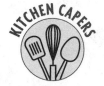

KITCHEN CAPERS

Don't pour leftover wine down the drain! Freeze in ice cube trays, and transfer to a freezer bag. Use the cubes to flavor casseroles, stews, soups, and sauces.

CULINARY Q & A

? Exactly what does it mean when a recipe says to "deglaze" a pan? And why is it such a big deal?

! When meat, poultry, fish, or vegetables are cooked, their natural sugars caramelize and stick to the bottom of the pan. By stirring a liquid, whether vinegar, wine, broth, or even water, into the pan to dissolve the browned fragments (a.k.a. "deglazing"), you can release a mother lode of flavor and health-giving nutrients.

SLOW COOKER PORK & CABBAGE

Red cabbage and pork are a match made in culinary heaven. In this recipe, the slow, easy cooking process brings out all the sweetness of the cabbage to complement the savory taste of the pork and the combined flavors of the brown sugar and thyme.

YIELD: 6 servings   **PREP:** 15 minutes   **COOK:** 7–8 hours

5 cups of chopped red cabbage

5 garlic cloves, minced

1 medium onion, chopped

⅔ cup of apple cider vinegar

⅔ cup of brown sugar

1 tsp. of dried thyme

3–4 lbs. of boneless pork shoulder roast

Salt and freshly ground black pepper to taste

1. Combine the cabbage, garlic, onion, vinegar, brown sugar, and thyme in a 4- or 5-quart slow cooker.

2. Sprinkle the pork with salt and pepper, and put it on top of the veggies. Cover, and cook on low until the pork's internal temperature registers at least 145°F (7 to 8 hours).

3. Remove the pork from the cooker. Cover, and let stand for 10 minutes. Then slice and arrange on a warmed serving platter with the cabbage mixture.

KITCHEN CAPERS For slow cooker pork recipes, always choose a shoulder roast. Pork tenderloin becomes unpleasantly overdone with very long cooking. If you're uncertain at shopping time, ask the butcher for help.

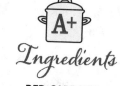

A+

Ingredients

RED CABBAGE
Promotes healthy vision

GARLIC
Fends off cold and flu viruses

PORK
Boosts the immune system

INSTANT GRATIFICATION

Fast-Cooker Ham with Apricots

Whip up this entrée in 20 minutes flat. Score the edges of a 2-pound slice of ham. Drain a 15-ounce can of apricots, reserving 1 cup of the syrup. Combine ¼ cup of packed brown sugar, 2 tablespoons of cornstarch, and ¼ teaspoon of ground nutmeg. Add 2 tablespoons of apple cider vinegar and the reserved apricot syrup, and stir until smooth. Then pour it over the ham. Cover, and cook in the microwave at 70 percent power for 5 minutes. Turn the ham over, and arrange the apricot slices on top. Cover, and resume heating at 70 percent power until the sauce has thickened (8 minutes). Let sit for 2 minutes before serving.

CRANBERRY CHICKEN

Cranberry vinegar, brown sugar, and ginger team up to give chicken a sweet-tart flavor that's perfect for fall and a tasty match for rice. Plus, it's a snap to make!

YIELD: 4 servings	**PREP:** 10 minutes	**COOK:** 30 minutes

4 skinless, boneless chicken breast halves

½ cup of soy sauce

¼ cup of cranberry vinegar

3 tbsp. of firmly packed brown sugar

1 tsp. of lemon juice

½ tsp. of ground ginger

½ red or yellow bell pepper, chopped

2 garlic cloves, chopped

Hot cooked rice

1. Arrange the chicken breasts in a shallow non-reactive pan or a heavy, sealable plastic bag.

2. In a medium bowl, mix the soy sauce, vinegar, brown sugar, lemon juice, ginger, pepper, and garlic. Pour the mixture over the chicken, cover, and refrigerate for at least an hour and no more than 24 hours.

3. Discard the marinade, and put the chicken in a baking dish. Bake until the juices run clear and a meat thermometer registers an internal temperature of 165°F (about 30 minutes). Serve over rice.

KITCHEN CAPERS Don't rinse chicken or any poultry. Rather than killing bacteria, as previously thought, the splashing water in the sink can actually spread the tiny terrors around. Simply cooking poultry to 165°F effectively destroys the most common culprits behind food-borne illness.

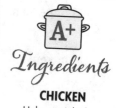

A+
Ingredients
CHICKEN
Helps weight loss
CRANBERRY VINEGAR
Helps promote cardiovascular health
BELL PEPPER
Boosts the immune system

CULINARY Q & A

? What's the best way to store chicken?

! Great job adding chicken to your repertoire! It contains essential vitamins and minerals; plus, it aids in losing weight, regulating healthy blood pressure, and supporting healthy eyes. Here's the best way to store it: Keep it in its original packaging, and tuck it into your refrigerator toward the back (which is generally the coldest part). It will keep for a day or two. For longer storage, freeze in its original packaging.

BALSAMIC BEEF SHORT RIBS

Balsamic vinegar teams up with an all-star collection of flavorful ingredients that give this hearty beef dish a winning taste and a knockout nutritional punch. Plus, the meat is so tender once it's cooked, it will fall right off the bones!

YIELD: 4–6 servings   **PREP:** 20 minutes   **COOK:** 1 ½–2 ½ hours

2 tbsp. of canola oil

4-5 lbs. of beef short ribs

2 medium onions, sliced

¼ cup of minced garlic

1 cup of orange juice

1 cup of red wine

½ cup of balsamic vinegar

½ cup of ketchup

2 tbsp. of grainy mustard

2 cups of beef stock (more or less)

Zest of 1 orange

Salt and freshly ground black pepper to taste

1. Heat the oil in a Dutch oven or large ovenproof skillet over medium-high heat. Brown the ribs on all sides (in multiple batches if necessary). Remove from the pan, and set aside.

2. Remove all but about 2 tablespoons of the fat from the pot, and reduce the heat to medium. Sauté the onions until they're translucent and just a tad crunchy (10 to 15 minutes). Stir in the garlic.

3. Mix in the orange juice, wine, vinegar, ketchup, and mustard. Simmer, then add the meat and enough stock to bring the liquid halfway up the side of the ribs. Return to a simmer, and skim the surface. Cover with foil and the pot lid.

4. Cook for 1 hour, then stir in the orange zest. Continue to cook until the meat is tender (for a total of 1 ½ to 2 hours). Transfer the ribs to a warm serving platter.

5. Bring the remaining sauce to a simmer until it's reduced to your desired thickness. Season with salt and pepper, and pour the sauce over the ribs.

A+

Ingredients

BEEF
Helps strengthen skin

ONIONS
Promote
oral health

ORANGE ZEST
Supports digestion

KITCHEN CAPERS Here's an easy way to make sure you always have orange or any other kind of citrus zest on hand when you need it: Before you squeeze the juice from the fruit, use a citrus zester to remove the colored portion of the peel. Then freeze it for up to six months.

ROASTED CHICKEN RISOTTO

This rich, dark risotto is a terrific use of leftover roasted chicken. And including fresh fennel is a major health plus. That's because it's chock-full of iron and the amino acid histidine, both of which are essential for rich, healthy blood.

YIELD: 6 servings	PREP: 15 minutes	COOK: 30 minutes

¼ cup of extra virgin olive oil

1 fennel bulb, trimmed and julienned, some fronds reserved for garnish

1 large onion, diced

1 ½ cups of carnaroli rice

¼ cup of balsamic vinegar

7 ½–8 cups of rich chicken stock, heated

2 cups of cubed roasted chicken

2 tbsp. of unsalted butter

1. Heat the olive oil in a medium-size pan over medium heat. Sauté the fennel and onion until softened but not browned (about 3 minutes).

2. Add the rice, and stir until it is opaque. Stir in the vinegar, and continue stirring until it is absorbed.

3. Add 1 cup of stock, and stir constantly until most of the liquid has been absorbed. Repeat with about 1 cup at a time until all but 1/4 cup of the stock has been used and the rice is al dente (about 18 to 20 minutes).

4. Stir in the remaining stock, chicken, and butter. Season with salt and pepper, and serve immediately, garnished with reserved fennel fronds.

KITCHEN CAPERS

The key to a successful risotto is to use either carnaroli or arborio rice. These short-grain, high-starch rices produce the creamy consistency that characterizes this classic Italian dish.

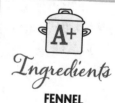

A+

Ingredients

FENNEL
Maintains healthy blood sugar

CARNAROLI RICE
Helps protect teeth and bones

CHICKEN
Boosts nervous system

CULINARY Q & A

? I love grilling, but I have very little prep time during the week. Do you have any tips for speeding up the process?

! A little planning ahead works wonders! On the weekends, freeze individual batches of various meats and their marinades in plastic bags. Then, before you leave in the morning, pull out a bag from the freezer and tuck it into the fridge to thaw. When you get home, your main dish will be ready to slap on the grill.

RIGATONI WITH SPICY MEAT SAUCE

In this hearty pasta recipe, cinnamon and cayenne pepper add an unexpected—but delicious and healthy—punch to traditional meat sauce. Paired with a simple green salad, it makes a quick, easy, and highly satisfying weeknight dinner.

YIELD: 4 servings	PREP: 10 minutes	COOK: 30 minutes

1 package (12 oz.) of rigatoni

1 lb. of ground pork or beef chuck

2 garlic cloves, minced

1 medium onion, finely chopped

Salt and pepper to taste

½ cup of tomato paste

½ tsp. of ground cinnamon

⅛ tsp. of cayenne pepper

1 ½ cups of water

1 tbsp. of red wine vinegar

Parmesan cheese

1. Boil pasta until al dente, according to the package directions. Drain, return it to the pot, and set it aside.

2. Brown the meat in a large pan over medium-high heat. Add the garlic and onion, and season with the salt and pepper. Cook, stirring occasionally, until the onion is tender.

3. Stir in the tomato paste, cinnamon, and cayenne pepper. Cook until fragrant (about 2 minutes). Add the water, and bring to a boil. Reduce to a simmer, and cook until slightly thickened (8 to 10 minutes). Stir in the vinegar.

4. Pour the sauce into the pot with the pasta, and combine. Serve with fresh Parmesan cheese for grating on top.

KITCHEN CAPERS Ignore advice you may read to rinse pasta after cooking it. That process removes all the surface starch—which is what adds texture and helps the sauce cling to the pasta.

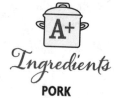

A+

Ingredients

PORK
Helps maintain skin health

ONION
Boosts immunity

CINNAMON
Promotes healthy blood sugar

INSTANT GRATIFICATION

3-Ingredient BBQ Chicken

This dish is another reason to add a slow cooker to your kitchen arsenal! Put 3 pounds of boneless, skinless chicken breasts in your slow cooker. Pour 2½ cups of Sweet-and-Tangy Barbecue Sauce (see page 54) on top. Then add 1 large chopped onion. Cover, and cook until the chicken reaches an internal temperature of 165°F (six to eight hours on low; three to four hours on high). Use two forks to shred the meat, and stir until it's evenly coated. Serve hot.

TASTY TURKEY MEATBALLS

Talk about healthy fast food! These marvelous meatballs are ready in a flash. Serve them with egg noodles, mashed red-skin potatoes, or roasted Yukon Gold potatoes (for a booster shot of beta-carotene), and you've got a cozy dinner that can't be beat.

YIELD: 4 servings	**PREP:** 10 minutes	**COOK:** 30 minutes

½ cup of brown sugar

½ cup of water

2 tbsp. of balsamic vinegar

2 tbsp. of soy sauce

1 tbsp. of cornstarch

1 lb. of ground turkey

1 egg, beaten

½ cup of bread crumbs

1 tbsp. of peanut or canola oil

2 tbsp. of unsalted butter

1 small onion, finely chopped

2 garlic cloves, minced

1. In a small bowl, mix the brown sugar, water, vinegar, soy sauce, and cornstarch. Set aside.

2. Mix the turkey, egg, and bread crumbs in a larger bowl. Form the mixture into balls roughly 2 inches in diameter.

3. Heat the oil in a heavy pan over medium heat. Cook the meatballs for 5 to 6 minutes on each side. Remove, and keep warm.

4. In the same pan, melt the butter, and cook the onion and garlic until soft. Add the sauce, and cook, stirring, until thickened. Add the meatballs, and heat until warmed through.

KITCHEN CAPERS After you wash your kitchen's greasy exhaust fans and air-conditioning grilles, wipe the exposed surfaces with white vinegar. It'll reduce the amount of potentially flammable grease that builds up in the future.

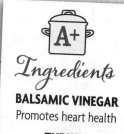

A+ Ingredients

BALSAMIC VINEGAR
Promotes heart health

TURKEY
Boosts immunity

EGG
Supports memory and cognition

CULINARY Q & A

? I'd like to roast a whole turkey more often, but the basting process is so tedious. Is there any way around it?

! Roasted turkey is full of iron, zinc, potassium, and phosphorus! While it does have to be basted while it's roasting, it will essentially do the job itself if you simply cover it with a double layer of cheesecloth that's been soaked in melted butter, olive oil, or canola oil. Remove the cloth 30 minutes before the bird is done.

CHICKEN BREASTS WITH BLUEBERRIES

This simple, delicious, and healthy recipe multiplies beautifully. What's more, it's just as tasty and nutritious whether you make it with fresh, frozen, or dried berries—so it's easy to have the ingredients already on hand.

YIELD: 2 servings	**PREP:** 5 minutes	**COOK:** 25 minutes

2 tbsp. of unsalted butter

2 whole skinless, boneless chicken breasts, cut in half

⅓ cup of peach or apricot jam

3 tbsp. of Dijon mustard

⅓ cup of blueberries (fresh, frozen, or dried)

½ cup of blueberry vinegar

1. Melt the butter over medium-high heat in a heavy skillet. Brown the chicken breasts on both sides (about 8 minutes).

2. Mix the jam and mustard, and spread it over the meaty side of the breasts. Put the blueberries on top. Reduce the heat and cook, covered, until the meat is no longer pink and the juices run clear (about 15 minutes). Transfer to a dish, and keep warm.

3. Add the vinegar, deglaze the pan, and boil on high heat until the liquid is thickened and reduced by about a third. Pour the sauce over the chicken, and serve.

KITCHEN CAPERS The key to success in sautéing chicken breasts is to use a heavy skillet that's just the right size to accommodate the pieces in one layer. If the pan is too big, the juices can burn; if it's too small, the overcrowded chicken will steam instead of brown.

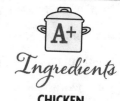

A+

Ingredients

CHICKEN
Boosts weight loss

MUSTARD
Eases asthma symptoms

BLUEBERRIES
Help support memory

INSTANT GRATIFICATION

Healthy Homemade Tartar Sauce

If you only think of tartar sauce as a tasty fish enhancer, think again. This sweet-and-tangy blend also perks up cold meats, and it makes a dandy, nutrient-packed dip for corn chips or raw vegetables. To make about 1½ cups, mix 1 cup of mayonnaise with 1 tablespoon each of chopped bread-and-butter pickles, chopped fresh tarragon, chopped green olives, and white balsamic vinegar; 1 teaspoon of freshly squeezed lemon juice; and ¼ teaspoon of celery seed. Chill for 20 minutes before using!

FAJITAS DIXIE STYLE

Pulled pork in a Carolina-style barbecue sauce puts a whole new spin on a Tex-Mex classic. If you prefer, use leftover roasted or deli rotisserie chicken (dark meat works best) in place of the pork. Either way, you're in for a Texas-size taste treat!

YIELD: 4 servings   **PREP:** 10 minutes   **COOK:** 20 minutes

⅓ cup of apple cider vinegar

2 tbsp. of sugar

2 tbsp. of Worcestershire sauce

1 ½ tsp. of salt

¼ tsp. of cayenne pepper

2 lbs. (or so) of leftover roasted pork or chicken

8 flour tortillas

Fresh cilantro leaves, chopped

1 avocado, diced

1 fresh, ripe tomato, chopped

1 red onion, chopped

1. Mix the first five ingredients in a medium saucepan. Heat to boiling over high heat. Reduce the heat to low, and simmer for 5 minutes.

2. Cut the meat into 1-inch-thick slices, then shred it by hand. Stir it into the sauce, cover, and heat through, stirring occasionally (about 5 minutes).

3. In a large dry skillet over medium-high heat, warm the tortillas one at a time until they're hot and slightly crisp around the edges but still soft in the center (1 to 2 minutes per side).

4. Spoon some meat mixture into the center of each tortilla. Top it with cilantro, avocado, tomato, and onion, and roll 'er up!

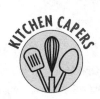

KITCHEN CAPERS For a recipe that needs fresh tomatoes when they're out of season—or when you can't get fresh-from-the-vine varieties—use grape tomatoes. All year round they offer up better flavor than many of the full-size versions.

CULINARY Q & A

? My dishwasher sometimes leaves chalky deposits on my dishes. What's the best way to remove them?

! Put the "victims" on the lower rack, and run the machine for about five minutes with 1 cup of vinegar—no soap. Follow up with a complete cycle using your regular detergent. Your dishes will come out sparkling clean with no elbow grease needed!

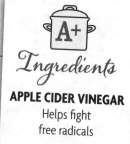

A+

Ingredients

APPLE CIDER VINEGAR
Helps fight free radicals

PORK
Boosts the immune system

AVOCADO
Supports heart health

POACHED SALMON WITH CHUTNEY

Salmon is an important part of any healthy diet. And you couldn't find a better entrée than this. The poaching process makes the fish as tender as butter, and the raspberry vinegar adds a subtle, fruity aroma. Pair it with a fruit chutney for a delicious meal.

YIELD: 4 servings	**PREP:** 15 minutes	**COOK:** 40 minutes

1 qt. of water

1 bottle of dry white wine*

½ cup of raspberry vinegar

Juice of 1 lemon

2 yellow onions, quartered

1 large carrot

1 medium leek, trimmed and cut into 2-inch lengths

3 sprigs of fresh parsley

2 sprigs of fresh thyme

1 bay leaf

1 tsp. of salt

4 (6–8 oz. each) salmon steaks or fillets

Sprigs of mint, cilantro, and thyme for garnish

Fruit chutney

* A dry Chardonnay is ideal. Don't use a sweet wine!

1. In a large nonreactive pot, combine the water, wine, vinegar, lemon juice, onions, carrot, leek, parsley, thyme, bay leaf, and salt. Bring it to a boil, and simmer for 30 minutes. Remove the pan from the heat, and let the liquid come to room temperature.

2. Arrange the salmon pieces on a poaching rack so that they are not touching each other. Lower the rack into the vegetable-broth mixture (a.k.a. court bouillon) until each piece of fish is surrounded by liquid.

3. Using an instant-read thermometer, slowly bring the liquid to about 160°F, and hold it there for 10 minutes. On a gas range, turn off the flame, and let the fish sit in the broth for 20 minutes. If you're using an electric stove, remove from heat.

4. Remove the salmon, and dry it on paper towels.

5. Serve immediately, garnished with fresh herb sprigs and a spoonful of fruit chutney (see Chapter Four). Or, refrigerate it for 2 hours, and serve chilled.

A+

Ingredients

ONIONS
Enhance digestion

SALMON
Promotes general wellness

FRUIT CHUTNEY
Provides nutrients essential for good health

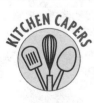

KITCHEN CAPERS

Any of the fruit chutneys in Chapter Four are delicious with salmon, but Mango Chutney (see page 136), Apricot & Almond Chutney (see page 139), and No-Wait Apple Cran-Peary Chutney (see page 140) are especially good, healthy choices.

STIR-FRIED FISH & PEPPERS

The next time you're in the mood for a terrific stir-fry, you could venture out to your favorite Chinese restaurant. Or, you could whip up this delicious version in no time flat.

YIELD: 4 servings	PREP: 15 minutes	COOK: 10 minutes

1 lb. of firm fish fillets, fresh or frozen and thawed

4 tbsp. of cornstarch, divided

1 can (20 oz.) of pineapple chunks in juice

¼ cup of honey

¼ cup of ketchup

¼ cup of soy sauce

3 tbsp. of dry sherry

3 tbsp. of white wine or sherry vinegar

3 tbsp. of peanut oil

1 medium red bell pepper, coarsely chopped (about ¾-inch squares)

Hot cooked rice

1. Cut the fish into 1-inch pieces. Put them in a bowl, toss with 3 tablespoons of the cornstarch, and set aside.

2. Drain the pineapple, reserving the juice. Mix juice with the remaining 1 tablespoon of cornstarch. Stir in the honey, ketchup, soy sauce, sherry, and vinegar; set aside.

3. Cook the fish in oil over high heat for about 1 minute per side. Remove the fish and set it aside. Stir-fry the bell pepper for 2 minutes in the same skillet, and remove.

4. Pour the juice mixture into the pan, and cook, stirring, until thickened and bubbly. Stir in the pineapple chunks, fish, and bell pepper. Cook for 1 minute. Serve over the rice.

KITCHEN CAPERS
If you overcook your stir-fry, add crunchy texture by mixing in sesame seeds, crushed peanuts, cashews, shredded carrot, or coarsely chopped raw cabbage.

A+ Ingredients

FISH
Promotes brain function

PINEAPPLE
Boosts immunity

KETCHUP
Helps support kidney health

CULINARY Q & A

? What exactly is the difference between a salmon steak and a salmon fillet?

! Both are rich in omega-3 fatty acids, protein, and potassium! But the difference is that a steak (salmon or otherwise) is a crosscut slice from a large dressed (that is, skinned, boned) fish. It's generally ½ to 1 inch thick. A fillet is a boneless piece of flesh cut from the side and away from the backbone. You can buy it with or without skin.

TUNA KABOBS

If you want to keep your blood pressure in check, here's a three-word solution: Eat more tuna. These skewered chunks are a fine way to tap into fish's pressure-lowering potent power. And they're just as tasty sautéed, broiled, or grilled.

YIELD: 4 servings   **PREP:** 15 minutes   **COOK:** 5 minutes

¼ cup of orange juice

⅛ cup of lime juice

1 small garlic clove, minced

1 tsp. of dried rosemary

Salt and black pepper to taste

⅓ cup + 2–3 tbsp. of canola oil, divided

1 lb. of yellowtail or albacore tuna steaks, cut into 1-inch chunks

1. In a bowl, mix the first five ingredients. Whisk in ⅓ cup of canola oil. Add the tuna, and stir gently to coat. Cover, and refrigerate for 45 minutes. Put four wooden skewers in a shallow pan, cover with water, and soak for 10 minutes.

2. Remove the tuna from the marinade and thread it onto the skewers. Put them in a shallow pan and pour the marinade over them. Cover, and refrigerate for 2 to 24 hours.

3. Cook the kabobs on a grill or under an oven broiler, or heat the remaining 2 to 3 tablespoons of canola oil in a skillet and sauté the kabobs over low heat. Cook until done, brushing frequently with the marinade. Serve immediately.

 KITCHEN CAPERS To make any kind of raw fish easier to cut, pop it into the freezer until it's partially frozen.

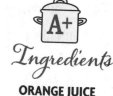
A+

Ingredients

ORANGE JUICE
Fights inflammation

LIME JUICE
Supports digestion

TUNA
Helps maintain heart health

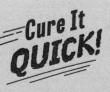 Cure It QUICK!

Trout's about Heart Health

One key to a healthy heart is a diet rich in omega-3 fatty acids. And trout is loaded with those nutrients. Deliver two servings of that firepower fast: Put two trout fillets on a sheet of oiled aluminum foil. Cover the fish with one quartered onion, one thinly sliced green pepper, 2 tablespoons of apple cider, and 1 teaspoon of dried tarragon. Season with garlic salt and black pepper. Seal the foil tightly around the trout. Then wrap the package in another piece of foil. Bake for 30 minutes at 350°F. Then open the wrappings, and dig in!

FISH WITH APPLES

This fish dish is tailor-made for early autumn, when apples are ripening on the trees and cider is rolling out of the presses. Thanks to the load of nutrients in Eve's favorite fruit, you couldn't ask for a healthier way to greet the start of the season.

YIELD: 5–8 servings   **PREP:** 15 minutes   **COOK:** 20 minutes

2 tbsp. of unsalted butter

2 medium onions, finely chopped

4 tart apples, cored and sliced

2 cups of apple cider

2 tsp. of apple cider vinegar

Salt and freshly ground black pepper to taste

6 white fish fillets (about 2 lbs. total)

1. Melt the butter in a large skillet, and sauté the onions until they're just soft but not brown.

2. Add the apples, apple cider, and vinegar. Season with salt and pepper. Cook, stirring, until warmed through (about 1 to 2 minutes).

3. Arrange the fish in a 9- by 13-inch baking dish. Pour the apple mixture on top. Cover, and bake until the fish flakes easily with a fork (12 to 15 minutes, depending on the thickness).

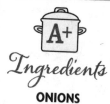

A+ Ingredients

ONIONS
Fight coughs and colds

APPLES
Help ease joint pain

FISH
Boosts immunity

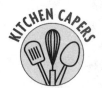

KITCHEN CAPERS
If fish bones drive you nuts, choose saltwater rather than freshwater species. The reason: Fresh water provides less buoyancy than salt water, so fish living in lakes and rivers have hundreds of tiny, filament-thin bones. Their seagoing counterparts have fewer bones that are thicker and therefore easier to dodge.

CULINARY Q & A

? What's the easiest way to scale a fish without making a mess of the kitchen?

! First, drop the fish into boiling water for 15 seconds. Then immediately plunge it into cold water. Wash it well, and put it, still wet, into a large plastic bag. Working inside the bag, scrape the skin with the blade of a knife against the direction of the scales. They'll fly off the fish, but they'll be trapped inside the bag. Finally, wash the fish once more in cold water to remove any remaining scales. That's all there is to it!

CLAMS WITH TOMATOES & ONIONS

Whether you dig your own clams or buy them from a local seafood dealer, you won't find a simpler or tastier way to enjoy them than in this delicious dish!

YIELD: 4 servings	PREP: 15 minutes	COOK: 10 minutes

5 ½ lbs. of clams, scrubbed

½ cup of dry white wine

1 tbsp. + ½ cup of extra virgin olive oil, divided

2 garlic cloves, minced

1 small red onion, finely chopped

2 tbsp. of lemon juice

2 tbsp. of white wine vinegar

5 large tomatoes, coarsely chopped

4 scallions, thinly sliced

2 tbsp. of coarsely chopped fresh cilantro

1. Rinse the clams under cold water. Drain, and cover with the wine in a pan. Cover, and bring to a boil. Reduce the heat, and simmer until the shells open (about 5 minutes). Drain. Discard the liquid, and any clams that didn't open.

2. Heat 1 tablespoon of the olive oil (more as needed) in a large saucepan over medium heat. Cook the garlic and onion until lightly browned. Then add the lemon juice, vinegar, and remaining ½ cup of olive oil. Cook until slightly thickened (about 2 minutes), stirring often. Stir in the tomatoes, scallions, and cilantro.

3. Gently toss the clams with the tomato-onion mixture. Serve immediately.

When buying clams, take them out of the bag as soon as you get home. Put them in a bowl, cover with a wet towel, and refrigerate. If they were fresh to begin with, they should keep for two days.

Ingredients

CLAMS
Help prevent anemia

TOMATOES
Promote brain health

CILANTRO
Helps build strong bones

INSTANT GRATIFICATION

Super-Simple Fish Topper

This wonderful white sauce takes just seconds to whip up, but its elegant appearance and fabulous flavor are worthy of the fanciest dinner party in town. To make it, just mix 2 teaspoons of white wine vinegar per ½ cup of unsweetened heavy (or whipping, not whipped!) cream. Serve it drizzled over baked, grilled, poached, or smoked fish.

FRESH TROUT WITH VINEGAR SAUCE

Attention, all you fly fishermen! This delicious recipe is especially dedicated to you, but you folks who buy your trout at the local fish market will love it, too.

YIELD: 4 servings   **PREP:** 10 minutes   **COOK:** 15 minutes

¼ cup of unbleached all-purpose flour

Salt and freshly ground black pepper to taste

4 rainbow trout with skin, heads removed

4 four-inch sprigs of rosemary

1 tbsp. of lemon zest, minced

3 tbsp. of extra virgin olive oil

2 garlic cloves, minced

¼ cup of rosemary white wine vinegar

¼ cup of dry vermouth

1. Mix the flour, salt, and pepper in a bowl. Lightly dredge the trout in the mixture. Tuck a sprig of rosemary and a pinch of lemon zest into each fish.

2. Warm the oil on medium heat in a nonreactive skillet, and sauté the trout until the fish is golden and flakes (about 5 minutes per side). Remove, and put on plate.

3. Add the garlic and 1 tablespoon of the seasoned flour to the skillet. Cook, stirring constantly, until the garlic and flour are golden. Pour in the vinegar and vermouth, and cook, still stirring, until the mixture is slightly thickened (about 5 minutes). Pour the sauce over the fish, and serve immediately.

A+ *Ingredients*

RAINBOW TROUT
Helps build strong muscles

ROSEMARY
Helps relieve stress

LEMON ZEST
Supports bone health

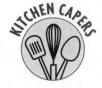

KITCHEN CAPERS

To store whole fish or fillets for up to two days (no longer!), put them in a large strainer, and set it over a bowl. Pile ice on top of the fish to keep the temperature close to 32°F.

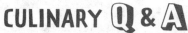

CULINARY Q & A

? Is there an easy way to clean the food grime that builds up in the microwave without using harsh chemical cleaners?

! Just pour 2 cups of water and ½ cup of vinegar into a microwave-safe bowl, and put it inside. Cook it on high for three to four minutes, or until the water starts to boil. Let it sit for another four minutes, with the door closed, so the steam can loosen the gunk. Remove the bowl, and wipe the interior clean with a damp sponge.

REAL-DEAL CRAB CAKES

The crab cakes most often served in restaurants contain more bread- or cracker-crumb filling than sweet, nutrient-rich crabmeat. This recipe is a delightful exception.

YIELD: 4 servings	**PREP:** 15 minutes	**COOK:** 20–25 minutes

1 lb. of cooked lump crabmeat

2 tbsp. of mayonnaise

1 egg, beaten

1 tbsp. of lemon vinegar

1 tsp. of seafood seasoning

1 tsp. of sharp prepared mustard

Dash of Worcestershire sauce

Hot-pepper sauce to taste

Salt and black pepper to taste

¼ cup of cracker crumbs

Canola oil

1. Put the crabmeat in a bowl, and sift through it with your fingers to remove any shell fragments. In another bowl, mix the next eight ingredients.

2. Slowly add the mayo mixture to the crabmeat, tossing it lightly with your hands until the crabmeat is coated (you may not need all the dressing). Add the cracker crumbs a little at a time (use just enough crumbs to bind the lumps together).

3. Gently divide the mixture into four loosely formed balls. Arrange them 2 inches apart in a lightly oiled 8-inch-square baking dish. Bake at 400°F until the crab cakes are delicately browned on top (about 20 to 25 minutes).

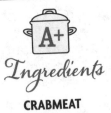

Ingredients

CRABMEAT
Fights inflammation

MAYONNAISE
Enhances digestion

MUSTARD
Aids weight loss

KITCHEN CAPERS

Refrigerating crab cakes, covered, for about an hour before baking will help them hold together better in the oven—and it won't affect the flavor in any way.

Cure It QUICK!

DOUSE THE FLAMES Cold-water fish like salmon and trout are renowned for their ability to help prevent heart disease, but they also have anti-inflammatory powers that can ease joint discomfort, digestive disorders, and acute traumas caused by injuries. This ultra-easy recipe works equally well with 1 ¼ pounds of either salmon or steelhead trout. To make four servings, lay the fish, skin side down, in a lightly oiled baking dish. Then pour in 2 tablespoons each of orange juice and soy sauce, 1 tablespoon of rice wine vinegar, and 1 teaspoon of sesame oil. Bake, covered, at 450°F until the thickest part of the fish is flaky (about 15 minutes).

GRILLED SALMON WITH NASTURTIUM VINAIGRETTE

If you're looking for a colorful—and flavorful—change of pace for your next backyard barbecue, reach for this recipe. The mild, peppery bite of nasturtiums blends with the sweetness of the honey and the rich flavor of the salmon to produce a tasty treat that'll become your new favorite go-to recipe.

YIELD: 4 servings   **PREP:** 15 minutes   **COOK:** 6–12 minutes

¼ cup of minced shallots

¼ cup of sherry vinegar

1 tbsp. of raw honey

½ cup + 2 tbsp. of extra virgin olive oil, divided

Salt and freshly ground black pepper to taste

½ cup of finely chopped fresh nasturtiums

1 tbsp. of chopped fresh chives

1 tbsp. of minced fresh tarragon

4 (5 oz. each) boneless salmon fillets with skin

6 cups of mixed baby greens

Whole nasturtiums for garnish

1. Blend the shallots, vinegar, and honey in a blender or food processor. With the motor still running, slowly add ½ cup of olive oil, and process until emulsified. Add salt and pepper, and pour into a glass jar. Stir in the nasturtiums, chives, and tarragon, and shake to mix thoroughly. Cover and refrigerate until serving.

2. Lightly brush the salmon with the remaining olive oil. Arrange the fillets on a grill rack, and grill, covered, on medium gas heat or medium coals until just barely cooked through (4 to 6 minutes per ½ inch of thickness, or until the fish begins to flake when tested with a fork). Turn once halfway through grilling time.

3. Toss half of the vinaigrette with the greens, and mound on individual plates. Set a salmon fillet on each one, drizzle with the remaining vinaigrette, and garnish with whole nasturtiums. Serve immediately.

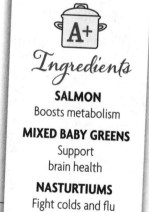

A+ Ingredients

SALMON
Boosts metabolism

MIXED BABY GREENS
Support brain health

NASTURTIUMS
Fight colds and flu

KITCHEN CAPERS

In addition to the fork test, you can check salmon for doneness using an instant-read thermometer inserted horizontally into the fish. It works especially well for thick steaks. The fish is done when the internal temperature reaches 140°F.

TUNA WITH OLIVES

In the hot climate of southern Spain, where this recipe hails from, folks prefer their food on the light side. Cooks in this region are especially noted for their way with fried fish.

YIELD: 4 servings	PREP: 15 minutes	COOK: 10 minutes

4 tuna steaks

¾ cup of dry white wine

2 garlic cloves, crushed

1 tsp. of white wine vinegar

1 bay leaf

1 sprig of fresh thyme

⅔ cup of extra virgin olive oil, plus more for cooking

1 cup of all-purpose flour

⅔ cup of chopped green olives

Salt and ground black pepper to taste

1. Arrange the tuna steaks in a shallow dish. Mix the next five ingredients in a bowl. Then slowly whisk in the olive oil and pour over the fish. Cover, and refrigerate overnight.

2. Put the flour into a shallow bowl. Remove the fish from the marinade and pat dry. Dip both sides of each steak into the flour, shake off the excess, and set aside on a plate.

3. Heat about 1 inch of olive oil in a deep pan. Fry the steaks until golden on both sides (4 to 6 minutes). Remove, and keep warm. Add the marinade to the pan, and boil until the liquid has reduced slightly. Strain it through a sieve into a bowl, and stir in the olives. Season with salt and pepper, pour the blend over the fish, and serve.

KITCHEN CAPERS

When a recipe calls for wine and you have none on hand, just substitute a mixture of 2 teaspoons of vinegar per 1 cup of grape or apple juice. Or use a blend of 1 part wine vinegar to 3 parts water.

A+

Ingredients

TUNA
Supports weight loss

WHITE WINE
Boosts immunity

GREEN OLIVES
Fight free radicals

Cure It QUICK!

GIVE YOUR LIBIDO A LIFT Medical pros tell us that an active sex life is one of the major secrets to health, happiness, and longevity. And one of the best aphrodisiacs of all is oysters. For a tasty way to enjoy them, arrange 24 oysters on top of a layer of coarse salt on a serving platter (so the oysters don't slide around). Then mix 4 tablespoons of dry white wine, 4 tablespoons of white wine vinegar, 2 tablespoons of pastis, and 1 minced shallot. Add a spoonful to each oyster, eat up, and enjoy the evening's entertainment!

POACHED FISH WITH BEAN SAUCE

This recipe contains fiber-rich chickpea dip mix (a.k.a. instant hummus), one of the handiest ingredients you can have. It's the perfect complement to lean, firm white fish.

YIELD: 4 servings   **PREP:** 10 minutes   **COOK:** 12 minutes

2 cups of water

1 bunch of scallions, thinly sliced

3 tbsp. of soy sauce

2 tbsp. of grated fresh ginger

1 tbsp. of rice vinegar

2 lbs. of white fish fillets*

⅓ cup of chickpea dip mix

1 large tomato, chopped

* Catfish, cod, halibut, and swordfish are good choices.

1. Combine the water, scallions, soy sauce, ginger, and vinegar in a large skillet. Boil for 1 minute.

2. Add the fish, and cook over very low heat until it is opaque (about 10 minutes). Set aside on a warm platter.

3. Bring the liquid back to a boil, add the dip mix, and stir until lightly thickened (about 1 minute). Add the tomato and heat through. Spoon the sauce over the fish and serve.

A+ Ingredients

SCALLIONS
Promote weight loss

GINGER
Helps relieve heartburn

FISH
Supports healthy vision

KITCHEN CAPERS Bowls of white vinegar neutralize odors from fish and other aromatic foods, but here's a neater idea: Fill a small spray bottle with water and 2 tablespoons of white vinegar, and keep it on a kitchen counter. Whenever the need arises, simply shoot a few puffs into the air.

CULINARY Q & A

? I'd like to start buying meat and fish in bulk because it's so much cheaper. What's the most efficient way to freeze it?

! First, put portions of the meat or fish into ziplock plastic bags, and use a permanent marker to write the date on each one. Then put these little sacks into a large freezer bag or a rigid plastic container, and label it with the contents. Then, whenever the time arises, take out the small bags you need and leave the rest in the freezer. With this double protection, your meat will fend off freezer burn much longer.

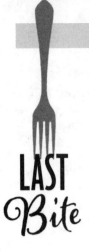

LAST *Bite*

PUT OUT THE FIRE

When a cooking fire erupts, your best plan of action depends on the location:

Oven. At the first sign of flames, turn off the oven and kill the juice to the circuit. Keep the oven door closed, and the fire will die from lack of oxygen.

Burning pan. Never try to carry a burning pan to the sink! Instead, turn off the range and exhaust fan, and slide a baking sheet over the flames. Leave it on until everything is completely cooled. If the burner or the oil in the pan is still hot, lifting the lid could supply enough oxygen to restart the fire.

Stove top. When oil or grease ignites, smother the flames with a thick layer of baking soda or salt. Do not douse any cooking fire with water or flour!

MEATY MATTERS

The acetic acid in vinegar can solve a trio of common carnivore conundrums:

Tough meat. Lean meat can be easier on your budget and your waistline, but it can also be chewy. Soak your meat in vinegar overnight before you cook it. You can rinse off the vinegar before cooking if you'd like, but it's not necessary. Either way, that meat will melt in your mouth!

Gamey game. Even folks who love venison, rabbit, and other wild game admit that the flavor can take some getting used to. If you're not fond of that distinctive bite, take the edge off by soaking the meat in a half-and-half mixture of vinegar and water for at least an hour before you cook it.

Overly salty ham. Add 2 tablespoons of white or apple cider vinegar to the water that you boil the ham in. It'll draw out some of the salty taste and perk up the flavor to boot!

Never station a fire extinguisher near a potential fire source. Avoid keeping it near your stove, clothes dryer, or any storage area that contains solvents and other flammable substances. Instead, hang the extinguisher by the door, so you can grab it quickly without getting close to the flames. Also, make sure that nothing blocks access to the extinguisher and everyone in your household can reach it easily.

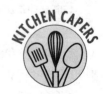

KITCHEN CAPERS

SOMETHING'S FISHY

Are you a seafood aficionado? If so, then make sure you keep plenty of vinegar on hand, and put it to work in these ways:

- To make scaling easier, rub white vinegar on the fish and let it sit for five minutes. The scales will practically fly off!

- When salmon, lobster, oysters, or clams are on the menu, soak them in vinegar for at least several hours (or even overnight). The acidic bath will tenderize the tough muscle fiber.

- For firmer, whiter fish fillets, soak them for about 20 minutes in a solution of 2 tablespoons of white vinegar per quart of water.

- Bring out the flavor of any kind of seafood by dousing it with a tablespoon or so of white wine or sherry vinegar while it's poaching or frying.

- After deep-frying fish, lightly spray each still-hot piece with apple cider vinegar. It'll moderate the fishy odor and also impart a slightly tangy taste that everyone will enjoy.

- Give canned fish or seafood a fresher taste by soaking it for 10 to 15 minutes in 2 tablespoons of white vinegar and 1 teaspoon of sherry, or 2 tablespoons of sherry vinegar—whichever you have on hand.

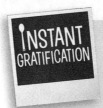

INSTANT GRATIFICATION

Infused Olive Oil

Just like infused vinegars, flavored olive oils are showing up at more and more specialty food stores, and online retailers, with flavors ranging from citrus fruits to truffles, hot peppers to mesquite and more. They can cost a small fortune to purchase, but it's easy to make your own. For starters, give this versatile blend a try: Put three peeled, sliced garlic cloves; one peeled, quartered onion; and ½ cup of high-quality extra virgin olive oil in a small pan over low heat. Heat just until the garlic starts to simmer, and then remove the pan from the burner. Let it cool for 10 minutes, then remove and discard the solids. Pour the oil into a sterilized, airtight glass container, and store it in the refrigerator for up to four days (no longer).

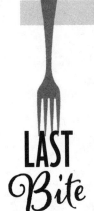

LAST Bite

FRY WITH CARE

Frying meat, fish—or anything else—on your stove top can lead to disaster in the blink of an eye. So always follow these six simple safety guidelines:

1. Always add oil to an unheated pan—and make sure it's dry and positioned away from any water source.

2. Never let water come into contact with hot oil. The water will vaporize into steam, which can make the oil splatter and cause serious burns.

3. Never leave a pan unattended when it's in use.

4. Make sure any pan is completely cool before you clean it.

5. Wait until all cooking oil is at room temperature before disposing of it. Then pour it into a sealable container, and toss it in the trash. Never pour oil or grease down the drain or into a compost bin.

6. Keep a kitchen fire extinguisher nearby (see the Kitchen Capers box on page 260) and learn how to use it effectively.

CULINARY Q & A

? I've heard that smoke from a charcoal barbecue can cause cancer. Is cooking meat on a charcoal grill really as dangerous as a lot of folks make it out to be?

! According to a great many medical experts, including those at the American Institute for Cancer Research, the answer is probably not. Having said that, it is true that cooking meat at overly high temperatures, or charring it over direct flames, causes the formation of two problematic substances, heterocyclic amines (HCAs) and polycyclic aromatic hydrocarbons (PAHs). Both have been linked to cancer in laboratory animals, but the jury is still out on the risk they pose for humans. Nutritional and health pros are unanimous in warning that consuming large quantities of red meat, no matter how it's cooked, is bad for you. But the consensus is that enjoying grilled foods in moderation is just fine.

HOW HOT ARE THE COALS?

A glance at the numbers will tell you the temperature of your oven and many gas grills. But when barbecuing, gauging the heat of charcoal briquettes is a more physical matter altogether. In this case, you can determine the approximate heat of the coals by the length of time you can hold your hand above the grill grate.

How Long You Can Stand the Heat	Heat Level	Temperature Range in °F
1–2 seconds	Hot	400°–500°
3–4 seconds	Medium	350°–375°
5–7 seconds	Medium-low	325°–350°

4 GREAT GUIDELINES FOR SAFER GRILLING

While the majority of health pros give two thumbs up to backyard barbecues, they also offer these four simple pointers for making your festivities safer and healthier for yourself and all others concerned:

1. Trim away excess fat to prevent it from dripping into and flaring up the flames, which can then cause the meat you're cooking to burn.

2. Brush coals to the sides, and grill your meat above the center of the barbecue. This will again reduce flame flare-ups. If necessary, use a drip pan, or cover the grill with punctured aluminum foil to avoid the problem entirely.

3. If you are using a gas grill, set the temperature at medium-high, and flip the meat frequently as it cooks to prevent charring.

4. Marinate your meat for at least 60 minutes in a vinegar- or lemon-based marinade that includes herbs like basil, mint, rosemary, sage, savory, marjoram, oregano, and thyme. These potent antioxidants will reduce HCA and PAH production by 99 to 100 percent. Chapter Two is chock-full of marinade recipes that will perform that prodigious feat (see page 30).

Chapter Eight

Pleasing Party Food

The vinegar-enhanced recipes in this chapter provide proof that appetizers and party food can be as healthy as they are festive. But you don't need to have a party—or even casual guests—as an excuse to serve the dips, spreads, and finger foods coming up. They're just as delicious, if not more so, when you enjoy them all by yourself, accompanied by a good book or your favorite movie.

TEXAS CAVIAR

No party in the Lone Star State would be complete without this kissin' cousin to bean salsa! But it doesn't just taste terrific. Thanks to the Texas-size load of fiber in black-eyed peas, it'll help ease any digestive woes you might have.

YIELD: about 3 cups	PREP: 20 minutes	CHILL: 2–48 hours

2 cans of black-eyed peas (15-oz. each), drained and rinsed

2 medium ripe tomatoes, chopped

1 small red bell pepper, finely chopped

1 or 2 jalapeño peppers, finely chopped

¼ red onion, finely chopped

¼ cup of fresh parsley, coarsely chopped

¼ cup of red wine vinegar

2 tbsp. of extra virgin olive oil

3 garlic cloves, minced

Salt and pepper to taste

1. Put all of the ingredients, except the salt and pepper, in a nonreactive bowl, and stir to combine thoroughly. Season with salt and pepper.

2. Cover with plastic wrap, and refrigerate for at least 2 hours and up to 48 hours.

3. Serve at room temperature with corn tortilla chips. For a festive presentation—and an added nutrient boost—use a combo of blue, red, and yellow corn chips.

 KITCHEN CAPERS

Mineral deposits and soap residue can badly damage your dishwasher. So twice a year, stand 1 cup of vinegar in the upper rack and lower rack, along with a load of dishes. The vinegar will be dispersed throughout the inner workings, removing the potential troublemakers.

 A+ Ingredients

BLACK-EYED PEAS
Help support your digestive system

TOMATOES
Promote cardiovascular health

ONION
Fights coughs and colds

 INSTANT GRATIFICATION

Easy Pleasin' Apricot Dip
Looking for a healthy and out-of-the-ordinary dip to serve with chicken wings or chicken strips? Look no further! Just mix 1 cup of apricot preserves, 2 tablespoons of balsamic vinegar, and 1 tablespoon of soy sauce in a glass bowl. You won't believe that anything so delicious could be so easy to make!

WONDERFUL WALNUT DIP

Do yourself a favor and tuck this simple, versatile, and highly healthy dip into your entertaining arsenal. You'll love the rich flavor—and so will your guests!

YIELD: 6–8 servings | **PREP:** 20 minutes

1 ½ cups of walnut pieces

1 tbsp. of extra virgin olive oil

1 tbsp. of sherry vinegar

Juice of 1 small lemon

1 tsp. of Dijon mustard

Salt and white pepper to taste

4–5 tbsp. of water

2 tbsp. of fresh chives, chopped

Toasted walnut pieces and chopped fresh chives for garnish

1. Preheat the oven to 350°F. Spread the walnuts in a single layer on a baking sheet, and bake, stirring twice, until lightly browned (10 to 12 minutes).

2. Put the nuts, olive oil, vinegar, lemon juice, mustard, salt, pepper, and 3 tablespoons of water in a food processor, and process until smooth. Add more water if necessary to get the desired consistency.

3. Stir in the chives, pour the dip into a bowl, and garnish with walnut pieces and chives. Serve with raw vegetables, apple slices, or your favorite crackers.

KITCHEN CAPERS Because of their fat content, nuts are at high risk for going rancid. Always buy them in small quantities. Also, choose nuts that are still in their shells. As a general rule (depending on how fresh they are when you get them), they'll keep twice as long as shelled versions.

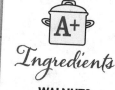

A+ Ingredients

WALNUTS
Help alleviate symptoms of SAD

OLIVE OIL
Promotes heart health

CHIVES
Support healthy bones

CULINARY Q & A

? Aren't nuts terribly fattening and bad for you?

! Absolutely not! Research has shown that nuts (including peanuts) contain vitamins, minerals, and plant compounds that help lower cholesterol, ward off cardiovascular disease, improve brain function, fight fatigue, and do much more. Furthermore, while it is true that nuts are high in fat, much of it is monounsaturated (a.k.a. good) fat that fills you up without filling you out. Studies show that folks who eat a handful of nuts each day are much less likely to be severely overweight than those who don't.

AVOCADO-CUCUMBER SALSA

Avocados exceed every other fruit in two plant compounds, beta-sitosterol and glutathione, that may help prevent heart disease and free radical damage. If you still think that salsa has to contain tomatoes, try this refreshing alternative.

YIELD: about 2 cups   **PREP:** 15 minutes

1 ripe avocado, peeled and diced

1 small cucumber, peeled and diced

1 chili pepper, minced (optional)

¼ cup of minced red onions

2 tbsp. of minced cilantro

2 tbsp. of lemon vinegar

1 tbsp. of freshly squeezed lime juice

Salt to taste

1. Put the avocado, cucumber, chili pepper (if desired), onions, and cilantro in a bowl. Add the vinegar and lime juice, and toss to coat the solid ingredients thoroughly. Add salt, and toss again.

2. If you prefer, pour the mixture into a food processor and pulse to get a guacamole-like consistency.

3. Serve immediately with crunchy tortilla chips (it's especially good with the blue corn variety), or refrigerate until ready to use. The salsa will stay fresh for up to 2 days, and thanks to the vinegar and lime juice, it should retain its full color.

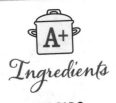

A+

Ingredients

AVOCADO
Supports heart health

CUCUMBER
Boosts hydration

CILANTRO
Helps calm anxiety

When you cut your finger, forget the first-aid kit! Just grab a small slice of avocado, and apply it to the wound. The fruit has antibiotic properties that will get right to work healing your skin, while the mellow pulp helps to ease your pain.

KITCHEN CAPERS

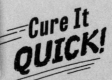

Cure It QUICK!

POUND-SHEDDING PEACH SALSA You can't ask for a healthier or tastier weight-loss aid than this sweet-and-tangy blend. Peaches not only make you feel full, but they're also rich in antioxidants called phenols that fight obesity-related and cardiovascular disease. Just mix 1½ cups of peeled, pitted, and diced peaches in a bowl with a small minced shallot, 1 tablespoon of balsamic vinegar, 2 teaspoons of lime zest, and 1 teaspoon each of minced jalapeño pepper and chopped fresh cilantro. Use it as a dip, or on grilled fish or chicken.

HAVE A BALL CHEESE BALL

Culinary warning: This cheese ball has been proven to disappear in a flash at any party. Plus, the ingredients are not just tasty—they're also chock-full of essential nutrients.

YIELD: 16 servings	**PREP:** 15 minutes	**CHILL:** 3–4 hours

8 oz. of grated Swiss cheese*

3 oz. of cream cheese, cubed and softened

½ cup of grated apple

3 tbsp. of apple cider vinegar, plus more as needed

3 tbsp. of minced fresh sage

½ cup of finely chopped pecans or walnuts

* *For more intense flavor, use Emmentaler or Gruyère.*

1. Combine the cheeses, apple, vinegar, and sage in a food processor, and blend until smooth.

2. Form the mix into a ball, adding more vinegar if it seems too dry, and roll it in the finely chopped nuts until thoroughly coated.

3. Cover and refrigerate for 3 to 4 hours. Serve paired with crackers, melba toast, or apple slices.

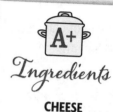

A+

Ingredients

CHEESE
Promotes strong bones

APPLE
Prevents colds and flu

PECANS
Help you lose weight

KITCHEN CAPERS

After you've used a food processor to mix sticky ingredients like cheeses, or even vegetable purees, the blade is left with a lot of good food on it. To prevent waste and save cleanup time, use this trick: Remove the contents from the processor bowl, put the blade section back in place, and pulse the power button for several seconds. The blade residue will fly onto the sides of the bowl. Use a rubber spatula to scrape the ingredients into your mixing bowl.

CULINARY Q & A

? Is it true that processed cheese is not as good for you as unprocessed types?

! Yes! Not only do these pseudo-cheeses lack the distinctive flavor and texture of the "real deal," they're also filled with things that won't benefit your health. They're pasteurized to extend their storage time, then mixed with emulsifiers to make them smoother, and finally "spiked" with preservatives and artificial colorings. In fact, according to USDA standards, only 51 percent of a processed cheese's final weight has to consist of cheese.

CHARRED CORN SALSA

This flavorful, easy-to-make salsa packs a medium heat level. To ramp it up or cool it down, simply use a hotter or milder pepper than the jalapeño called for below.

YIELD: 2 cups	PREP: 30 minutes	WAIT: 1 hour

2 ears of fresh-picked corn

4 tbsp. of extra virgin olive oil, divided

1 cup of chopped cherry tomatoes

¼ cup of coarsely chopped fresh cilantro

¼ cup of finely chopped red onions

1 garlic clove, chopped

1 small jalapeño pepper, finely chopped

½ tsp. of dried cumin

¼ tsp. of salt

1 tbsp. of freshly squeezed lime juice

1 tbsp. of white wine vinegar

1. Rub the corn with 2 tablespoons of the olive oil. Roast at 425°F, until the kernels are lightly browned on the outside and tender on the inside (about 20 minutes). Turn occasionally so they brown evenly on all sides.

2. Remove the corn from the oven. When it's cool enough to handle comfortably, cut the kernels from the cobs, and set them aside to cool completely.

3. In a bowl, combine the remaining ingredients, the corn, and the remaining olive oil. Mix thoroughly. Cover and set aside at room temperature for 1 hour to let the flavors blend. Serve with your favorite corn chips.

 KITCHEN CAPERS

Here are three simple secrets to cooking tender corn on the cob: Never boil it in salted water, which makes it tough. Keep the time between 3 and 10 minutes, depending on the size and age of the ears. Finally, add a little milk and sugar to the cooking water.

A+
Ingredients

CORN
Helps maintain vision

CHERRY TOMATOES
Support healthy bones

CILANTRO
Promotes cardiovascular health

INSTANT GRATIFICATION

Delightful DIY Chili Seasoning Mix

While this blend is ideal for any kind of chili, it also gives a delightful kick to taco meat, grilled burgers, or meatloaf. To make about ¾ cup, combine ¼ cup each of chili powder and paprika, 2 tablespoons of dried minced onion, 4 teaspoons of dried cumin, 2 teaspoons each of dried oregano and salt, and 1 teaspoon of garlic powder. Seal and store away from light and heat.

FOODS FOR THE LONG HAUL

Most food and drink go bad eventually. They either become unsafe to eat or simply lose their original flavor and nutrient punch. These long keepers are exceptions to that rule. As long as they're stored properly, they'll last indefinitely, even after they've been opened.

Food with Staying Power	How to Keep It Fresh
Cornstarch	Store in a cool, dry place, ideally in an airtight container.
Distilled liquor	Store in a cool, dark place; keep tightly closed between uses.
Distilled white vinegar	Store in a cool, dark place, and cap the bottle tightly after each use.
Honey	Store tightly closed in a cool area; if it crystallizes, set the opened jar in warm water and stir until the honey is smooth again.
Pure maple syrup	Refrigerate after opening; for long-term storage, freeze in airtight containers.
Pure vanilla extract	Store in a cool, dark place, and cap the bottle tightly after each use.
Brown rice	Store at room temperature; it will stay fresh for 3 to 6 months, 12 to 18 months in the freezer.
All other rice	Store in a cool, dry area; once opened, transfer to a sealed, airtight container, ideally in the refrigerator or freezer.
Salt	Store in a cool, dry place.
Sugar	Store in a cool, dry place; to prevent hardening, transfer to an airtight container.

CULINARY Q & A

? What's the secret to getting really good corn at the supermarket?

! If you don't care to grow your own crop, buy your supply from a reputable produce market that does a brisk business, so you'll be getting the freshest corn possible. Look for ears with bright green, tight-fitting husks and silk that's dry (not soggy!) and pale gold to golden brown in color. Never buy corn that's been husked. Without that protective covering, the sugar flies out of the kernels even faster than usual.

BEET, CHICKPEA, & ALMOND DIP

Greek cuisine is renowned for its appetizer dips, and this one is a classic. It also happens to be a delectable and nutritious addition to any menu, whether you serve it as a prelude to a backyard barbecue or as part of a cocktail-party buffet.

YIELD: about 2 cups   **PREP:** 20 minutes   **COOK:** 25 minutes

1 large (8 oz.) beet, peeled and cut into ¾-inch cubes

½ tsp. of salt

1 cup of canned chickpeas

¾ cup of extra virgin olive oil, plus more for brushing

¼ cup of slivered almonds

5 garlic cloves, peeled

1 ½ tbsp. of red wine vinegar

Salt and black pepper to taste

6 seven-inch-diameter pita bread slices

1. Cook the beet cubes in a pan of boiling salted water until tender (about 12 minutes). Drain and chop.

2. Combine the beets, chickpeas, olive oil, almonds, and garlic in a food processor. Blend until smooth. Add the vinegar, and blend again. Taste, and mix in salt, pepper, and additional vinegar if desired. Transfer the mix to a bowl.

3. Brush the pita bread on both sides with olive oil, and sprinkle with salt and pepper. Cut slices into 8 wedges and arrange on rimmed baking sheets. Bake at 400°F until lightly brown and crisp (about 12 minutes). Let cool to room temperature.

4. Put the dip in the center of a platter, surround with pita chips, and serve.

 KITCHEN CAPERS Make a simple, nutritious dip by blending whipped cream cheese or mayo with the fortified vinegar of your choice. Find delicious DIY vinegar recipes in Chapter One.

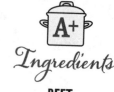 A+ *Ingredients*

BEET
Boosts heart health

CHICKPEAS
Help control blood sugar levels

ALMONDS
Support weight loss

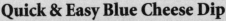

INSTANT GRATIFICATION

Quick & Easy Blue Cheese Dip
This recipe is tailor-made for busy days. Grab a bowl and mix together ¾ cup of mayonnaise, 4 ounces of crumbled blue cheese, ¼ cup of sour cream, 1 tablespoon each of red wine vinegar and lemon juice, and ½ teaspoon of garlic powder. Season to taste with salt and pepper, cover the bowl, and stash it in the refrigerator. Let it chill for at least two hours. It makes 10 servings and goes well with crackers, chips, apple slices, or raw vegetables.

TANGY TROPICAL FRUIT SALSA

You'd be hard-pressed to find a salsa that's as packed full of health power as this refreshing blend. In the summer, you may want to depart from the "tropical" moniker and substitute fresh, ripe nectarines and peaches for the mango and papaya.

YIELD: 3 cups	PREP: 15 minutes	CHILL: 1–48 hours

1 cup of diced mango
(¼-inch cubes)

1 cup of diced papaya
(¼-inch cubes)

1 cup of diced pineapple
(¼-inch cubes)

½ cup of Marvelous Mango
Vinegar (see page 20)

1 tbsp. of diced chili peppers

1 tbsp. of finely chopped
fresh cilantro

1 tbsp. of minced red onions

1 tbsp. of toasted pine nuts*

½ tsp. of grated fresh ginger

*See toasting guidelines
on page 57.*

1. Mix the fruits, vinegar, chili peppers, cilantro, onions, pine nuts, and ginger in a nonreactive bowl.

2. Cover, and refrigerate for at least 1 hour before serving. Use it as a dipping sauce for shrimp cocktail or chicken strips, or serve it as a topping for grilled chicken or fish. Tightly covered, it will keep for about 48 hours before the fruits' texture deteriorates.

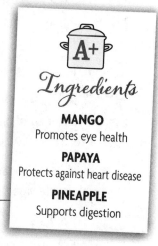

Ingredients

MANGO
Promotes eye health

PAPAYA
Protects against heart disease

PINEAPPLE
Supports digestion

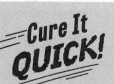

KITCHEN CAPERS If you use papaya in a recipe, don't toss the seeds! They have a peppery-mustardy flavor that make 'em great in marinades and salad dressings (just whirl a few teaspoons of seeds in a blender with the other ingredients). They also enhance the digestion of meat and high-protein foods.

Cure It QUICK! **PEEPER-PLEASING PEPPER SPREAD** Red peppers are rich in nutrients that support healthy eyesight—especially night vision—and also help protect against both macular degeneration and cataracts. To make this delicious defensive weapon, drain two jars of roasted red peppers and chop them coarsely. Put the chunks in a food processor with 1½ cups of extra virgin olive oil, 8 ounces of crumbled feta cheese, 1½ teaspoons of chopped fresh thyme leaves, and 2 peeled garlic cloves. Add salt and freshly ground black pepper to taste, and pulse until smooth. Serve as a spread for crackers or bread, or use it atop pasta or potatoes.

VANISHING BLUE CHEESE SPREAD

Why "vanishing"? Because when you serve this delectable spread at a party, it disappears before your very eyes! Also worth mentioning is that one of the key ingredients in this recipe, parsley, contains more protein than any other member of the vegetable kingdom.

YIELD: about 2 ½ cups	PREP: 15 minutes

¼ cup of shelled walnuts

2 tbsp. of chopped chives

2 tbsp. of chopped fresh parsley

½ cup of blue cheese, crumbled

1 package (8 oz.) of cream cheese, cold

2 tsp. of white balsamic or white wine vinegar

1. Finely chop the walnuts, chives, and parsley in a food processor, and pour the mixture into a small bowl. Stir in the blue cheese, and set aside.

2. Place the cream cheese and vinegar into the bowl of the food processor, and puree until smooth. Add the nut-herb mixture, and process until well blended.

3. Serve the spread in a bowl, surrounded by crackers, toast rounds, or raw vegetables. Or use it as a topping for finger-size ham, roast beef, or chicken sandwiches.

KITCHEN CAPERS

If you enjoy using cottage cheese in dips, or even on its own, this tip is for you: You can keep it fresher longer by stirring a teaspoon of vinegar into the container. Any kind will do. The acetic acid in the vinegar will prolong the life of the cheese without altering the flavor one iota.

A+

Ingredients

WALNUTS
Support healthy weight

PARSLEY
Promotes strong bones

BLUE CHEESE
Boosts nervous system function

INSTANT GRATIFICATION

Quick Italian Bread Dip

When you have the gang over for a hearty Italian dinner—or you simply want a luscious, healthy snack—mix up this traditional dipping oil. Simply whisk 2 tablespoons of balsamic vinegar, 2 tablespoons of shredded Parmesan cheese, and a dash of salt in a bowl. Then slowly whisk in ½ cup of extra virgin olive oil. That's all there is to it. Serve it with a loaf of crusty, rustic Italian bread, and enjoy!

CHEESY CUCUMBER DIP

When summer barbecue season rolls around, this simple, cooling dip can be one of your best assets. It goes together in a flash, it's filled with healthy ingredients, and it tastes great with everything from potato chips to fresh vegetables.

YIELD: 2 cups	**PREP:** 10 minutes	**CHILL:** 3–4 hours

1 medium cucumber, peeled, seeded, and diced

2 tbsp. of minced fresh dill

2 tbsp. of minced fresh salad burnet*

2 tbsp. of dill or salad burnet white wine vinegar

1 garlic clove, minced

Salt and black pepper to taste

1 cup of ricotta cheese

½ cup of plain yogurt

* Use young leaves; old ones tend to have a bitter flavor.

1. In a nonreactive bowl, combine the cucumber, dill, salad burnet, vinegar, and garlic. Season with salt and pepper.

2. Stir in the ricotta cheese and yogurt. Add vinegar as needed to achieve the desired consistency. Cover, and refrigerate for at least 3 to 4 hours.

3. Let the dip come to room temperature before serving with chips, crackers, or veggies.

A+ Ingredients

CUCUMBER
Promotes healthy skin

DILL
Supports digestion

YOGURT
Fends off colds and allergies

KITCHEN CAPERS To make fast, easy work of removing cucumber seeds, first cut the cuke in half widthwise. Push an apple corer down through the center of each half. Then either dice or slice the seed-free tubes, as needed.

CULINARY Q & A

? I've been hearing a lot about the health benefits of an herb called salad burnet. My grandmother used to grow a plant by that name. Is this the same plant?

! Indeed it is! Salad burnet is an old-time herb that's staging a big-time comeback in nutritional circles, and for good reason: The whole plant is rich in bioflavonoids, along with iron; potassium; and vitamins A, B, and C. Plus, the leaves have a refreshing, cucumber-like taste that makes them perfect for salads or sandwiches. Salad burnet also makes a flavorful and versatile infused vinegar.

RASPBERRY–POPPY SEED DIP

This dip is festive-looking enough to dress up any occasion—and you can make it up to three days ahead of time without sacrificing one iota of flavor, appearance, or nutrition.

YIELD: 1 ½ cups	PREP: 15 minutes	CHILL: 1 hour–3 days

½ pint of fresh raspberries

¼ cup of freshly squeezed orange juice

¼ cup of raspberry vinegar

1 tsp. of dry mustard

1 tsp. of sugar

Salt and pepper to taste

¾ cup of vegetable oil

2 tbsp. of poppy seeds

1. Puree the raspberries, orange juice, vinegar, mustard, and sugar in a food processor. Taste, and add salt and pepper as desired. With the motor running, slowly pour in the oil.

2. Strain through a fine sieve into a bowl (to remove the berry seeds). Stir in the poppy seeds. Cover, and refrigerate for at least 1 hour or up to 3 days.

3. Whirl the mixture briefly in the food processor, or whisk by hand to recombine. Serve chilled or at room temp with fruits, vegetables, or crackers.

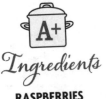

A+

Ingredients

RASPBERRIES
Support brain function

VINEGAR
Aids weight loss

POPPY SEEDS
Promote skin health

If you can't use raspberries right away, don't wash them before you refrigerate. If they are damp, they'll mold quickly. If kept dry in a lidded container, they'll keep for three days in the fridge or 12 months in the freezer. Just before you use the berries, rinse them gently with clear, cool water and pat them dry.

KITCHEN CAPERS

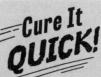

Cure It QUICK!

BERRY FINE STRAWBERRY-TOMATO SALSA When it comes to helping fight or prevent illnesses of all kinds, strawberries and tomatoes are a genuine dream team. Get the dynamic duo playing on your side with this super-easy salsa. To make 24 servings, quarter 2 pints of cherry tomatoes, and chop 1 pint of fresh strawberries. Combine them in a large bowl with 8 chopped scallions (white and green parts) and ½ cup of minced fresh cilantro. Whisk 2 tablespoons of balsamic vinegar into 6 tablespoons of extra virgin olive oil. Season with salt to taste, and gently stir the dressing into the tomato-berry mixture. Cover, and chill until serving time. Then set it out with a big bowl of tortilla chips, and watch it disappear!

SWEET & SPICY RED PEPPER DIP

If you or your guests are watching your weight, this recipe has your name written all over it. It's packed with flavor (and nutrients) but is also very low in calories.

YIELD: 2 cups   **PREP:** 15 minutes   **CHILL:** 1 hour–2 days

2 tbsp. of extra virgin olive oil

1 jalapeño pepper, seeded and minced

1 large onion, chopped

4 garlic cloves, minced

6 red bell peppers, roasted, peeled, and seeded

1 tbsp. of balsamic vinegar

1 tbsp. of red wine vinegar

1 tbsp. of light brown sugar

1 tsp. of ground cumin

Salt to taste

1. Heat the olive oil in a large skillet over medium heat. Add the jalapeño pepper and onion, and sauté until the onion has browned. At the 5-minute mark, stir in the garlic. Remove from the heat, and let cool slightly.

2. Combine the jalapeño-onion mix in a food processor with the red peppers, balsamic and red wine vinegars, brown sugar, and cumin until smooth. Taste, and add salt as desired.

3. Pour the puree into a bowl, and let cool completely. Cover tightly, and refrigerate for at least 1 hour or up to 2 days.

A+ Ingredients

JALAPEÑO PEPPER
Fights colds and flu

ONION
Supports oral health

RED BELL PEPPERS
Promote youthful skin

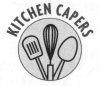

KITCHEN CAPERS

To keep chopped onions from turning bitter when you mix them into dips and spreads, soak them for about 5 minutes in a mixture of 4 cups of water and 1½ tablespoons of vinegar. Stir every minute or so, and drain well before adding them to the other ingredients.

CULINARY Q & A

? A friend of mine says that chemicals in food make you fat, and if you simply switch to an all-organic diet, your poundage will plummet. Is there any truth to this claim?

! None whatsoever. While it is true that eating organically grown food will help you avoid a lot of harmful toxins, shoveling down (for instance) a pint of double-chocolate fudge ice cream will have the same effect on your waistline regardless of whether the originating cows ate pesticide-free grass or genetically modified grain.

SMOKED-FISH PÂTÉ

This creamy mixture pairs beautifully with savory crackers or bread—for example, classic party rye or toasted baguette slices. The flavor reaches its peak after an overnight stay in the refrigerator, so plan ahead if you want to serve it at a party.

YIELD: 2 cups	**PREP:** 10 minutes	**CHILL:** 8–24 hours

1 cup of smoked fish, skinned, deboned, and flaked

1 package (8 oz.) of cream cheese, softened

1 stick of unsalted butter, softened

¼ cup of minced onions

2 tbsp. of balsamic vinegar

1 tbsp. of lemon juice

1 small garlic clove, minced

Ground black pepper to taste

2 tbsp. of chopped chives

1. Combine the fish, cream cheese, butter, onions, vinegar, lemon juice, garlic, and pepper in a food processor. Pulse until well mixed but not completely pureed.

2. Transfer the mixture to a serving bowl, cover tightly, and refrigerate for 8 to 24 hours.

3. Bring the mix to room temperature, top with chives, and serve.

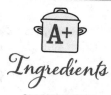

Ingredients

SMOKED FISH
Helps weight loss

ONIONS
Boost oral health

LEMON JUICE
Supports digestion

KITCHEN CAPERS Cooking enthusiasts know that nothing beats copper pans when it comes to conducting heat. To keep your cookware shiny, fill a spray bottle with vinegar and 3 tablespoons of salt, shake until the salt dissolves, and give the copper a good spritzing. Let the pans sit for 12 minutes, and then scrub them clean.

CULINARY Q & A

? My kitchen sink always seems to clog up, but I don't want to fill my house with the smell of chemicals. Is there a safer alternative to commercial drain cleaners?

! Yes! Pour ½ cup of baking soda into the drain, and then add ½ cup of white vinegar. Let it sit for 15 minutes. (You may hear noise, but don't be alarmed.) Rinse with hot water. Don't use this method if you've already tried a commercial de-clogger. The vinegar can react with the drain cleaner to create dangerous fumes. To prevent future buildups, pour a cup of white vinegar down the drain every month or so.

BOSTON BAKED BEAN DIP

Centuries ago, New England pilgrims originated the nutritious casserole that we now know as Boston baked beans. This dip is a variation of that classic dish.

YIELD: 4–8 servings	**PREP:** 15 minutes	**COOK:** 30 minutes

5 slices of bacon, chopped

½ cup of chopped onions

1 can (16 oz.) of navy beans, drained and rinsed

½ cup of ketchup

½ cup of lager beer

3 tbsp. of packed brown sugar

1 package (1.25 oz.) of chili seasoning mix*

1 tbsp. of apple cider vinegar

1 tbsp. of molasses

1 tbsp. of Worcestershire sauce

1 ½ tsp. of brown mustard

¼ cup of sour cream (optional)

* Or 2 to 3 tablespoons of a DIY version (see Instant Gratification, page 270).

1. In a large, heavy pan over medium heat, cook the bacon and onions until the bacon is crisp (10 to 15 minutes).

2. Stir in the beans, ketchup, beer, brown sugar, chili seasoning mix, vinegar, molasses, Worcestershire sauce, and mustard.

3. Bring to a boil, then reduce heat to a simmer. Cover the pan and simmer, stirring occasionally, until the beans are tender and the mixture is thickened (about 15 minutes). Stir in the sour cream if desired.

4. Garnish with various toppings. Grated cheese, scallions, bacon, and/or sour cream are good options. Serve warm with crackers, toasted mini bread slices, or baked pita bread triangles.

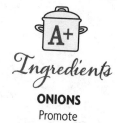

A+ Ingredients

ONIONS
Promote cardiovascular health

NAVY BEANS
Support metabolism

KETCHUP
Boosts eye health

KITCHEN CAPERS
A packet of commercial chili seasoning contains about 5 tablespoons of mix that generally includes flour and other worthless fillers. Generally speaking, 2 to 3 tablespoons of a good homemade version provides the equivalent of flavoring power—with fresher and healthier ingredients. As with any seasoning, though, use whatever amount suits your taste. Your best bet: Start with a tablespoon or so, and add more until you reach your desired heat level.

MAGICAL MELON SALSA

This cool and hot blend is a natural partner for tortilla chips, but it also makes a terrific topping for tacos, grilled chicken, or pulled pork—and the list goes on!

YIELD: about 2 ½ cups	PREP: 20 minutes

1 cup of cubed seedless cucumber

½ cup of cubed cantaloupe

½ cup of cubed honeydew melon

½ cup of diced red onions

1 jalapeño pepper, diced

1 tbsp. of chopped flat-leaf parsley

1 tbsp. of white balsamic vinegar

1 tbsp. of extra virgin olive oil

Kosher or sea salt to taste (optional)

1. Combine the cucumber, cantaloupe, honeydew, onions, pepper, and parsley in a bowl until everything is mixed thoroughly.

2. Pour the vinegar into another bowl. Slowly whisk in the olive oil. Add salt if desired.

3. Drizzle the vinegar and olive oil mix over the chopped ingredients, and toss gently to coat. Serve immediately, or cover and refrigerate until ready to use. It should keep well for up to 24 hours.

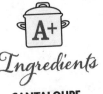

A+ Ingredients

CANTALOUPE
Relieves bloat

HONEYDEW
Ensures healthy hydration

RED ONIONS
Help mantain blood glucose levels

KITCHEN CAPERS

To get rid of all those unhealthy chemical additives on fruits or veggies, give fresh produce a good spritz of this DIY cleanser: In a spray bottle, mix 1 cup of white vinegar, 1 tablespoon of baking soda, the juice of ½ lemon, and 1 cup of water. Shake well. Spray produce, and let it sit for five minutes. Rinse thoroughly.

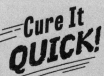

Cure It QUICK!

WONDERFUL WATERMELON SALSA This summertime classic is chief among the world's disease fighters, or at least high on the list. In fact, cup for cup, watermelon delivers one-third more brain-boosting lycopene than tomatoes. For a delicious way to make 16 servings of that firepower, first chop half of a large, seeded watermelon; one seeded red chili pepper; half of a red onion; and a handful of fresh cilantro. Mix it all in a large bowl with 2 tablespoons of balsamic vinegar, and season with salt to taste. Cover and refrigerate for an hour or longer to meld the flavors. Then serve it with corn tortilla chips.

POSITIVELY PLEASING PEANUT DIPPING SAUCE

If you think that peanut butter is only good for sandwiches and cookies, think again. In this easy recipe, it takes center stage in a luscious, healthy dip that'll be a hit at any party.

YIELD: 1 ⅔ cups	**PREP:** 10 minutes

¾ cup of peanut butter

⅓ cup of soy sauce

¼ cup of rice vinegar

¼ cup of water

3 tbsp. of raw honey

1 ½ tsp. of grated fresh ginger
  or ½ tsp. of ground ginger

1 garlic clove, minced

¼ tsp. of red pepper flakes,
  plus more for garnish

1. Combine all of the ingredients in a medium-size mixing bowl. Whisk until creamy and well blended. Add more water, as needed, to thin out the mixture.

2. Dip a cracker into the blend, and take a bite. If it's not sweet enough to suit you, stir in more honey. To ramp up the heat or spiciness, add more garlic, ginger, and/ or red pepper flakes.

3. Transfer the mix to a serving bowl, and garnish with red pepper flakes. Serve with crackers, melba toast, or apple slices.

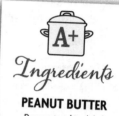

A+ Ingredients

PEANUT BUTTER
Promotes healthy weight loss

HONEY
Boosts memory

GINGER
Soothes acid reflux

KITCHEN CAPERS Natural peanut butter may be better for you than the popular emulsified brands, but the healthy stuff has one flaw: It separates after it sits for a while. To solve that problem, store the jar upside down. Once you flip the jar upright, the oil will flow downward, passing through the pureed nutty part along the way.

CULINARY Q & A

? What's the big deal about using "raw" honey in recipes? Won't any kind of honey work?

! Not by a long shot. While any kind of honey will add sweetness to a recipe, it won't deliver the rich, more complex flavor of pure, raw (a.k.a. unprocessed) honey. More importantly, the brands you find next to the peanut butter and jelly in most grocery stores have been put through a heating and filtering process that kills off the health-giving enzymes and nutrients. You can find the good stuff in farmers' markets, the organic/natural food sections of most major supermarkets, and online.

A DILLY OF A PICADILLO DIP

Traditional picadillo, popular in many Latin American countries, is made with ground meat, tomatoes, and other regional ingredients. It's generally served with rice or beans.

YIELD: 16 servings   **PREP:** 20 minutes   **COOK:** 3–8 hours

1 lb. of ground beef

1 jar (16 oz.) of salsa

½ cup of chopped onions

½ cup of raisins

¼ cup of sliced pimento-stuffed olives

2 tbsp. of red wine vinegar

3 garlic cloves, minced

½ tsp. of ground cinnamon

½ tsp. of ground cumin

½ cup of slivered almonds, toasted, plus more for garnish

1. Brown the ground beef in a large, heavy skillet (8 to 10 minutes), using a wooden spoon to break up the meat as it cooks. Drain off the fat.

2. In a 4-quart slow cooker, combine the beef, salsa, onions, raisins, olives, vinegar, garlic, cinnamon, and cumin. Cook for 6 to 8 hours on low or 3 to 4 hours on high.

3. Stir in the almonds. Transfer to a serving bowl and garnish with additional almonds. Serve immediately or keep warm, covered, for up to 2 hours.

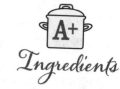

Ingredients

GROUND BEEF
Helps maintain healthy muscles

RAISINS
Fight tooth decay

ALMONDS
Support healthy metabolism

KITCHEN CAPERS Toast slivered almonds by spreading them in a single layer on a shallow, rimmed baking pan. Bake at 350°F until light brown. Stir once or twice, and keep an eye on them so they don't burn.

INSTANT GRATIFICATION

Malt Vinegar–Tarragon Dip

If you love malt vinegar on fish and chips, you'll love it in this creamy dipping sauce. To make it, bring ⅔ cup of malt vinegar to a boil in a small pan, and continue boiling until the vinegar is reduced by half. Remove it from the heat and let it cool for five minutes. Mix in another 1 teaspoon of malt vinegar, 1½ cups of mayonnaise, and 1 tablespoon of chopped fresh tarragon (or ½ tablespoon of dried). Season with salt and freshly ground black pepper, then cover and refrigerate for half an hour. Serve it with chicken, fish, or potatoes.

BAKED RICOTTA-TOMATO SPREAD

Whether you want an easy but elegant appetizer for a sit-down dinner party, or a warm delicious addition to a cocktail-party buffet, this cheesy, wholesome spread is a winner.

YIELD: 8 servings   **PREP:** 15 minutes   **COOK:** 25 minutes

16 oz. of whole-milk ricotta cheese

2 tbsp. of unsalted butter

1 cup of diced onions

6 garlic cloves, minced

1 cup of halved grape tomatoes

1 tbsp. of balsamic vinegar

Salt and black pepper to taste

1. Strain the ricotta cheese into a bowl (see the Culinary Q & A box, below), and let it drain for 30 minutes or so.

2. Press the drained cheese into a broiler-safe baking dish. Put the pan on a rimmed baking sheet, then into the oven on the middle rack. Broil until the cheese is heated through and just beginning to brown. Remove, and set the pan on a rack to cool slightly.

3. Melt the butter in a skillet. Add the onions and garlic, and sauté until beginning to brown. Stir in the tomatoes and cook until they are softened and starting to caramelize. Add in the vinegar, and cook until reduced slightly. Remove from the heat, and season with salt and pepper.

4. Transfer the baked cheese to a serving dish, and spoon the tomato mix on top. Serve with crusty baguette slices.

Ingredients

RICOTTA CHEESE
Helps build muscle

GARLIC
Fends off cold and flu viruses

TOMATOES
Support cardiovascular health

KITCHEN CAPERS

To remove rainbow marks inside aluminum pots, fill it with a solution of 1 tablespoon of vinegar per quart of water, and heat on low for four minutes—but no longer! Then rinse with clear water.

CULINARY Q & A

? What's the best way to strain ricotta cheese?

! Line a strainer with fine-mesh cheesecloth, paper towels, or coffee filters. Set it over a bowl that supports the lip of the straining device, leaving room at the bottom. Gradually spoon the cheese into the strainer. Cover the cheese with a plate that fits inside the strainer, and top the plate with a can of food or other object of similar weight. The cheese should be ready within half an hour.

BLACK OLIVE TAPENADE

Tapenade hails from the Mediterranean region, where it's typically spread on crusty, rustic bread, which absorbs all its delightful flavors. It's become widely available online and in specialty-food shops, but it takes just minutes to make your own.

YIELD: about 1 ½ cups	**PREP:** 5 minutes

1 ½ cups of chopped black olives

2 anchovy fillets

2 garlic cloves

3 tsp. of capers

2 tsp. of dried thyme

1 tsp. of Dijon mustard

1 ½ tbsp. of lemon vinegar

Black pepper to taste

5 tbsp. of extra virgin olive oil

1. Combine the olives, anchovies, garlic, capers, thyme, mustard, vinegar, and pepper in a blender or food processor. Process for 1 minute, or until well blended.

2. With the motor still running, slowly add the olive oil to the blended mixture until you have a smooth, creamy paste.

3. Transfer the finished product to a bowl, and serve with rustic country French or Italian bread, crunchy crackers, or fresh raw veggies.

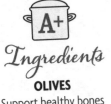

A+

Ingredients

OLIVES
Support healthy bones

ANCHOVIES
Help relieve anxiety

OLIVE OIL
Promotes heart health

A food processor is one of the handiest kitchen tools you could have, but they do have their limits. Never use a food processor to chop anything that's hard, like coffee beans or ice. These will damage the blades. Also, avoid gummy or sticky foods, such as dried fruits, which can clog up the works and strain the motor.

KITCHEN CAPERS

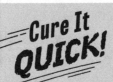
Cure It QUICK!

NOURISHING CRANBERRY DIP This recipe is a tasty way to up your intake of fruits and their potent load of immunity-boosting antioxidants. What's more, it couldn't be easier to make. Just combine a 14-ounce can of cranberry sauce, ¾ cup of sugar, ⅓ cup of vegetable oil, and ½ teaspoon of dry mustard in a blender with ½ cup of Christmassy Cranberry Vinegar (recipe on page 17). Whirl it all until smooth, then pour it into a bowl, cover, and refrigerate until chilled. Serve it with any of your favorite fruits. It's especially good with bananas, apples, kiwi, grapes, and oranges.

SPINACH-ARTICHOKE DIP

Up your intake of Popeye's favorite power food with this classic dip. It's a perfect recipe to have at your fingertips for impromptu entertaining because it goes together in a flash and uses ingredients that are easy to keep on hand.

YIELD: 12–14 servings   **PREP:** 5 minutes   **COOK:** 20 minutes

2 cups of freshly grated Parmesan cheese

1 can (14 oz.) of artichoke hearts, chopped

1 package (10 oz.) of frozen spinach, thawed and drained

1 carton (8 oz.) of whipped cream cheese

2/3 cup of sour cream

1/2 cup of feta cheese

1/3 cup of mayonnaise

2 tsp. of minced garlic

1 tbsp. of white wine vinegar

1. In a large bowl, combine the Parmesan cheese, artichokes, and spinach.

2. In another bowl, mix the cream cheese, sour cream, feta cheese, mayonnaise, garlic, and vinegar. Add the blend to the spinach-artichoke mixture, and stir to mix thoroughly.

3. Bake in a 9- by 13-inch baking dish at 375°F for 20 minutes. Serve with crackers, toast triangles, or toasted baguette slices.

KITCHEN CAPERS To lessen the calories or fat in dips, use low- or nonfat versions of mayo, sour cream, and so on, but don't expect the result to taste the same. For a less dramatic change, mix low-fat products with their full-fat counterparts.

A+

Ingredients

PARMESAN CHEESE
Helps maintain the digestive system

ARTICHOKE HEARTS
Promote healthy liver function

SPINACH
Supports eyesight

CULINARY Q & A

? I was recently gifted a fancy new bread box. Will it really keep my bread fresher for longer than keeping it in the pantry will?

! A bread box doesn't make much of a difference. At room temperature, bread stays fresh and tasty for about three days, whether it's in a drawer, a cabinet, or a bread box. If you really want to keep bread at its peak, stash it in the freezer. Remove however much you need at a time and put the rest back. It'll keep for three months or so and taste as fresh as it was the day you bought it.

ONE-SIZE-DOES-NOT-FIT-ALL GUACAMOLE

If you've only ever had creamy guacamole, give this chunkier version a try. It couldn't be easier to make, it delivers the full five-star nutrition of alligator pears (a.k.a avocados), and it gives you room to adjust the heat to suit your taste.

YIELD: about 3 cups   **PREP:** 10 minutes

3 large avocados, chopped

1 ½ cups of chopped scallions

1 ½ cups of halved grape tomatoes

2 cans (4 oz. each) of diced green chili peppers

1 tbsp. of extra virgin olive oil

1 tbsp. of hot-pepper vinegar

Kosher or sea salt to taste

1. Combine half of the chopped avocados in a large bowl with the scallions, grape tomatoes, chili peppers, olive oil, vinegar, salt, and pepper. Stir well to combine.

2. Add the remaining avocados, stirring gently to retain their chunkiness, until everything is well mixed.

3. Serve immediately with your favorite chips, or cover tightly and refrigerate for up to 5 days.

 KITCHEN CAPERS When your cooler smells stale, don't panic. And don't run out and buy a replacement. Just wash the chest with hot soapy water, and dry it with a towel. Then set a small bowl of white vinegar into the container, close the lid, and let it sit overnight. It'll be fresh-smelling and ready by morning!

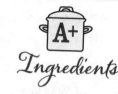 **A+** *Ingredients*

AVOCADOS
Support metabolism

TOMATOES
Help boost kidney health

CHILI PEPPERS
Fight inflammation

 INSTANT GRATIFICATION

Guacamole Italiano

This fresh take on the Tex-Mex classic combines avocados with the famous Italian Caprese salad plus (the real punch) white balsamic vinegar. The result: a brand-new—and ultra-healthy—tasty treat. To make it, combine two mashed avocados, ½ cup each of diced grape tomatoes and fresh mini mozzarella pearls, 2 tablespoons of chopped fresh basil (or more to taste), and 1 tablespoon of white balsamic vinegar in a bowl. Stir well to mix. Then season with salt to taste, and serve it with chips, crackers, or crusty Italian bread.

TUNA-BASIL CAPONATA

In this fresh take on the classic Sicilian dish, tuna, with its boatload of omega-3 fatty acids, stands in for eggplant, while the basil-parsley dressing gives it a whole new flavor twist.

YIELD: 8 servings	**PREP:** 15 minutes	**COOK:** 20 minutes

2 tbsp. plus ¾ cup of extra virgin olive oil

3 large onions, chopped

2 jars (24 oz. each) of pasta sauce

6 oz. of anchovies, drained and chopped

2 ½ cups of sliced black olives

1 can (12 oz.) of water-packed tuna, drained

10 oz. of small capers, drained

¾ cup of white wine vinegar

½ cup of chopped basil

½ cup of chopped parsley

6 large garlic cloves, minced

1. Heat 2 tablespoons of the olive oil in a large pan. Add the onions, and sauté over medium heat until limp (8 to 10 minutes), stirring frequently.

2. Add in the pasta sauce and anchovies, and simmer, partially covered, for 10 minutes, continuing to stir.

3. Combine the olives, tuna, capers, remaining ¾ cup of olive oil, vinegar, basil, parsley, and garlic in a large bowl. Pour in the pasta sauce mix, and combine thoroughly. Season with salt and pepper, and chill, covered, until serving time. Serve with crusty Italian bread.

KITCHEN CAPERS

To clean the oily buildup on your range hood, wipe it down with a spray made from 1 cup of white vinegar and ½ cup of baking soda per 2 cups of hot water. Spritz it onto the hood, and wipe the greasy film away. Rinse off the residue with a damp cloth, and your hood will sparkle!

A+ Ingredients

ANCHOVIES
Support healthy weight loss

TUNA
Encourages healthy blood pressure

PARSLEY
Promotes strong bones

CULINARY Q & A

? Lately, scads of healthy-food websites are claiming that parsley—that frilly garnish—is some kind of superfood. Are they nuts?

! Nope—not by a long shot. According to scientific studies, eating even as little as 1 tablespoon of parsley a day (about the size of a typical garnish) can help fight fatigue, prevent colds and flu, relieve muscle and joint pain, boost immunity, eliminate allergy symptoms, improve the health of your skin, and do much more.

FESTIVE FRUIT DIP

Appetizers don't come any healthier—or tastier—than this. Serve it in one of two ways: in a bowl as a dipping sauce or poured over a platter of fresh fruits.

YIELD: about 3 cups	PREP: 15 minutes	CHILL: 1–24 hours

¾ cup of orange juice

½ cup of cubed mango

¼ cup of citrus-infused vinegar

1 can (11 oz.) of mandarin oranges, drained

1 cup of cubed pineapple

1 banana, peeled

1 kiwi, peeled

¾ cup of sugar

2 tsp. of coconut extract

1 tsp. of poppy seeds

1. Combine the orange juice, mango, and vinegar in a blender or food processor, and whirl until thoroughly blended. Add the mandarin oranges, pineapple, banana, and kiwi, and process again.

2. Add the sugar, coconut extract, and poppy seeds, and blend to achieve the consistency of a thick syrup. Cover, and chill from 1 to 24 hours.

3. Pour the sauce into a bowl, set it on a platter, and arrange your choice of fruit pieces around it. Or, if you prefer, drizzle the sauce directly over the fruit.

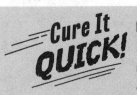

KITCHEN CAPERS

Clean a blender by pouring in 1 cup of white vinegar and ¼ cup of baking soda. After bubbles subside, add 2 cups of water, and blend for six minutes. Use a small brush on any stubborn residue. Rinse, add a cup of water and a few drops of dishwashing liquid, and blend again.

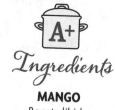

A+

Ingredients

MANGO
Boosts libido

BANANA
Supports skin health

KIWI
Enhances sleep time and quality

Cure It QUICK!

DOUSE THE FLAMES DIP Onions fight inflammation, and that can help prevent many major illnesses. Start the show by slicing a medium sweet onion. Melt 1 tablespoon of unsalted butter in a skillet over medium heat, and cook, stirring occasionally, until the onion has softened and caramelized (10 to 15 minutes). Remove from the heat, and stir in 2 tablespoons of apple cider vinegar. Scrape the mixture into a blender, add 1 cup of mayonnaise, 2 tablespoons of raw honey, and 1 tablespoon of prepared mustard, and blend until smooth. Season with salt and pepper to taste, pour the mixture into a bowl, and refrigerate, covered, until you're ready to serve.

MUSHROOM DIP WITH GUINNESS

Don't wait till St. Patrick's Day to surprise guests with this unconventional blend. At any time of the year, it makes a festive addition to a party spread. Serve it with your choice of crackers or—better yet—chunks of Irish soda bread.

YIELD: about 2 cups   **PREP:** 30 minutes   **COOK:** 20 minutes

2 tbsp. of unsalted butter

3 large garlic cloves, chopped

4 cups of sliced white mushrooms

Salt and freshly ground black pepper to taste

1 cup of Guinness® stout

3 tbsp. of plain yogurt

1 tsp. of balsamic vinegar

1. Melt the butter in a large pan. Add the garlic, and sauté until fragrant. Stir in the mushrooms, and cook until soft and browned. Season with salt and pepper.

2. Pour in the beer, and bring to a boil. Reduce the heat to medium, and simmer, stirring occasionally, until most of the liquid has gone. Remove from the heat.

3. Let the mushrooms cool to room temp, then put them into a blender. Pulse until finely crumbled. Add the yogurt and vinegar, and process to a creamy consistency. Taste, and add more salt, pepper, or vinegar as desired.

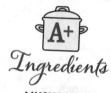

A+

Ingredients

MUSHROOMS
Help prevent anemia

GUINNESS
Promotes healthy heart function

YOGURT
Fends off colds and allergies

KITCHEN CAPERS To keep bugs away when you're entertaining outdoors, mix 2 parts apple cider vinegar and 1 part honey or molasses in a bowl and pour the mix into disposable aluminum pie pans. Set them around the perimeter of your yard. The bugs'll go to the sweet stuff and leave you alone.

CULINARY Q & A

? Whenever I buy mushrooms, I put them in the fridge, but they always turn slimy within a day or two. Am I doing something wrong?

! From the sound of it, you're storing your mushrooms in the packaging they came in. Instead, as soon as you get them home, line the bottom of a brown paper bag with a folded paper towel, and arrange a single layer of mushrooms on it. Cover them with another paper towel, and continue layering the mushrooms until the bag is almost full. Then fold down the top, secure it with a binder clip, and tuck the sack into the fridge.

DEEP-FRIED BEETS WITH HORSERADISH DIP

In nutritional circles, beets are noted for their ability to deliver long-lasting energy. So if you're having your pals over before heading out on a hike—or a day of marathon flea marketing—serve up this flavor-rich fuel for the journey.

YIELD: 24 beets   **PREP:** 15 minutes   **COOK:** 1 ¼ hours

24 baby beets

2 tbsp. plus ¼ cup of extra virgin olive oil

½ cup of water

1 tbsp. of red wine vinegar

2 tsp. of Dijon mustard

1 shallot, finely chopped

Kosher or sea salt and freshly ground black pepper to taste

½ cup of sour cream

1 ½ tbsp. of prepared horseradish

1 cup of all-purpose flour

3 large eggs

2 cups of fine dried bread crumbs

Vegetable oil for frying (about 6 cups)

1. Arrange the beets in a single layer in a shallow baking dish. Drizzle with 2 tablespoons of olive oil. Add water, cover with foil, and roast for 40 to 50 minutes. Let cool, then remove the skins.

2. Whisk the vinegar, mustard, shallot, and remaining ¼ cup of olive oil in a bowl. Add the salt, pepper, and beets and toss to coat. Set aside. Mix the sour cream and horseradish in another bowl, and refrigerate.

3. Pour the flour into a shallow dish. Lightly beat the eggs in a separate bowl. Put the bread crumbs in another dish.

4. Fit a large pot with a thermometer, and pour in enough vegetable oil to measure about 2 inches. Heat until the thermometer registers 350°F.

5. Dredge each beet in flour, dip it in eggs, then roll it in bread crumbs. Fry, turning occasionally, until the breading is golden brown all over. Transfer to paper towels to drain. Serve with the chilled horseradish dip.

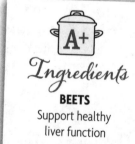

A+ Ingredients

BEETS
Support healthy liver function

HORSERADISH
Enhances bone health

EGGS
Promote memory

KITCHEN CAPERS Some dips thicken when chilled. If necessary to improve "scoopability," thin the dip with a liquid that's used in the recipe, or another appropriate fluid. For example, a splash of milk works perfectly for sour cream–based blends. Broth, water, or olive oil can also make fine thinners.

BLUE CHEESE & CRANBERRY CROSTINI

A platter of these hors d'oeuvres all but shouts "Merry Christmas!" But don't limit these taste treats to winter holiday parties. They're just as good at any time of the year.

YIELD: 12–15 crostini   **PREP:** 15 minutes   **COOK:** 10 minutes

- 8 oz. of blue cheese, crumbled
- ½ cup of chopped toasted walnuts
- ½ cup of dried cranberries
- 1 baguette, cut into ¼-inch slices
- 4 tbsp. of walnut oil, divided
- 8 cups of arugula, torn into bite-size pieces
- 2 tbsp. of balsamic vinegar
- Finely ground sea salt to taste

1. Mix the cheese, nuts, and berries in a bowl. Brush the baguette slices with 2 tablespoons of walnut oil, and spread them out on a baking sheet. Bake at 400°F until lightly toasted (about 5 minutes), turning them over at about the halfway point.

2. Remove from the oven, and top each slice with about 1 tablespoon of the cheese mixture. Return to the oven to melt the cheese (about 5 minutes).

3. Meanwhile, toss arugula with vinegar and the remaining 2 tablespoons of the walnut oil. Season with salt. Remove the crostini from the oven, top each one with a bit of arugula, and serve immediately.

KITCHEN CAPERS

When chopping dried fruit, the pieces tend to cling to the knife and to each other. Nix the togetherness by rolling the fruit in your hands with just a dab of flour before you start cutting.

A+ Ingredients

BLUE CHEESE
Ensures proper muscle contraction

CRANBERRIES
Support heart health

WALNUT OIL
Fights inflammation

CULINARY Q & A

? I serve my dips with crackers and breads, but I've been hearing that gluten is horribly unhealthy. Is this true?

! For people with celiac disease or similar conditions, gluten can be deadly, but for the vast majority of the population, it's perfectly harmless. While gluten itself does not offer any particular health benefits, the whole-grain foods that contain it deliver heaps of them. Their rich assortment of vitamins, minerals, and fiber can help lower cholesterol, regulate blood sugar, fight inflammation, and protect your teeth and gums—not to mention keeping your internal "plumbing" running smoothly.

PANCETTA-WRAPPED FIGS

Figs are one of the world's healthiest foods. In this recipe, the soft, savory sweetness of vinegar-poached figs is complemented by meaty, salty pancetta for a truly delectable dish.

YIELD: 36 pieces	PREP: 15 minutes	COOK: 35 minutes

½ cup of red wine vinegar

½ cup of water

1 tbsp. of juniper berries

1 tbsp. of light brown sugar

10 whole black peppercorns

2 whole cloves

18 dried Black Mission figs, stemmed

12 oz. of pancetta

1. Combine the first six ingredients in a pan. Bring to a boil. Add the figs, reduce the heat, and simmer gently for 5 minutes. Remove from the heat, and let stand, covered, until the mixture comes to room temperature.

2. Using a slotted spoon, transfer the figs to a cutting board, and cut each fruit in half. Slice the pancetta into ⅛-inch-thick rounds, and cut into ½-inch-wide strips. Wrap a pancetta strip around each piece. Put the bundles, seam side down, on a wire rack set on a baking sheet.

3. Bake at 350°F until the pancetta is brown (30 minutes). Secure each wrapped fruit with a toothpick, move them all to a warmed platter, and serve immediately.

Ingredients

JUNIPER BERRIES
Enhance kidney health

FIGS
Aid weight loss

PANCETTA
Boosts memory

KITCHEN CAPERS

If you can't find pancetta in your local supermarket, substitute bacon, Canadian bacon, or prosciutto. Any one of them will deliver the same hearty, salty flavor.

Cure It QUICK!

BONE-BOOSTING STUFFED APRICOTS Apricots are rich in minerals essential for bone health. Add that to the hefty load of calcium in goat cheese (considerably greater than in other types), and you've got one powerful weapon in the fight against osteoporosis! To make the dish, first cut 10 apricots in half, and remove the pits. Arrange the fruits on a plate, and fill the center of each half with goat cheese (you'll need 6 to 8 ounces total). Drizzle 3 to 4 tablespoons of balsamic vinegar over the top, and sprinkle with ¼ cup of chopped, toasted pistachios. For extra flavor, use apricot-infused balsamic vinegar. You can find it online, or make your own. (See Peachy Keen Vinegar on page 16. Replace the peaches with apricots and the white wine vinegar with white balsamic.)

SALT & VINEGAR POTATOES WITH YOGURT-SCALLION DIP

If you just can't get enough of salt and vinegar potatoes, you'll love this version, which stars Yukon Gold taters—one of the tastiest and most nutritious spuds of all.

YIELD: 6 servings	PREP: 10 minutes	COOK: 40 minutes

8 medium Yukon Gold potatoes, cut into 1-inch cubes

4 tsp. of salt, divided

1 stick of unsalted butter, melted

2 tbsp. of white balsamic vinegar

½ cup of Greek yogurt

¼ cup of heavy cream

1 garlic clove, minced

1 scallion (white and green parts), chopped

1. Put the potatoes and 3 teaspoons of salt in a large pot, and cover with water. Bring to a boil, cook for 3 minutes, then drain.

2. Spread the still-hot potatoes in a single layer on a lightly oiled, rimmed baking sheet. Sprinkle with the remaining salt, and drizzle with the butter and vinegar. Toss to combine, then spread back into one layer. Bake at 425°F until browned and crispy (20 to 30 minutes). Transfer to a serving platter.

3. Mix the yogurt, cream, garlic, scallion, and a pinch of salt in a bowl. Serve the warm potatoes with the dip and a supply of sturdy toothpicks.

A+

Ingredients

YUKON GOLD POTATOES
Fight inflammation

BALSAMIC VINEGAR
Supports healthy blood pressure

YOGURT
Aids digestion

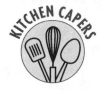

KITCHEN CAPERS Yogurt, sour cream, and cottage cheese keep longer if you store them upside down. Just make sure the lids are on good and tight. To be safe, put each one in a plastic bag and set it into a storage container with the lid off.

CULINARY Q & A

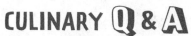

? Yukon Gold potatoes go bad before other types. What's the best way to store them?

! Store the gold potatoes in a paper bag in the refrigerator crisper drawer, away from any onions. Don't wash them before storing, as this removes their natural protective coating. Use them within a week. Also, when you shop for potatoes, select ones that feel firm to the touch and have no bruises, cuts, sprouts, or green spots. One potato with even a small damaged area will make the rest go downhill fast.

BRUSSELS SPROUT & PROSCIUTTO SKEWERS

Thanks to a colossal load of vitamin C, Brussels sprouts just happen to rank as one of the top immune-system boosters of all. Here's a delicious and elegant way to serve them.

YIELD: 32 skewers	PREP: 20 minutes	COOK: 45 minutes

1 lb. of small Brussels sprouts, rinsed

6 tbsp. of extra virgin olive oil, divided

Kosher or sea salt and freshly ground black pepper to taste

2-4 tbsp. of balsamic vinegar

¼ lb. of thinly sliced prosciutto

1. Slice the Brussels sprouts in half and spread them in a single layer on a lightly oiled baking sheet. Pour 4 tablespoons of olive oil over them, and sprinkle with salt and pepper.

2. Roast at 400°F until the sprouts are tender-crisp (about 20 minutes). Toss them with the vinegar, spread the sprouts again to a single layer, and bake for another 20 minutes.

3. Cut the prosciutto into roughly ¼-inch squares. Heat 2 tablespoons of olive oil over medium heat. Add the prosciutto, and sauté until it's crispy (about 5 minutes). Set aside.

4. Remove the sprouts from the oven. When they're cool enough to handle, slide a sprout half onto a toothpick, followed by 2 squares of prosciutto, then another sprout. Place on a platter, and serve.

Brussels sprouts aren't the only healthy tidbits that pair well with prosciutto. For a sweet-and-salty flavor, use chunks of cantaloupe, honeydew, or pineapple (fresh or canned) in place of the sprouts.

KITCHEN CAPERS

A+

Ingredients

BRUSSELS SPROUTS
Enhance immune system

OLIVE OIL
Fights inflammation

BALSAMIC VINEGAR
Supports weight loss

INSTANT GRATIFICATION

Sun-Dried Tomato Pesto

Pesto is best known as a topping for pasta, but this version is just as tasty spread on crackers or toasted bread. To make it, combine 3 cups of sun-dried tomatoes (not in oil); 1 ¼ cups of balsamic vinegar; 1 cup of extra virgin olive oil; 1 cup of minced fresh oregano, parsley, or basil (or a combo); and 3 peeled garlic cloves in a food processor. Add salt and pepper to taste, and pulse until the mix has the texture of traditional pesto. Serve immediately, or refrigerate, covered, and bring to room temperature before serving.

PEPPER-WRAPPED SAUSAGES

Red peppers deliver a dynamite load of immune-system and anti-inflammatory benefits. Combine them with the sausages' offering of essential protein, and you've got an appetizer that's as nutritious as it is colorful and delicious.

YIELD: 8 sausages **PREP:** 15 minutes **COOK:** 45 minutes

8 spicy sausages

Juice of 1 lemon, divided

½ tsp. of crushed red pepper flakes

1 ½ tbsp. of white wine vinegar

½ tsp. of dried oregano

¼ tsp. of freshly ground black pepper

4 roasted red bell peppers, halved

1 scallion, chopped

1. Spread the sausages in a single layer in a shallow baking dish. Sprinkle with half the lemon juice and the pepper flakes. Bake at 375°F, turning occasionally, until browned and crisp on the outside (about 45 minutes). Drain, set aside, and keep warm.

2. Mix the remaining lemon juice, vinegar, oregano, and black pepper in a bowl.

3. Wrap each sausage in a red pepper half. Arrange them on a platter, and pour the lemon juice mixture over them. Garnish with the chopped scallion, and serve immediately.

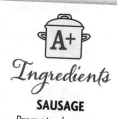

Ingredients

SAUSAGE
Promotes hormone balance

LEMON JUICE
Helps boost liver health

RED BELL PEPPERS
Help maintain youthful skin

KITCHEN CAPERS For an extra-colorful—and equally healthy—presentation, use a combination of red, yellow, orange, and green roasted peppers to wrap your sausages. (Some excellent jarred brands come in mixtures of red and yellow.)

CULINARY Q & A

? What's the secret to getting the most juice as possible from fresh lemons?

! Choose the right lemons. The juiciest fruits tend to have thin skins. So when you're shopping, look for small to medium-size lemons with skin that's smooth, rather than textured. These are the most likely to be productive juicers.

MARINATED OLIVES

These tasty tidbits beat anything you'll find in a fancy food shop. They're terrific either as healthy snacks or added to your favorite recipes—and they're simple to make.

YIELD: about 1 quart	PREP: 25 minutes

4 cups of assorted olives

2 garlic cloves, minced

1 tbsp. of diced red bell peppers

1 tbsp. of grated lemon zest

1 tbsp. of grated orange zest

1 sprig of fresh oregano

½ cup of balsamic vinegar

½ cup of extra virgin olive oil

1. Drain off any brining liquid, and rinse the olives well. Put them in a large, sterilized glass jar with the garlic, diced peppers, lemon and orange zest, and oregano.

2. Whisk the vinegar and oil in a bowl, and pour just enough of the mixture into the jar to completely cover the olives. Put the lid on the jar, and shake it to mix the contents. Then stash it in the refrigerator.

3. If necessary (say, when you've just learned that unexpected guests will be arriving within the hour), it's fine to serve the olives right away. But wait longer if you can because the morsels reach their peak of flavor after chilling for two weeks or so.

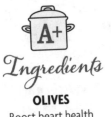

A+

Ingredients

OLIVES
Boost heart health

RED BELL PEPPERS
Promote eye health

ORANGE ZEST
Supports healthy blood pressure

When you want to pull some olives out of a jar without emptying it, just use a melon baller. It's the perfect size for snagging the fruits, and the little hole in the gadget's bottom drains the brine.

KITCHEN CAPERS

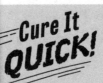

Cure It **QUICK!**

DYNAMITE KALE CHIPS Nutritionists give kale top marks for promoting the health of your liver. These are tasty enough that even gung ho tater chip fans will gobble them up. First cut the leaves away from one bunch of kale and discard the ribs. Tear the leaves into your desired size—they will shrink while baking. In a bowl combine the leaves with 2 tablespoons of apple cider vinegar, 1 tablespoon of extra virgin olive oil, and ¼ teaspoon of salt. Then use your hands to toss the kale for a minute or so until it's soft and a little darker. Spread the kale out in a single layer on a lightly oiled baking sheet. Bake until the kale is crunchy (7 to 10 minutes). Serve immediately, or store in a sealed container.

EASY MINI MEATLOAF BITES

When you're entertaining a crowd, reach for this recipe. If you're staging a cocktail buffet, serve the protein-packed morsels in a chafing dish to keep them warm.

YIELD: 42 balls	**PREP:** 15 minutes	**COOK:** 15 minutes

¾ lb. of ground ham

¾ lb. of ground pork shoulder

½ cup of seasoned fine bread crumbs

1 egg

1 can (10.75 oz.) of tomato soup

½ cup of packed brown sugar

¼ cup of red wine vinegar

½ tsp. of dry mustard

1. Mix the first four ingredients in a bowl. Shape the mixture into approximately 1-inch-diameter meatballs.

2. Arrange the balls in a layer in an 8- by 12-inch microwave-safe baking dish, and cover with vented plastic wrap. Cook on high until firm (about 8 minutes), turning them over at the midpoint. Skim off the fat, and let stand, covered. Repeat if necessary.

3. Mix the next four ingredients in a bowl. Microwave, uncovered, on high until bubbly (about 3 minutes), stirring once. Pour over the meatballs. Cover, and cook until heated (about 3 minutes).

4. Serve immediately, accompanied by cocktail forks or sturdy toothpicks.

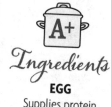

A+

Ingredients

EGG
Supplies protein

TOMATO SOUP
Delivers essential antioxidants

RED WINE VINEGAR
Aids weight loss

KITCHEN CAPERS A social gathering is an ideal opportunity to use your favorite silver flatware and serving trays. But whether the pieces are sterling or silver plate, wash them soon after they come into contact with vinegar because it will make the metal tarnish faster. So will eggs, olives, or salt.

CULINARY Q & A

? I have friends who still insist that microwave ovens are dangerous. Is this true?

! No—with one "but." The reason these devices are safe is that the potentially troublesome microwaves are trapped inside their steel enclosure, where they bounce around. The waves are too small to fit through the screen in the door, and the mechanism that generates the waves turns off instantly when the door opens. However, if your microwave has been damaged, and the door doesn't close tightly, you're best off replacing it.

BAKED RED PEPPER DUMPLINGS

These nifty nuggets will win you five-star accolades from your guests. Not only do the neatly wrapped packages look amazing on a serving tray, but they're also delicious—and filled with some of the healthiest ingredients on the planet.

YIELD: 16 servings	**PREP:** 20 minutes	**COOK:** 25 minutes

½ cup of finely diced red bell peppers

3 tbsp. of finely chopped red onions

1 tbsp. of extra virgin olive oil

3 tbsp. of peach-mango preserves

1 ½ tbsp. of apple cider vinegar

¼ tsp. of hot-pepper sauce

3 tbsp. of chopped fresh cilantro, divided

1 tsp. of freshly squeezed lime juice

¼ tsp. of finely grated lime zest

1 (14.1 oz.) refrigerated piecrust

2 oz. of cream cheese, cut into 16 cubes

Water

1. Sauté the peppers and onions in the oil until tender. Add the preserves, vinegar, and hot-pepper sauce. Cook, stirring, until thick, breaking up chunks. Stir in 2 tablespoons of the cilantro and the lime juice and zest.

2. On a lightly floured surface, roll out the dough to form an 11- by 11-inch square, patching corners and trimming edges as needed. Then cut the square into 4 rows and each of those into 4 pieces (winding up with 16 squares, each measuring 2 ¾ by 2 ¾ inches).

3. Spoon 1 teaspoon of the vinegar mixture into the center of each square, and top with a cream cheese cube. Moisten the edges with water. Press the four corners of the square together at the top. Set the pouches 1 inch apart on a lightly oiled baking sheet. Bake at 400°F until golden brown (14 to 17 minutes).

4. Remove from the oven. Top the pouches with the remaining vinegar mix. Cool slightly, and sprinkle with the remaining cilantro.

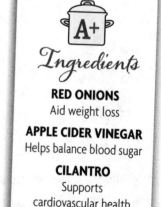

A+

Ingredients

RED ONIONS
Aid weight loss

APPLE CIDER VINEGAR
Helps balance blood sugar

CILANTRO
Supports cardiovascular health

KITCHEN CAPERS

To make cutting the dough easier, overlap two sheets of 8 ½- by 11-inch paper to make an 11-inch-square template. To create the smaller "package" pieces, fold the paper square in half, then in half again. The pattern will be exactly the size you need to form 2 ¾- by 2 ¾-inch squares.

CHEESE & CIDER FONDUE

This fondue version gets an added kick from apple cider vinegar, hard cider, and brandy. Enjoy it in front of a roaring fire with good company and your choice of beverages.

YIELD: 4–6 servings   **PREP:** 25 minutes   **COOK:** 20 minutes

8 oz. of sausage, cut into ½-inch-thick slices

4 cups (about 1 lb.) of grated Gruyère cheese

1 tbsp. plus 2 tsp. of cornstarch

1 cup of hard apple cider

1 tbsp. of apple cider vinegar

2 tbsp. of clear pear brandy

Black pepper to taste

2 firm, tart apples, cored and cut into ½-inch-thick slices

1 baguette, cut into ¾-inch cubes

8–10 bite-size new potatoes, steamed

1. In a large, heavy skillet, sauté the sausage over high heat until browned on both sides (2 to 3 minutes). Transfer to a baking sheet and put it in a 300°F oven to keep warm.

2. Combine the cheese and cornstarch in a bowl. Pour the hard cider and vinegar into a heavy pan over medium heat. Simmer, then reduce the heat to medium-low. Add a handful of cheese, and stir until it's melted. Repeat the process until all the cheese has been melted.

3. Raise the heat to medium, and cook until the fondue begins to bubble, stirring constantly. Stir in the brandy. Season with pepper.

4. Transfer the mixture to a fondue pot. Arrange the sausage and apple slices, bread cubes, and potatoes in bowls around the pot.

KITCHEN CAPERS To keep cheese from going moldy, wrap it in a paper towel that's damp with apple cider vinegar. Refrigerate in a ziplock bag. Remoisten every few days if necessary.

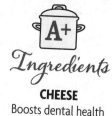

A+

Ingredients

CHEESE
Boosts dental health

HARD APPLE CIDER
Supports cardiovascular health

APPLES
Help prevent colds

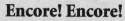

INSTANT GRATIFICATION

Encore! Encore!

When you serve fondue, give your guests a treat: When the fondue has dwindled to a thin layer of cheese on the bottom of the pot, lower the flame, and let the coating turn into a brown crust. Break it into pieces, and share it with your pals. In Switzerland, this final attraction is considered a great delicacy.

PICKLED PINK DEVILED EGGS

Deviled eggs are classic—some would even say "ho-hum"—party fare, but this version rises to new heights from both visual and flavor standpoints. And the beet juice, olive oil, and parsley add a nutritional kick to the already-healthy eggs.

YIELD: 24 servings	**PREP:** 15 minutes

12 hard-boiled eggs

¼ cup of pickled-beet juice

2 tbsp. of extra virgin olive oil

2 tsp. of white wine vinegar

Salt and freshly ground black pepper to taste

Pickled beet strips for garnish

Flat-leaf parsley sprigs for garnish

1. Slice the eggs in half. Put the yolks in a food processor, and blend until smooth. Add the beet juice, olive oil, vinegar, salt, and pepper. Process again until the consistency is smooth.

2. Pour the mixture into a small ziplock plastic bag.* Snip ¼ inch off a bottom corner and squeeze filling into each egg half.

3. Poke a beet strip into the mound of filling on each egg, and put a small sprig of parsley on top.

If you prefer your deviled eggs chilled, put the eggs and filling in the fridge for 20 minutes.

A+ Ingredients

EGGS
Promote skin health

BEET JUICE
Helps support healthy liver function

OLIVE OIL
Boosts metabolism

KITCHEN CAPERS

Serve your deviled eggs on a bed of olives, grape tomatoes, or a mix of greens and chopped veggies. The textured nest will keep the eggs from rolling and provide additional healthy tidbits to munch on.

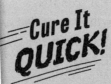

Cure It QUICK!

FLU-FIGHTING CHICKPEAS Thanks to their potent load of zinc and copper, humble little chickpeas (a.k.a. garbanzo beans) are among the most powerful immunity boosters around. Here's how to add them to your diet: Rinse and drain a 15-ounce can of chickpeas, and boil them with 2 cups of white vinegar for about 15 minutes. Then turn the burner off, and let the pot sit for 30 minutes. Drain and pour the chickpeas onto a lightly oiled, rimmed baking sheet. Add 1 tablespoon each of garlic powder and parsley flakes, and 1 teaspoon of sea salt. Stir the mixture around to coat. Bake at 400°F, stirring every 15 minutes, until crunchy (45 to 60 minutes). Remove from the oven, let cool, and serve.

SOUTHERN BOILED PEANUTS

You can't go wrong serving this southern favorite at a tailgate party or backyard barbecue. It multiplies like a dream, so if you're entertaining the whole neighborhood, simply grab the biggest stockpot you can possibly find and ramp up the numbers.

YIELD: about 8 servings	PREP: 5 minutes	COOK: 2–4 hours

1 cup of coarse kosher or sea salt

1 ½ cups of vinegar

2 lbs. of raw peanuts in the shell

2 tbsp. of raw honey

1 or 2 hot peppers, fresh or dried (optional)

1. Fill an 8-quart nonreactive pot two-thirds of the way with water and add the salt. Bring to a simmer over medium-high heat, and stir until the salt has dissolved.

2. Add the vinegar, peanuts, honey, and pepper(s) if using. Bring to a boil over medium-high heat. Then lower to a simmer, and loosely cover the pot.

3. Simmer, stirring occasionally and tasting periodically, until the nuts reach your preferred texture (2 to 4 hours). Remove from the heat, leave the nuts in water for 1 hour, then drain. Serve warm or store in the refrigerator for up to 2 weeks.

KITCHEN CAPERS When you're shopping for unshelled peanuts, look for ones that don't rattle when you shake them. The shells should be clean and unblemished, with no cracks or breaks. Store the nuts, tightly wrapped, in the refrigerator, where they'll keep for up to six months.

CULINARY Q & A

? I do a lot of impromptu entertaining. Can I make a big batch of these Southern Boiled Peanuts and freeze them?

! Absolutely! Drain the boiled nuts, and let them come to room temperature. Then pack them into airtight, freezer-safe containers, getting as much air out as possible before you seal the packages. Tuck them into the freezer. At a temperature of 0°F or lower, they'll keep almost indefinitely. Be aware that once you've thawed the nuts, any leftovers won't keep long, so to avoid waste, freeze your supply in small batches.

A+

Ingredients

PEANUTS
Support weight loss

HONEY
Helps healthy digestion

HOT PEPPERS
Stimulate the immune system

ROBUST ROASTED MUSHROOMS

The combo of peanut butter, soy sauce, and ginger lends a hint of Asian flavor—and a boatload of nutritious goodness—to these tasty nuggets. They're tailor-made for advance party planning because you need to prep them a day or two in advance.

YIELD: 16 servings   **PREP:** 10 minutes   **COOK:** 15 minutes

¼ cup of Pinot Grigio wine

2 tbsp. of freshly squeezed lemon juice

2 tbsp. of white wine vinegar

1 tbsp. of creamy peanut butter

1 tbsp. of soy sauce

2 tsp. of raw honey

1 tsp. of grated fresh ginger

16 fresh mushrooms (about 1 lb.)

1. Mix the wine, lemon juice, vinegar, peanut butter, soy sauce, honey, and ginger in a bowl. Add the mushrooms, and stir to coat thoroughly. Cover, and refrigerate for 8 to 48 hours.

2. Line a rimmed baking sheet with aluminum foil. Arrange the mushrooms, cap side down, on the sheet. Drizzle with the marinade, and bake at 450°F for 10 minutes.

3. Remove from the oven, and turn the mushrooms over. Baste with marinade, return to the oven, and bake for another 5 minutes. Serve hot or at room temperature.

 KITCHEN CAPERS If you have leftover mushrooms, cooked or raw, whirl them in a blender, adding a little vegetable broth. Then freeze the puree in ice cube trays and use it to flavor soups, stews, or casseroles.

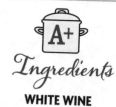 **A+** *Ingredients*

WHITE WINE
Aids weight loss

PEANUT BUTTER
Increases energy level

MUSHROOMS
Help prevent anemia

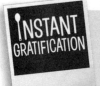 **INSTANT GRATIFICATION**

As You Leek It Dip

This mild, creamy dip puts often-overlooked—and highly healthy—leeks in the spotlight. Serve it with crackers, and it's sure to be a big hit at your next party or get-together. To make enough to feed 20 munchers, mix 1 cup of creamy salad dressing, 8 ounces of softened cream cheese, ¾ cup of chopped leeks, half of a 12-ounce jar of bacon bits, and 1 tablespoon each of white vinegar and white sugar in a bowl. Season with salt and freshly ground black pepper to taste. Cover and refrigerate for 2 to 3 hours before serving.

STUFFED SWEET MINI PEPPERS

If you've ever seen those bags of mini peppers in the supermarket produce aisle and wondered how to use them, here's your answer: Turn them into festive finger food! These colorful and nutritious gems are sweet with just a hint of bite.

YIELD: about 24 servings   **PREP:** 20 minutes

1 bag (32 oz.) of sweet mini peppers

1 can (15 oz.) of chickpeas, drained

¼ cup of mayonnaise

1 tbsp. of apple cider vinegar

½ tsp. of dry mustard

2 scallions, finely sliced

Sea salt to taste

Pinch of cayenne pepper

1. Cut the stem ends off the peppers, slice them in half lengthwise, and remove the seeds. Set aside.

2. Put the chickpeas, mayonnaise, vinegar, mustard, scallions, salt, and cayenne pepper in a food processor. Pulse four or five times, so the ingredients are mixed together but the chickpeas are still chunky.

3. Pour the mixture into a bowl, and stir to make sure it's well blended. Stuff each pepper half with 2 tablespoons of the mixture. Arrange them on a plate, and serve immediately, or cover tightly with plastic wrap and refrigerate for up to 3 days.

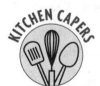

KITCHEN CAPERS

While the mini peppers need to be fresh from the store, the chickpea stuffing will freeze for up to three months in a container. To use, thaw the mix overnight in the fridge, then stuff the peppers as described above.

A+

Ingredients

SWEET PEPPERS
Help keep skin healthy and youthful

CHICKPEAS
Boost eye health

MAYONNAISE
Promotes brain health

CULINARY Q & A

? Do you have any ideas for keeping crudités and other vegetable finger foods cool without using ice? It makes such a mess when it melts!

! Here's one neat trick: Round up a supply of small white stones—smooth river rocks or beach stones are ideal. Scrub them well with hot, soapy water, followed by a rinse in a vinegar-water solution. Then freeze the stones in sturdy containers. At serving time, layer the ice-cold rocks in a bowl or on a platter, and arrange your nibbles on top. It makes an eye-catching presentation and, best of all, the stones won't melt!

BEEF & BLUE CHEESE SLOW-COOKED SLIDERS

Beef and blue cheese are a match made in heaven. And this recipe also has an added twist! The balsamic reduction lightens the richness of the beef and cheese, brightens the flavor, and adds an impressive collection of health benefits.

YIELD: 12 sliders   **PREP:** 25 minutes   **COOK:** 4–10 hours

5 tbsp. of extra virgin olive oil, divided

1 medium yellow onion, finely diced

5 garlic cloves, minced

3 lbs. of boneless chuck roast

⅓ cup of hot water

1 cup of balsamic vinegar

12 slider buns

1 cup of crumbled blue cheese

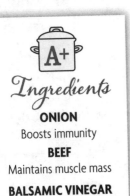

A+
Ingredients
ONION
Boosts immunity
BEEF
Maintains muscle mass
BALSAMIC VINEGAR
Supports weight loss

1. Heat 2 tablespoons of the olive oil over medium heat in a sauté pan that's large enough to hold the chuck roast. Add the onion and garlic, and cook, stirring, until soft and just beginning to caramelize. Pour the mixture into a slow cooker.

2. Add the remaining oil, raise the heat to medium-high, and sear the roast on each side until golden brown (2 minutes per side). Put the meat into the slow cooker on top of the onion-garlic mixture. Pour the hot water into the pan, deglaze it, and pour the enriched liquid into the slow cooker. Cook on low for 8 to 10 hours or on high for 4 to 6 hours. Remove the beef from the pot, and shred with two forks.

3. While the beef is cooking, bring the vinegar to a boil in a small pan over medium-high heat. Reduce to a heavy simmer, and cook, stirring continuously, until the vinegar has thickened and reduced by about half. Remove from the heat, cool slightly, and refrigerate in an airtight container until ready to use.

4. To make the sliders, put the desired amount of shredded beef on the bottom of each bun, top with blue cheese, drizzle with the balsamic reduction, and add the "lid." Serve warm or at room temperature.

When you cut yourself as you're prepping for a party and some blood gets onto your clothes, don't take the time to change. Instead, dab full-strength white vinegar onto the red spot. Let it soak in for 10 minutes, then blot with a clean cloth. Repeat as necessary (but it probably won't be).

KITCHEN CAPERS

HAPPY, HEALTHY NEW YEAR SLIDERS

These mini sandwiches are delicious any time of the year, especially for your annual New Year's Eve party! And they are full of healthy nutrients to boot.

YIELD: 8 servings	PREP: 20 minutes	COOK: 15 minutes

1 tbsp. of extra virgin olive oil

1 medium sweet onion, chopped

1 cup of frozen cranberries

¼ cup of orange juice

2 tbsp. of balsamic vinegar

2 tbsp. of brown sugar

1 tbsp. of coarse-grain mustard

4 red-leaf lettuce leaves, torn in half

8 potato slider buns

8 oz. of roasted turkey breast, sliced

1. Heat the olive oil in a pan over medium heat. Sauté the onion until it's softened. Add the cranberries, orange juice, vinegar, sugar, and mustard. Simmer, stirring, until the ingredients are combined and the berries have softened.

2. Remove from the heat, and pour into a bowl. Let it cool before building the sliders, or cover and refrigerate for up to 2 days. Return it to room temp before using.

3. To build the sliders, lay a lettuce leaf half on the bottom of each bun and add a spoonful of the cranberry mix. Follow with a slice of turkey and another spoonful of the berry blend. Pop the top on.

KITCHEN CAPERS Put a silicone baking mat under your cutting board before you start chopping. It provides a perfect non-slip surface that keeps the board in place—thereby helping you avoid cutting yourself.

A+

Ingredients

CRANBERRIES
Support heart health

ORANGE JUICE
Helps fight free radicals

TURKEY
Promotes thyroid health

CULINARY Q & A

? What's the best way to store leaf lettuces? I know they're healthier than other types, but the leaves seem to wilt or rot in the blink of an eye.

! To give these softies the longest-possible life span, put the entire bunch into a jar full of water, just as you'd do with cut flowers. Then put a big plastic bag over the whole thing and set it in the fridge. **Note:** *If you grow your own leaf lettuce, pull up the whole plant and put it, roots and all, into the water.*

MINI CAPRESE BITES

This classic Italian combo of fresh tomatoes, basil, mozzarella cheese, and balsamic vinegar is a flavor-filled showstopper. In this case, the conventional salad version appears instead as mini skewers that look almost too cute to eat.

YIELD: 32 skewers   **PREP:** 20 minutes

1 pint of grape or small cherry tomatoes, halved

10–14 small, fresh mozzarella cheese balls, sliced into thirds

1 bunch of fresh basil

¼ cup of extra virgin olive oil

2 tbsp. of balsamic vinegar

Salt and freshly ground black pepper to taste

1. Thread 1 tomato half onto a 4-inch wooden skewer, followed by 1 piece of cheese, 1 basil leaf (cut in half if too large), and another tomato half.

2. Lay the skewers in a single layer on a shallow serving dish. The sides of the skewers can touch.

3. Whisk the oil and vinegar together in a bowl, and drizzle the mixture over the skewers. Season with salt and pepper, and serve.

For maximum flavor, let cheese sit at room temperature for 30 to 60 minutes (depending on how warm the room is) before serving. The exception is cottage cheese, which should be kept chilled until you're ready to use it.

Ingredients

CHERRY TOMATOES
Support healthy blood pressure

MOZZARELLA CHEESE
Promotes healthy prostate function

BASIL
Maintains eye health

Easy Chicken Bites

For a protein-rich addition to a cocktail buffet, cut two boneless, skinless chicken breasts into bite sizes and sprinkle them with paprika, salt, and pepper to taste. Mix the chunks in a bowl with 1 tablespoon of red wine vinegar, or more if needed for complete coverage. Cover and refrigerate for at least an hour (or up to 24 if you're prepping in advance). Heat ⅓ cup of extra virgin olive oil in a skillet over medium heat, and sauté the chicken bits until golden brown on both sides (about 3 minutes). Let cool slightly, then thread on wooden toothpicks, and serve.

CINNAMON NACHOS WITH BALSAMIC STRAWBERRIES

The sweet, fragrant blend of cinnamon, strawberries, and balsamic vinegar makes a platter of these nachos a natural—and nutritious—treat to serve guests. But they're also the perfect accompaniment to a relaxing evening all by yourself at home.

YIELD: 8 servings	PREP: 10 minutes	COOK: 10 minutes

8 (6-inch) whole-grain flour tortillas

4 tbsp. of unsalted butter, melted

¼ cup plus 2 tsp. of sugar

2 tsp. of ground cinnamon

2 cups of chopped fresh strawberries

2 tsp. of balsamic vinegar

2 tsp. of minced fresh thyme

1. Brush one side of each tortilla with melted butter. Mix ¼ cup of sugar and the cinnamon in a bowl, and sprinkle the mixture over the tortillas.

2. Cut each tortilla into 6 evenly sized triangles. Put them on a rimmed baking sheet and bake at 350°F until lightly golden and crisp (about 10 minutes).

3. Toss the strawberries in a bowl with the vinegar, thyme, and remaining 2 teaspoons of sugar. Set the bowl and the fresh-from-the-oven chips on a serving platter and enjoy!

KITCHEN CAPERS The secret to keeping strawberries at their peak of freshness longer begins the moment you get them home from the market. Put the unwashed berries into a bowl lined with dry paper towels and cover them with another paper towel. Then tuck the bowl into the refrigerator, where your healthy stash should last for about a week.

A+ Ingredients

TORTILLAS
Support healthy digestion

CINNAMON
Fights inflammation

STRAWBERRIES
Promote healthy vision

CULINARY Q & A

? Is it okay to freeze butter? And is it true that you shouldn't store it in the refrigerator's butter compartment?

! Yes on both counts. You can simply freeze it, in its original packaging, where it should keep just fine for about a year. After that, it will still be safe to eat, but the flavor may begin to deteriorate. In the fridge, store butter, tightly wrapped, at the back of a shelf—not in the compartment on the door, where the temperature fluctuates. Add a layer of foil for extra protection, if you'd like.

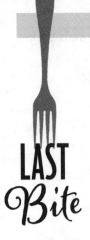

POINTERS FOR PLEASING PARTY FOOD

THE QUESTION OF QUANTITY...

can be tough when serving a crowd. So keep these three rules in mind:

- When you're serving only hors d'oeuvres, plan on 12 per person.

- If you will be serving dinner as well as appetizers, you should be fine with eight hors d'oeuvres per guest.

- Hedge your bets by making more than you think you'll need. How many more is up to you, but it's better to have leftovers than be hungry!

DIP DYNAMICS

Making a dip is a simple two-part process: Mix and serve. But here are some things you want to keep in mind to make them even more delicious:

1. Base the quantity on the mood of the dippers. Most likely, cheering fans at a Super Bowl bash will dip a lot more chips than a more subdued crowd at a cocktail party. In general, though, figure on about ¼ cup of dip per person.

2. Combine the ingredients in a bowl, then transfer the finished product to an attractive serving bowl. The reason: Few serving bowls are large enough to allow for thorough blending without making a mess of your prep surface.

3. While most dips benefit from a pre-serving resting period to blend the flavors, there are exceptions. Guacamole and some salsas are best served as soon as possible after making. If they sit too long, the flavors get muddled.

4. When you do refrigerate a dip, cover the bowl tightly with plastic wrap. This way, unwanted odors won't mingle with the chilling dip—and vice versa.

CULINARY Q & A

? What's the difference between portobello, crimini, and baby bella mushrooms?

! Mushrooms sold as portobellos are larger, and they've been allowed to ripen after picking, so the gills are exposed and dark. Criminis are smaller and fresher. Their gills are covered with a thin veil of mushroom skin. Baby bella is simply another name for criminis. Both criminis and portobellos are more intensely flavored than traditional white button mushrooms, but they're all equally healthy.

DIP THOSE VEGGIES!

But in some cases, give them a little TLC first. Many vegetables, like baby carrots and cherry tomatoes, simply need to be cleaned before you arrange them around a bowl of dip. But these types require a little pretreatment to perk up their flavor and appearance:

Broccoli and cauliflower. Cut the florets into bite-size pieces. Cook in a saucepan of lightly salted water for about one minute—no longer!

Potatoes. Look for tiny, marble-size new potatoes—a combo of red, white, and blue varieties looks especially festive. Scrub them well, then cook them in a pan of lightly salted water for about 15 minutes, or until tender when pierced with the tip of a small knife.

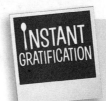

Delicious Dip Done Two Ways

For an instant sweet dip, mix 4 tablespoons of fruit-infused vinegar with a 12-ounce container of whipped cream cheese, and sweeten to taste with honey. It's scrumptious with gingersnaps or vanilla wafers. When you want a savory version to use with vegetables or tortilla chips, omit the honey and use garlic or onion vinegar.

In each case, drain the cooking pan, and immediately rinse the vegetables under cold running water to stop the cooking. Spread the pieces out on paper towels and pat them completely dry. When they're cool, wrap in fresh paper towels, and refrigerate in ziplock plastic bags for up to 24 hours, or until you're ready to use them.

SALSA—BEYOND THE DIP DISH

We know salsa is great for dipping chips! But there are many other ways you can put it to good use. Here's a handful of ways to take it beyond the party:

- Serve it with scrambled eggs for breakfast or lunch.
- Use it as a condiment to perk up your favorite sandwiches and wraps.
- Spoon it over chicken breasts, grilled or fried fish, or even mix it into tuna salad!
- Stir it into mayonnaise or sour cream for a snappy tartar sauce.
- Add a spoonful or so to the blender to jazz up your favorite smoothies (more about smoothies coming up in Chapter Nine).

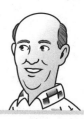

Chapter Nine

Bracing Beverages

In no other culinary category does vinegar pack a stronger and more direct health punch than it does in beverages. The possibilities range from potent but tasty tonics like Lively Liver Libation to the liquid meals we call smoothies to—yes—cocktails worthy of the fanciest party in town. This chapter presents a motley menu of simple, delicious, and nutrient-packed drinks, old and new. So get ready to hoist a glass to good health and long life!

GREEN AND FRUITY SMOOTHIE

A green smoothie serves up an enormous load of health-giving nutrients in one quick-to-make, eat-on-the-go "package." But the taste can take some getting used to. So if you haven't tried these jolly green drinks before, make your first one with baby spinach. It packs a full load of nutrients, but adds virtually no taste to the blend.

YIELD: 1 serving	PREP: 5 minutes

1 ½ cups of frozen mango chunks

1 ½ cups of water (or more as needed)

¼ cup of pineapple juice

2 tbsp. of white balsamic vinegar

1 banana, peeled and sliced

3-4 handfuls of baby spinach

1-2 handfuls of flat-leaf parsley

1. Combine all the ingredients in a blender.

2. Whirl until smooth. If necessary, add more water to achieve the desired consistency and pulse again.

3. Pour the smoothie blend into a glass and drink up!

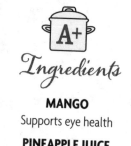

A+ Ingredients

MANGO
Supports eye health

PINEAPPLE JUICE
Aids digestion

BANANA
Builds strong bones

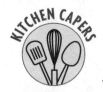

KITCHEN CAPERS Many smoothie recipes include ice cubes. Ignore that listing. When you incorporate ice into a smoothie, it melts and simply dilutes the flavor. So instead, freeze portions of fresh fruit for later use in smoothies. In this case, the recipe's 1 ½ cups of frozen mango is all you'll need to ensure that the resulting drink will be ice cold, thick, and incredibly flavorful. If by chance the blend is too thick to suit you, add a little water or, better yet, more of a juice that's called for in the recipe.

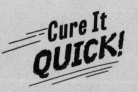

Cure It QUICK!

TUMMY-TAMING TEA Fennel seeds are renowned for their ability to quickly quell nausea and stomach upsets as well as postmeal indigestion. So the next time you're suffering from a case of the midsection miseries, give this tasty tea a try: Bring 2 cups of water to a boil in a nonreactive pan. Remove it from the heat, and add 1 tablespoon of fennel seeds and 1 cinnamon stick. Cool slightly, and stir in 1 tablespoon of apple cider vinegar and raw honey to taste. Sip the brew slowly, and make more during the day as needed.

APPLE-PEAR SMOOTHIE

This remarkable recipe supplies a big percentage of your daily nutrient needs in a single tasty, easy-to-whip-up drink. Enjoy it for breakfast, lunch, dinner—or as an ultra-healthy snack any time that your heart desires.

YIELD: 1 serving	PREP: 10 minutes

1 medium cucumber, chopped

½ avocado, chopped

½ medium apple, chopped

½ medium ripe pear, chopped

¾ cup of chopped kale

2 tbsp. of apple cider vinegar

1 tbsp. of freshly squeezed lemon juice

Water as needed

1. Combine the first seven ingredients in a blender.

2. Whirl until smooth. If necessary, thin the blend with water to achieve a pleasing consistency.

3. Enjoy your power-packed treat!

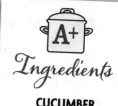

A+ Ingredients

CUCUMBER
Boosts immunity

PEAR
Helps support a healthy heart

KALE
Aids weight loss

KITCHEN CAPERS

When you bring home pears that aren't quite ripe, put them in a brown paper bag with an apple. Poke the sack in several places with the tip of a knife. Then keep a close eye on it, and give the pears the gentle-squeeze test every day. Unlike most fruits, pears are ripe when they're still fairly firm. You'll know they're ready for eating when your fingers produce only a very slight give to the flesh.

CULINARY Q & A

? I love to use freshly squeezed lemon juice in drinks of all kinds, but the arthritis in my hands makes it all but impossible to juice the fruit, even with an electric juicer. Is there any way to make the job slightly easier?

! One way is to slice the lemon into wedges, then use a nutcracker to squeeze and mangle them. Or simply jab a fork into the flesh and squeeze both ends of the wedge inward toward the fork. Then twist it every which way. Either method will give you lots of juice to use in future recipes with far less (if any) discomfort.

CRANBERRY–SWEET POTATO SMOOTHIE

On the morning after Thanksgiving or Christmas—or any other time you've got leftover sweet potatoes on hand—whip them up into this creamy smoothie. It's filled to the brim with both flavor and tons of power-packed nutrients.

YIELD: 1 16-ounce smoothie	PREP: 5 minutes

1 ½ cups of orange juice

½ cup of cooked sweet potatoes, chilled and chopped

½ cup of frozen cranberries

½ avocado, chopped

3 tbsp. of Christmassy Cranberry Vinegar*

2 tbsp. of raw honey

* Recipe on page 17. Or substitute balsamic vinegar.

1. Mix all of the ingredients thoroughly in a blender.

2. Process until smooth.

3. Transfer the blend to a glass and drink a toast to many more happy, healthy holidays!

Ingredients

ORANGE JUICE
Fights inflammation

SWEET POTATOES
Help regulate blood pressure

CRANBERRIES
Support urinary tract health

To keep a supply of sweet potatoes always on hand for smoothies, cook up a batch and freeze it. Wash, peel, and boil the tubers until tender. Mash them, and sprinkle them with a teaspoon of freshly squeezed lemon juice to prevent discoloration. Let cool, divide them among single-serving, airtight containers, and freeze. They will keep for 12 months.

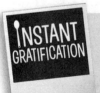

KITCHEN CAPERS

Chocolate-Vinegar Cooler

INSTANT GRATIFICATION

For years, scientists have been singing the praises of dark chocolate for its ability to perform health-giving feats. And balsamic vinegar is loaded with compounds that can help strengthen your immune system and fight the free radicals that cause premature aging. Put 'em together, and you've got one delicious powerhouse of a beverage! Mix 1 cup of dark chocolate chips and ¼ cup of balsamic vinegar in a pan, and warm the mix over medium heat until the chocolate melts. Whisk until smooth. Put 2 to 3 tablespoons of the blend into an ice-filled glass, and add 1 to 2 ounces of vodka if you like. Fill the balance with sparkling water, and stir.

PEANUT BUTTER & BANANA SMOOTHIE

If you like peanut butter, you'll love this protein-packed drink. Have it for breakfast, and it'll get your day off to a rousing start. Or enjoy it as a quick but nourishing lunch.

YIELD: 2 servings **PREP:** 5 minutes

1 ½ cups of almond milk (plus more as needed)

1 cup of frozen strawberries

¼ cup of peanut butter

1 frozen banana, peeled and sliced

2 tbsp. of raw honey

1 tbsp. of apple cider vinegar

1 tbsp. of ground flaxseed

1. Combine all the ingredients in a blender, and process until smooth, adding more almond milk, if necessary, to achieve the desired consistency.

2. Pour into two tall glasses, and serve immediately. Or refrigerate the second serving for later. In a tightly closed nonreactive container, it will keep well for 24 hours.

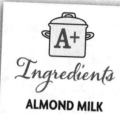

A+ Ingredients

ALMOND MILK
Boosts immunity

BANANA
Encourages healthy sleep

FLAXSEED
Helps balance hormones

KITCHEN CAPERS

Don't toss out overripe bananas. Instead, peel them, and whirl them in a blender with 1 teaspoon of freshly squeezed lemon juice per banana. Then freeze the puree in airtight containers. Straight from the freezer, it makes a flavorful, nutrient-rich addition to just about any smoothie recipe, as well as frozen daiquiris and similar blended drinks, alcoholic or otherwise.

CULINARY Q & A

? I love my aluminum cookware, but it's so hard to keep clean—and that's important to me because I keep all my pots and pans hanging from a ceiling rack rather than stashed in a cupboard. What's the best way to clean this stuff?

! Simply combine ½ cup each of cream of tartar and baking soda in a bowl. Add ½ cup of white vinegar, and mix to form a paste. Stir in ¼ cup of soap flakes (such as Ivory Snow®). Apply the paste with a plain steel wool pad, and rinse with clear water. It'll keep your aluminum pots and pans looking brand-spankin' new. Store any leftover cleanser in a glass jar with a tight-fitting lid. Use as needed.

STRAWBERRY-KIWI SMOOTHIE

You can almost think of this nutrient-rich concoction as a fruit salad in a glass. It's perfect as a quick and ultra-healthy lunch or snack on a warm summer day. And, like any smoothie, it couldn't be simpler to make.

YIELD: 1 serving   **PREP:** 5 minutes

¾ cup of halved frozen strawberries

½ cup of coconut milk

½ cup of peach nectar

1 fresh kiwi, peeled and chopped

3 tbsp. of peach vinegar

2 tbsp. of toasted coconut

1 tbsp. of raw honey

1 tsp. of pure vanilla extract

1. Mix all of the ingredients thoroughly in a blender.

2. Process until the consistency is smooth and creamy.

3. Pour the blend into a glass, and drink to good health!

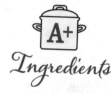

A+

Ingredients

COCONUT MILK
Helps prevent anemia

PEACH NECTAR
Supports cardiovascular health

KIWI
Promotes skin health

Kiwis can be the very dickens to skin with a knife or peeler, but the job is a snap when you use an ordinary spoon instead. Start by cutting the fruit in half. Then, in one of the halves, insert the spoon between the skin and the flesh at one end. Turn the kiwi as you gently push the spoon in until you hit the other end. Rotate the fruit once to make sure that all but a tiny bit of the flesh at the end has separated from the skin. Then simply scoop out the flesh. Repeat the process with the other half, and you're in business!

KITCHEN CAPERS

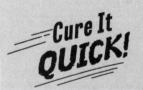

Cure It QUICK!

LIVE LONG AND PROSPER Before General Sam Houston became president of the Republic of Texas (and later a governor of the state), he enjoyed a long and illustrious military career. Despite serious battlefield injuries and the strains of public life, he stayed healthy and spry well into old age. He credited that feat to a potion he whipped up daily, made from 5 parts grape juice, 3 parts apple juice, and 1 part apple cider vinegar. In case you want to give it a try, Sam's recommended dose is ½ cup of the tasty tonic each day.

ALOE-BLUEBERRY SMOOTHIE

This tasty treat combines the potent healing power of aloe vera with antioxidant-rich fruits to deliver a major boost to your immune system. It may also help alleviate skin conditions such as psoriasis—one of the most miserable autoimmune diseases of all.

YIELD: 1 serving   **PREP:** 5 minutes

1 ½ cups of fresh or frozen blueberries

1 cup of water

1 large apple, peeled and chopped

1 medium banana, peeled and sliced

4 tbsp. (2 oz.) of pure, food-grade aloe vera gel*

1 tbsp. of apple cider vinegar

* Equal to 8 ounces of aloe vera juice. Aloe vera gel is available in health-food stores and supermarkets.

1. Mix all the ingredients thoroughly in a blender.

2. Process until smooth and creamy.

3. Pour the potion into a glass, and drink to a new ramped-up immune system!

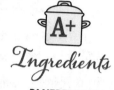

Ingredients

BLUEBERRIES
Help support memory

BANANA
Boosts skin health

ALOE VERA GEL
Promotes healthy blood sugar

KITCHEN CAPERS If you buy aloe vera leaves, or have a plant at home, remove the spiky edges from a leaf, then slice it in half lengthwise and use a spoon to scrape out the gel. If you get more than you need for a recipe, refrigerate any extra in a lidded container; it'll keep for a week. To keep it longer, freeze the gel in ice cube trays, then transfer the cubes to a freezer-safe container.

CULINARY Q & A

? I've always known that aloe vera was good for treating scratches, scrapes, and burns, but I've recently heard that it's also good for internal problems. Is this true?

! It sure is! Aloe vera juice is packed with health-giving vitamins and minerals that can solve or prevent some of the most nagging health problems around. It can help soothe heartburn and stomachaches. And it can even help fight inflammation throughout your body, hydrate your skin, soothe damage to internal tissues, and detoxify your system. You can buy aloe vera juice, or add 2 teaspoons of the gel to a smoothie or a glass of juice.

ROSEMARY-BERRY SMOOTHIE

Talk about a health-giving superstar! In addition to offering up a boatload of anti-aging antioxidants, rosemary can (among other feats) improve your memory and concentration, lift your spirits, aid your digestion, relieve muscle pain, and boost your immune system. This fruity treat is a delicious way to tap into that powerhouse.

YIELD: 1 serving	PREP: 5 minutes

1 cup of frozen raspberries

1 cup of milk or water

½ cup of frozen blackberries or blueberries

½ fresh or frozen banana, sliced

1 tbsp. of balsamic vinegar

Leaves from 2 sprigs of fresh rosemary, chopped

Raw honey to taste (optional)

1. Mix all the ingredients thoroughly in a blender or food processor.

2. Process until smooth and creamy.

3. Serve in a glass, and sip it down to enjoy all the nutritious benefits!

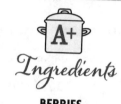

A+ Ingredients

BERRIES
Support brain function

BANANA
Builds strong bones

ROSEMARY
Boosts memory

To make sure you always have rosemary and raw honey on hand for this or any other smoothie recipe, turn the combo into a syrup. Combine ¼ cup of fresh rosemary leaves and 2 tablespoons of raw honey in a heat-proof container. Pour in ½ cup of boiling water, and stir to dissolve the honey. Let it steep for 20 minutes, then strain out the rosemary. Refrigerate the syrup for up to a week, or freeze it in ice cube trays.

KITCHEN CAPERS

INSTANT GRATIFICATION

Fruit Salsa Smoothie

When you've mixed up a fruity salsa (like the Tangy Tropical Fruit Salsa on page 273), and you have some left over, don't let it go to waste. Instead, mix it into this scrumptious and ultra-healthy drink. Just combine 2 to 3 cups of the salsa, two peeled, chopped bananas, and a handful or so of torn romaine lettuce in a blender, and let 'er rip. If the final product is too thick to suit you, add a little water, and blend to achieve your ideal consistency.

FABULOUS FAT-BURNING SMOOTHIE

If you're packing more pounds than you should—as the majority of Americans are these days—one of the best things you can do for your health is to drop your excess baggage. This luscious, slimming superstar can help you do just that.

YIELD: 2 servings　　　**PREP:** 5 minutes

2 green tea bags

¾ cup of boiling water

2 cups of blueberries, fresh or frozen*

12 oz. of vanilla full-fat yogurt

2 tbsp. of ground flaxseed

2 tbsp. of unsalted almonds

1 tbsp. of apple cider vinegar

* Or substitute other berries of your choice.

1. Steep the tea bags in the water for 5 minutes. Then remove and discard them.

2. While the tea cools, whirl the other ingredients in a blender until smooth.

3. Add the tea, and blend for a few more seconds. Then pour the potion into a tall glass, and drink to your good looks, good health, and happiness. Cheers!

A+

Ingredients

GREEN TEA
Boosts stamina and endurance

FLAXSEED
Promotes healthy skin and hair

APPLE CIDER VINEGAR
Enhances digestion

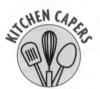

KITCHEN CAPERS

To give fruit juices an extra flavor kick, just add a dash of infused vinegar. Basil vinegar is a perfect match for tomato juice (or Bloody Marys). Lemon vinegar livens up pineapple juice. And apple juice gets a breath of fresh air—so to speak—from a shot of herb vinegar.

CULINARY Q & A

? I've been trying to lose weight by drinking apple cider vinegar in water before each meal. I thought the fat would just flow off like magic, but I haven't dropped a pound!

! From the sound of it, you've been relying on ACV alone to make you lose weight. But it doesn't work that way. While apple cider vinegar will ramp up your body's fat-burning processes and your overall metabolism, you need to combine that power with healthier eating habits and more exercise. Once you do that, you will start to see the pounds flow off.

BANANA-WALNUT SMOOTHIE

Numerous studies show that adding ½ to 1 teaspoon of cinnamon to your diet every day can help maintain healthy blood sugar levels, which could prevent type 2 diabetes.

That same dose can also help lower your LDL (bad) cholesterol and reduce inflammation throughout your body. This delicious drink is one fine way to get your daily dose—along with all the other numerous health benefits of apple cider vinegar.

YIELD: 1 serving	**PREP:** 5 minutes

1 ½ cups of whole milk

1 banana, peeled and sliced

¼ cup of chopped walnuts

2 tbsp. of honey

1 tbsp. of apple cider vinegar

½ tsp. of ground cinnamon

1. Combine all six of the ingredients in a blender.

2. Puree until smooth.

3. Pour the blend into a glass, and drink it down!

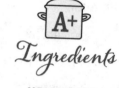

A+
Ingredients

WHOLE MILK
Boosts heart health

WALNUTS
Support healthy weight

CINNAMON
Helps fight free radicals

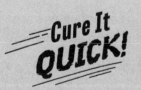

KITCHEN CAPERS

Walnuts retain their nutrients and flavor longer when you buy them with the shells on. But even when you use a nutcracker, those coverings can be tough to crack. To make the job easier, put the nuts in a pan, cover them with water, and bring them to a boil. Remove the pan from the heat, cover, and let it cool to room temperature (about 15 minutes). Blot the shells dry, then crack each of them from end to end. No muss, no fuss!

Cure It QUICK!

A WEIGHT-LOSS WONDER Trying to shed a few pounds? This cocktail should help: Before each meal, mix 1 teaspoon of unprocessed apple cider vinegar in a glass of warm water (make sure it's warm!). Add a teaspoon of raw honey if you'd like. Then drink up. If you're like most folks, this elixir will decrease your appetite, so you'll just naturally want to eat less. **Note:** *Proponents of this tonic claim that in addition to curbing your appetite, it'll also improve your memory. How's that for a versatile aperitif?*

MIGHTY MULTINUTRIENT SMOOTHIE

With this simple recipe at your fingertips, there's no excuse for depriving yourself of essential nutrients, no matter how much your action-packed agenda keeps you on the go. Believe it or not, this tasty beverage delivers nearly all of the vitamins and minerals needed each day for you to stay at tip-top health.

YIELD: 1 serving   **PREP:** 5 minutes

1 ½ cups of fresh spinach

1 cup of green grapes

1 cup of vanilla yogurt (preferably full-fat)

1 banana, peeled and sliced

½ apple, chopped (but not peeled)

1 tbsp. of apple cider vinegar

1 tbsp. of ground flaxseed

Water as needed

1. Combine all the ingredients, except water, in a blender.

2. Process until smooth. Add water if necessary to achieve the desired consistency.

3. Pour the tasty treat into a glass, and sip away! Or, save in the freezer for later use.

A+

Ingredients

SPINACH
Supports healthy blood pressure

GRAPES
Enhance brain health

FLAXSEED
Increases nutrient absorption

KITCHEN CAPERS When you spill something greasy—like cooking oil, melted butter, or a big glob of peanut butter—it's all but impossible to clean it up thoroughly. Somehow, there's always a slick, shiny residue. Enter white vinegar, the world's heavy-weight grease-cutting champ. Just pour some of the acidic marvel onto a sponge or clean cloth and wipe the unwanted film away.

CULINARY Q & A

? I've heard that vinegar can interact with some drugs. Is this true?

! Yes. While vinegar is generally one of the safest ingredients, it does have adverse reactions with some medications, including digoxin (Lanoxin®), insulin, and diuretic drugs. If you're taking any of those meds, check with a doctor before you use vinegar in large quantities—in smoothies, tonics, or other beverages. If you are pregnant or think you might be pregnant, ask your obstetrician how much vinegar is safe for you to consume.

LEMON-GINGER TONIC

Gung ho fans of apple cider vinegar wouldn't dream of beginning the day without a dose of their favorite tonic: 1 tablespoon of ACV mixed in warm water. If you'd rather get your morning off to a tastier start, give this version a try. Besides easing the full-frontal flavor force of ACV, the other ingredients add their own health-giving kick.

YIELD: 1 serving	**PREP:** 5 minutes

1 cup of warm (not hot) water

1 tbsp. of apple cider vinegar

1 tbsp. of freshly squeezed lemon juice

½ tbsp. of pure maple syrup

½ tsp. of ground ginger

1. Combine all of the ingredients in a blender.

2. Process on high for about 30 seconds.

3. Pour the potion into a glass and drink to your good health!

A+

Ingredients

LEMON JUICE
Supports digestion

MAPLE SYRUP
Helps fend off free radicals

GINGER
Fights inflammation

KITCHEN CAPERS In this or any other tonic or smoothie recipe that calls for ground ginger, substitute the fresh version whenever you have enough of it on hand. It will give your smoothie or other beverages more potent flavor as well as higher anti-inflammatory and other health benefits. Use about 1 ½ teaspoons for every ½ teaspoon of the ground spice. For best results, either use a high-powered blender or increase the blending time as needed to make sure the ginger mixes in well.

INSTANT GRATIFICATION

Zip-a-Dee-Do-Da!

To start your day off with a zip and a pow, pour a shot of vinegar into your morning glass of tomato juice or your favorite smoothie recipe. It's your choice what kind of vinegar you'd like to use, but ACV is always a good choice. Or, if you're looking to be more adventurous, why not instead use a vinegar that's infused with herbs, fruits, or vegetables that complement your drink? A high-quality commercial version is fine, or make your own custom blend using any of the simple DIY recipes in Chapter One, starting on page 2.

SUPER JUICE

Don't be fooled by the delicious, sweet-tart taste of this beverage. It's actually a powerful cold killer as well as a crackerjack hangover cure, and because it's full of apple cider vinegar, it contains numerous other health benefits.

YIELD: 6 servings **PREP:** 5 minutes

½ cup of apple cider vinegar

¼ cup of organic 100 percent grape juice

1 tbsp. of freshly squeezed lemon juice

1 tsp. of raw honey (or more to taste)

½ tsp. of ground cinnamon

2 cups of water

1. Mix all of the ingredients thoroughly in a pitcher or large jar until well combined.*

2. Store it, tightly covered, in the refrigerator.

3. Serve it in ice-filled glasses anytime that you want a super-refreshing and super-healthy pick-me-up.

   * *Double this recipe if you like; it'll keep for several weeks in the fridge.*

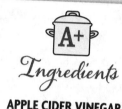

Ingredients

APPLE CIDER VINEGAR
Encourages healthy weight loss

GRAPE JUICE
Supports cardiovascular health

CINNAMON
Promotes healthy blood sugar

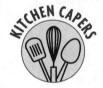

KITCHEN CAPERS

To intensify the health-giving impact and the flavor of Super Juice, freeze a batch of the blend in ice cube trays. Then pour your drink over those super cubes instead of the kind made from plain water.

CULINARY Q & A

? I've always read that you should drink eight glasses of water every day, but recently a friend told me that theory has been debunked. Is she right?

! Yep. While it is true that a steady supply of H_2O is essential for your well-being, no scientific research supports the magic number eight. On the contrary, studies now tell us that there's no need to count because your body will tell you when it's time to drink up. Clue: You'll feel thirsty (surprise!). What's more, you don't have to guzzle water to keep your body healthily hydrated. Beverages of all kinds, including juice, milk, tea, and (yes, nutritionists now tell us) even coffee, deliver the elixir of life. So do fruits, vegetables, and plenty of other foods as well.

SUMMER SWITCHEL

Before commercial sports drinks, folks quenched their hot-weather thirst with this highly healthy DIY beverage. If you're accustomed to drinking sweet drinks, this formula might take some getting used to—but if you give it a chance, it'll grow on you—guaranteed.

YIELD: 1 gallon	**PREP:** 5 minutes

1 cup of apple cider vinegar

1 cup of raw honey or pure maple syrup

¼ cup of molasses

1 tbsp. of ground ginger (or less to taste)

2–3 cups of warm water

Cold water

Fresh lemon slices (optional)

1. Put the vinegar, honey or maple syrup, molasses, and ginger in a 1-gallon jar or jug.*

2. Add 2 or 3 cups of warm water and stir to thoroughly dissolve the honey and molasses.

3. Fill the balance of the container with cold water. Stir or shake to combine the ingredients, and pour the libation into ice-filled glasses. Garnish with lemon slices if you like, and drink a toast to the good old summertime!

With a shot of dark rum added to it, switchel makes a dandy—and healthy—cocktail at any time of the year.

A+ Ingredients

MAPLE SYRUP
Boosts immune system

MOLASSES
Supports sexual health

GINGER
Helps relieve heartburn

Adding a teaspoon of ginger concentrate to drinks and smoothies can give your immune system a boost. To make, put a 3- to 4-inch piece of peeled fresh ginger in a blender with a tablespoon of water, and blend until smooth. Strain the mix into a pint-size glass jar and add enough water to fill. Keep it, covered, in the fridge for up to a week.

KITCHEN CAPERS

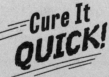

Cure It QUICK!

NIX NIGHTTIME MUSCLE MISERIES Muscle cramps are bad enough any time of day, but—like any other physical or mental problem—they seem a thousand times worse when they strike in the wee hours of the morning. Fortunately, this remarkable remedy can usually save the day, er, night: Mix 1 tablespoon of calcium lactate (available at pharmacies and health-food stores) with 1 teaspoon of apple cider vinegar and 1 teaspoon of honey in half a glass of warm water. Drink it down, and the pain should back off within 20 minutes or so. Repeat as needed.

LIVELY LIVER LIBATION

Your liver performs more than 200 crucial functions in your body, including eliminating toxic substances from your blood, converting food into chemicals that your body needs, and more. Making fresh parsley a regular part of your diet, such as with this tasty cocktail, will help keep that vital organ running smoothly.

YIELD: 1 serving   **PREP:** 5 minutes

½ cup of fresh parsley leaves, finely chopped

½ cup of organic beet juice

½ cup of organic carrot juice

1 tbsp. of apple cider vinegar

1. Put all of the ingredients together in a blender.

2. Pulse the button until everything is thoroughly combined and smooth.

3. Pour the potion into a glass and get ready for a cleaner, meaner liver!

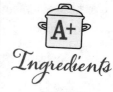

A+

Ingredients

PARSLEY
Promotes strong bones

BEET JUICE
Helps ease asthma symptoms

CARROT JUICE
Boosts immunity

KITCHEN CAPERS While parsley, beets, and carrots are all heavy-weight liver-cleansing champs, they're not the only tasty drink ingredients that can keep this vital organ humming merrily along. Garlic, grapefruit, green tea, leafy greens, and avocados also rank among the top half-dozen liver detoxifiers. Add them to compatible smoothies and other drinks every chance you get.

CULINARY Q & A

? I have a friend who is constantly guzzling carrot juice. She calls it the "king of juices" and claims it can cure just about every ailment under the sun. Is she exaggerating?

! A bit. After all, nothing cures everything. But it's true that drinking an 8-ounce glass of carrot juice several times a week can work wonders for your health and well-being. It helps fortify your blood, fend off respiratory ailments, prevent water retention, strengthen your immune system, and guard against the effects of secondhand smoke. You can get all of these benefits from bottled 100 percent carrot juice, but you'll get a far more potent product by making it at home or buying it fresh from your local juice bar.

ANTI-VIRUS COCKTAIL

This mighty beverage gets its firepower from elderberries. Recent scientific studies have proven that these humble-looking, great-tasting berries pack both immunity-boosting anthocyanins and anti-viral compounds. Here, they also join forces with apple cider vinegar for even more potent protection.

YIELD: 1 ½ cups	**PREP:** 15 minutes	**CHILL:** 24 hours

1 cup of fresh elderberries, washed and dried

2 cups of apple cider vinegar

1 ½ cups of raw honey

2 tbsp. of ground ginger

1 tsp. of ground cinnamon

½ tsp. of ground cloves

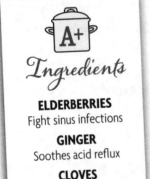

A+

Ingredients

ELDERBERRIES
Fight sinus infections

GINGER
Soothes acid reflux

CLOVES
Help relieve nausea

1. Put the berries in a nonreactive pan, and lightly mash them with a fork. Stir in the vinegar, and bring to a boil over medium heat. Boil for 5 minutes, stirring frequently. Remove from the heat, and let the liquid cool until it is lukewarm.

2. Strain the liquid into a nonreactive bowl. Discard the berries, and stir in the honey, ginger, cinnamon, and cloves. Mix well to thoroughly combine.

3. Transfer the mixture to a sterilized glass bottle or jar, and refrigerate, tightly covered, for 24 hours before serving. It will keep for up to 1 year.

4. Once or twice a day, mix the syrup with your choice of still or sparkling water, and drink to a virus-free winter. The preventive dose is 1 ½ teaspoons to 1 tablespoon per day for an adult; for a child, it's ½ to 1 teaspoon per day.*

  * *Because this formula contains honey, it should never be given to children under two years of age.*

Unripened elderberries are mildly toxic. So if you're picking them from your own bushes or from the wild, make sure you only snag the ripe ones. Avoid any berries that are green or pale purple. Instead, pluck the light blue ones (the berry skin is actually very dark purple, but a waxy white "bloom" makes it appear blue). If there is any doubt in your mind, keep an eye on the local birds: If they're passing the berries by, you know the fruits need more "cooking" time.

KITCHEN CAPERS

APPLE PIE POWER DRINK

Among devotees of apple cider vinegar as a health tonic, the optimum dose is 2 tablespoons a day. But as healthy as it is, the standard mix of ACV in water can get old after a while. Here's one way to jazz it up—and add an even bigger boost to your health.

YIELD: 1 serving   **PREP:** 5 minutes

2 tbsp. of apple cider vinegar

2 tbsp. of organic 100 percent apple juice

6 oz. of cold water*

4 drops of pure vanilla extract (or more to taste)

Sprinkling of ground cinnamon

Raw honey to taste

* *To add more pizzazz, use sparkling water instead of still.*

1. Combine the vinegar, apple juice, water, vanilla extract, and cinnamon in a jar or pitcher. Shake or stir to mix well.

2. Taste and stir in honey as desired.

3. Pour the potion into an ice-filled glass, and drink to your health!

A+ Ingredients

APPLE CIDER VINEGAR
Enhances digestion

APPLE JUICE
Promotes intestinal health

PURE VANILLA EXTRACT
Helps fight free radicals

KITCHEN CAPERS If you use a thermos bottle to tote a beverage to work, here's a trick you need to know: When you get home at the end of the day, pour ¼ cup of vinegar into the bottle, and fill 'er up the rest of the way with hot tap water. Then whisk the inside with a bottle brush, and rinse with clear water. Bingo—good as new!

CULINARY Q & A

? I like to use herbal tinctures to make healing teas, but the commercial versions all have alcohol as the base. I've heard that vinegar works just as well. Is that true?

! It sure is! Just put ½ cup of herbs into a sterilized, lidded glass jar. Pour in warmed apple cider vinegar until it reaches 2 to 3 inches above the top of the herb layer. Cover and put it in a warm, dark place for at least four to six weeks—the longer, the better. Shake the jar often. Strain out the solids, pour the liquid into clean bottles, and store them in a cool, dark place. The tincture will retain its full potency for about a year. After that, its medicinal effect will start to decline.

APRICOT-BALSAMIC FIZZ

Apricot nectar and balsamic vinegar give a flavorful and healthy kick to this festive cocktail. It makes a refreshing addition to a backyard barbecue— or you can simply enjoy it as you relax on your deck before dinner.

YIELD: 1 cocktail	PREP: 5 minutes

4 oz. of sparkling water

2 oz. of vodka

1 oz. of apricot balsamic vinegar

1 ½ tbsp. of apricot nectar

2 tsp. of freshly squeezed lime juice

Thin lime slice (optional)

1. Combine the sparkling water, vodka, vinegar, nectar, and lime juice in a cocktail shaker.

2. Stir well or shake vigorously to combine, and pour the mixture over ice cubes in a chilled 12-ounce glass.

3. Garnish the glass with a slice of lime if you like, and get ready to say "aaahhh…"

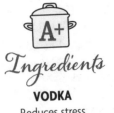

A+ Ingredients

VODKA
Reduces stress

APRICOT NECTAR
Supports digestion

LIME JUICE
Promotes stomach health

Fruit-infused vinegar makes a jazzy substitute for fruit juice in any cocktail recipe. To try it in your favorite drink, simply replace about a third of the juice with vinegar. Then take a sip. If you'd like a little more snap, add more vinegar. If the taste is too acidic to suit you, add more juice, sparkling water, or other sweet ingredient.

KITCHEN CAPERS

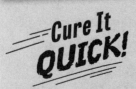

Cure It QUICK!

SOOTHE JOINT DISCOMFORT Whether it goes by the name of housemaid's knee, tennis elbow, or weaver's bottom, joint discomfort is a royal pain in the you-know-what! There are plenty of topical remedies that can ease your suffering. But here's a simple routine that works from the inside to help reduce achy-breaky inflammation, strengthen your joints, and boost your immune system: One hour before breakfast, drink 12 ounces of water with ½ cup of apple cider vinegar, 2 tablespoons of honey, and 1 teaspoon of cayenne pepper mixed into it. Repeat each morning until your joints are back in business.

PEACHY KEEN SHRUB SYRUP

In colonial times, people used vinegar to preserve fruit. These vinegar concoctions (dubbed *shrub syrups* or *shrubs*) were then repurposed for use in cocktails and other beverages.

YIELD: about 3 cups   **PREP:** 15 minutes   **COOK:** 15 minutes

2 cups of peeled
and mashed
ripe peaches

2 cups of sugar

2 cups of white
balsamic vinegar

1. Mix the fruit, sugar, and vinegar in a pan. Bring it to a very brief boil, then simmer it for about 15 minutes while stirring frequently and tasting occasionally.

2. Once the sugar has melted and the vinegar has a very strong peach flavor, remove from heat. Strain the mix thoroughly —two or three times—through a sieve or cheesecloth.

3. Let the syrup cool to room temp, pour it into a sterilized bottle, and store it in the fridge, where it'll keep for a month. Use it in shrub cocktails, or add a tablespoon of the syrup to a tall glass. Fill it up with fizzy water and ice and enjoy!

A+ *Ingredients*

PEACHES
Maintain skin health

SUGAR
Helps low
blood pressure

BALSAMIC VINEGAR
Promotes skin health

If don't want to make your own vinegar shrub syrups, an Internet search will bring up specialty shops and online retailers offering an array of choices. You'll find flavors like strawberry, cranberry, and cherry, exotic versions like tamarind and turmeric, as well as combos like carrot-beet and lemon-ginger.

KITCHEN CAPERS

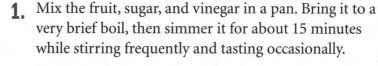

CULINARY Q & A

? I made peach shrub and I'd like to serve it at a party. Do you have good drink ideas?

! Here are two easy—and healthy—winners that your guests will love:
Peach & bourbon cocktail. Mix 2 ounces of bourbon, ¾ ounce of cherry liqueur, ¾ ounce of peach shrub syrup, and a dash of absinthe in an ice-filled cocktail shaker. Shake well, and strain into a chilled cocktail glass for serving.
Peach mocktail. Put 3 Key limes (quartered) and 8 fresh mint leaves in a cocktail shaker, and muddle them. Add 1 ounce of peach shrub syrup and ice, and shake, shake, shake. Strain into a tall, ice-filled glass, and top with ginger ale for serving.

STRAWBERRY-RHUBARB SHRUB

This shrub belongs in your collection! Besides delivering a delicious and nostalgic taste treat, it offers up the nutritional clout of these two classic summertime fruits.

YIELD: about 3 cups	PREP: 20 minutes	WAIT: 8 days

¾ cup of chopped fresh strawberries

¾ cup of chopped rhubarb stalks

1 ½ cups of sugar

¾ cup of apple cider vinegar

¾ cup of balsamic vinegar*

Or substitute Berry Lovely Vinegar (recipe on page 18).

1. Combine the strawberries and rhubarb in a bowl. Sprinkle the sugar on top, and mix well until the fruit is thoroughly coated. Cover and let sit at room temperature for 1 hour.

2. Mash the fruit, cover and let sit at room temperature until most of the fruits' juices have been released (about 1 hour). Mash the fruit again until it's completely mushy. Let it sit, covered, at room temperature for 24 hours. Add the vinegars, cover again, and let it sit for 7 days, stirring once a day.

3. Strain the mixture into a sterilized glass bottle or jar, cover it tightly, and store it in the refrigerator for up to 3 weeks. Use it in a cocktail (see the Strawberry-Rhubarb Collins, below), or simply mix it with sparkling wine or club soda.

KITCHEN CAPERS

To give drinks an elegant yet simple garnish, put fresh berries into ice cube trays filled with water and freeze. Pop 'em out and use them in fruit-flavored cocktails or plain sparkling water. The berries will dress up the beverage and add vitamins at the same time.

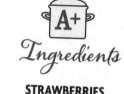

A+ Ingredients

STRAWBERRIES
Boost immunity

RHUBARB
Helps promote healthy vision

APPLE CIDER VINEGAR
Enhances digestion

INSTANT GRATIFICATION

Strawberry-Rhubarb Collins

This up-to-the-minute cocktail is all but guaranteed to launch a flood of way-back-when stories at your next backyard barbecue. Or simply sip it on your deck on a warm summer evening as you reminisce about the good old days. To make it, combine 1 ½ ounces each of lemon vodka and strawberry-rhubarb shrub in a collins glass. Fill the glass with ice, top it with club soda, and stir. Perch a slice of strawberry on the rim if you like.

CRANBERRY–BLACK PEPPER COCKTAILS

This delightful drink gets its sweet-and-tangy flavor from a shrub made with cranberries spiced with black pepper. It's tailor-made for cool-weather entertaining—the combo all but shouts "Fall is here!" And because the shrub keeps for up to 30 days, you can make a supply to have on hand all through the holidays.

YIELD: 12 servings   **PREP:** 15 minutes   **CHILL:** 8–12 hours

2 cups of cranberries (fresh or frozen)

1 cup of apple cider vinegar

½ cup of sugar

½ cup of water

1 tbsp. of whole black peppercorns, lightly crushed

2 bottles of chilled sparkling wine

20 dashes of orange bitters

Whole cranberries for garnish

1. Combine the cranberries, vinegar, sugar, water, and peppercorns in a nonreactive pan. Stir to mix thoroughly.

2. Cover and cook over medium-high heat, stirring occasionally, until the sugar dissolves and the berries begin to pop open (about 10 minutes). Remove from the heat, uncover, and let the mixture cool to room temperature (about 30 minutes).

3. Pour the mixture into an airtight, nonreactive container and refrigerate for 8 to 12 hours. Strain through a fine-mesh strainer into another airtight container and refrigerate for up to 30 days.

4. To make the cocktails, slowly pour the wine into a large pitcher. Add the cranberry mix and bitters, and stir. Serve in glasses garnished with cranberries.

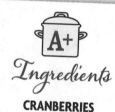

A+ Ingredients

CRANBERRIES
Maintain oral health

BLACK PEPPER
Increases nutrient absorption

SPARKLING WINE
Promotes good skin health

KITCHEN CAPERS When you're getting ready for a big party, and you discover that your wine and cocktail glasses are all looking hazy and dull, don't fret! Just fill a pan with vinegar, and heat it until it's almost—but not quite—too hot to put your finger in. Soak the glasses for about three hours, and then wash them as usual. (Depending on the depth of the "cloud cover," you may need to scrub with a plastic scouring pad.) When you're done, they'll sparkle like stars!

FIGGY BOURBON COCKTAIL

The earthy flavor of the figs combines with the mild sweetness of the whiskey and maple syrup to produce a drink that's perfect for the first cool days of autumn. Plus, figs are some of the world's healthiest foods—so you can indulge guilt-free!

YIELD: 1 serving	PREP: 15 minutes	COOK: about 15 minutes

12 ripe figs, halved

¼ cup of balsamic vinegar

Ice

1 ½–2 oz. of bourbon

1 ½ tsp. of freshly squeezed lemon juice

1 ½ tsp. of pure maple syrup

Dash of orange bitters

1. Arrange the fig halves in a 9- by 9-inch baking pan, and pour the balsamic vinegar over them. Bake at 350°F for 12 minutes, stirring three times. Remove from the oven, and let cool for 10 minutes.

2. Pour the figs, with liquid, into a blender, and process until smooth. Store the puree in an airtight container in the refrigerator for up to 1 week, or freeze it in ice cube trays for up to 3 months.

3. To make one drink, fill a cocktail shaker with ice. Add the bourbon, lemon juice, syrup, bitters, and 1 heaping teaspoon of fig puree. Shake, strain, and serve.

A+ Ingredients

FIGS
Aid weight loss

BALSAMIC VINEGAR
Supports healthy blood pressure

BOURBON
Promotes healthy brain function

KITCHEN CAPERS

When shopping for fresh figs, give each one a gentle squeeze. It should give to the touch without being mushy. Also, the stem should stay firmly in place when wiggled. Refrigerate them in a tightly covered container, where they'll keep for up to three days.

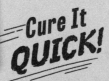

Cure It QUICK!

JOINT-SOOTHING NECTAR Legions of joint-pain sufferers have found blessed relief by consuming a little apple cider vinegar each day. And tart cherry juice is jam-packed with anthocyanins that help reduce pain in joints and muscles. To put this dynamic, delicious duo to work, simply mix 1 cup each of ACV and 100 percent tart cherry juice in a glass jar with a tight, non-metallic lid. Then once or twice a day, stir 2 teaspoons of the mixture into a tall glass of water, and drink it up. Store the blend in the refrigerator, where it will keep for up to two weeks.

SUPERPOWERED PUNCH

You could think of this drink as gazpacho in a glass—or maybe a Bloody Mary on steroids. With or without vodka, it makes a flavorful, festive—and nutrient-packed—addition to any brunch, lunch, or group gathering.

YIELD: 8 servings   **PREP:** 15 minutes   **CHILL:** 1–4 hours

1 qt. of tomato juice

1 bottle (12 oz.) of cocktail sauce

2 cans (4.25 oz. each) of tiny shrimp, rinsed and diced

2 cups of finely diced celery

½ cup of diced green pepper

2 scallions, finely diced

¼ cup of sugar

3 tbsp. of Garden Harvest Vinegar*

1 tbsp. of lemon juice

1 tsp. of horseradish

½ tsp. of garlic salt

½ tsp. of salt

Vodka (optional)

* Recipe on page 23.

1. Combine all the ingredients, except the vodka, in a nonreactive mixing bowl. Cover and chill for 1 to 4 hours.

2. Transfer the mixture to a large chilled pitcher.

3. Add vodka to taste, or serve with a bottle or decanter of vodka on the side so guests can add it if they like.

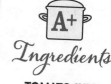

Ingredients

TOMATO JUICE
Fights inflammation

SHRIMP
Help build healthy bones

CELERY
Promotes heart health

KITCHEN CAPERS A big bowl of punch makes a festive addition to any cocktail table, but keeping the blend cool without diluting it presents a challenge. So try this slick trick: Freeze some of the punch in a ring mold, and float the frozen circle in the bowl. It'll keep the libation cool without diluting it, as the customary block of ice does.

CULINARY Q & A

? Lately, my leg muscles have been cramping up throughout the day. I'm at a loss on what to do. Can vinegar help me out with this?

! It sure can—and it's so easy! Before each meal, drink a glass of water with 2 teaspoons each of apple cider vinegar and honey mixed into it. Within a short time, you should be footloose and cramp-free all day long.

SLOW COOKER MULLED WINE

Mulled wine is a classic treat at any cold-weather gathering. In this version, balsamic vinegar lends a flavorful and healthy kick to the usual blend of vino and spices.

YIELD: 8 serving	PREP: 15 minutes	COOK: 30–60 minutes

1 bottle (750 ml) of red wine*

4 cups of apple cider

½ cup of raw honey

¼ cup of balsamic vinegar

Juice of 1 orange

1 (2-inch) piece of fresh ginger, peeled

4 cinnamon sticks, plus more for garnish

4 whole cloves

3 allspice berries

3 star anise

Orange slices for garnish

* Choose one that's fruity but not too sweet.

1. Add the wine, cider, honey, vinegar, and orange juice to a 3-quart or larger slow cooker, and stir to combine. Stir in the ginger, cinnamon, cloves, allspice, and star anise.

2. Cook on low until warm (30 to 60 minutes). Ladle into mugs, and serve each with an orange slice and cinnamon stick.

3. To keep the wine warm, leave the slow cooker on its "warm" setting. If it doesn't have that option, switch between "low" and "off."

A+

Ingredients

RED WINE
Supports cardiovascular health

ALLSPICE
Boosts blood circulation

STAR ANISE
Fights fungal infections

KITCHEN CAPERS Anyone who spends time in the kitchen knows how easy it is to get burned. So stop right now and grab the white vinegar. Pour some into a spray bottle, and stash it in the fridge. Then, the next time you need relief from a minor burn, just spritz yourself with the chilled vinegar.

INSTANT GRATIFICATION

Vim & Vinegar Manhattan

Legend has it that the famous Manhattan cocktail was conceived by none other than Winston Churchill's mother for a party she was throwing. But this version has a vinegar twist! To make two drinks, pour 3 ounces of rye whiskey and 1½ ounces each of sweet vermouth, dry vermouth, and apple cider vinegar into an ice-filled cocktail shaker. Shake or stir, as you prefer, and divide the liquid between two cocktail glasses. Garnish each drink with a maraschino cherry or two.

HOT CHOCOLATE WITH A BITE

After a day of sledding, skating, or cross-country skiing with your pals, invite the gang back to your place and serve up this warming treat. To ensure that the beverage is as healthy as it is delicious, use the purest, darkest chocolate you can find.

YIELD: 1 quart   **PREP:** 5 minutes   **COOK:** 5 minutes

2 cups of light cream

2 cups of milk

1 ½ tbsp. of sugar

½ tsp. of pure vanilla extract

½ tsp. of ground cinnamon

¼ tsp. of cayenne pepper

⅛ tsp. plus a pinch of ground nutmeg

6 oz. of high-quality dark chocolate

1 tbsp. of cinnamon balsamic vinegar*

Marshmallows for garnish

Or substitute plain balsamic vinegar.

1. Combine the cream, milk, sugar, vanilla, cinnamon, cayenne pepper, and nutmeg in a pan.

2. Heat the mixture on medium to just below the boiling point, stirring occasionally to prevent burning. Don't let the mixture boil!

3. Add the chocolate, and cook, stirring, until melted.

4. Stir in the vinegar, and serve in warmed mugs, garnished with marshmallows if you like.

Ingredients

MILK
Helps build healthy bones

CINNAMON
Fights inflammation

DARK CHOCOLATE
Promotes skin health

KITCHEN CAPERS Ground spices lose flavor and aroma in the blink of an eye. When you can, buy them whole, and grind or grate only as much as you need at one time. Whether ground or whole, spices will stay fresh longer if you keep them in the fridge.

CULINARY Q & A

? I don't use marshmallows often, but I like to keep them on hand for hot chocolate or for toasting at summertime barbecues. Is there a secret to keeping them fresh?

! Yep! Slice open the top of the original bag, put inside a ziplock bag, and freeze. Take out as many as you need for a recipe and let them thaw. To save a bag of marshmallows that have gone hard in the pantry, put a slice of bread in the bag and seal it up. Then check back in a few days. They should be soft again.

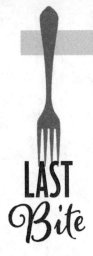

LAST
Bite

DELIGHTFUL DRINKS

WHEN YOUR BEVERAGE (OR FOOD) IS HOT TO TROT

Under ideal circumstances, you should try to let all ingredients come to room temperature, or close to it, before you toss them into a blender jar. If that's not feasible, follow these guidelines to ensure that you don't wind up with a mess—or what could even result in severe burns—on your hands:

- Fill the jar no more than a third to halfway. More hot stuff than that is likely to build up steam that will blow the lid off.

- Remove the feeder cap and put the blender lid securely on the jar.

- Cover the opening loosely with a clean dish towel that's folded to be slightly larger than the lid. This will allow the hot steam to escape through the edges of the towel, while still keeping the contents from splattering.

- Holding the lid on tightly, start blending on the lowest speed, gradually increasing it as needed. Never remove the lid while the motor is running.

Note: *Many newer blenders have lids that vent steam pressure without the need to remove the center part—but it still pays to proceed with extreme caution.*

TWO WAYS TO CLEAN YOUR CRYSTAL...

And any other treasured glassware. Here's your two-part TLC plan:

1. Dodge the dishwasher. Over time, minerals in the hard-hitting spray will etch the glass and wear away any painted designs. So play it safe, and wash the glasses in a sink full of hot water instead. Add 1 cup of vinegar and a few drops of dishwashing liquid to the water to really get your glassware sparkling.

2. Spray and rinse. Spritz each glass with full-strength vinegar, and then rinse it quickly in hot water. After that, you can either dry it with a soft, clean dish towel, or simply let it drip-dry on a rack or mat.

Although you can use rubber spatulas and wooden-spoon handles to de-clog blender blades efficiently and safely, you do run the risk of having these essential kitchen tools nicked in the process. So here's a less damaging idea: Use a stalk of celery to clear up the jam. Then simply bite off the tasty—and healthy—end of the "utensil."

FIGHT FATIGUE

We all get tired every now and then. But if you feel constantly fatigued, the reason may be that lactic acid has built up in your system. (The buildup tends to occur during periods of stress or strenuous exercise.) If that's the case, this simple trick may help: At bedtime each night, take 3 teaspoons of apple cider vinegar mixed into ⅛ cup of honey. Continue the routine until you feel like your old bouncy self again.

BLENDING 101

Whirling vinegar and other ingredients into delicious and healthy drinks may seem like a straightforward process—and, to a large degree, it is. But here are some basic guidelines that can make the job go more smoothly and also prolong the life of your lean, mean, drink-making machine:

Load with care. Add liquid and soft ingredients to the jar first, followed by solids. And make sure that solids are no larger than about 1 inch across.

Avoid jump starts. Skipping right away to a high speed puts undue strain on the blender's motor. Instead, begin at a slow speed and gradually build up to a faster pace.

Stop for "traffic" jams. When food becomes lodged in the blades, stop the motor immediately. Once the blades have come to a complete stop, remove the cover and use a rubber spatula or the handle of a wooden spoon to clear out the clog. Never try to ease a food jam by jiggling the jar of a running blender.

Prevent jams. When you're adding frozen fruit or ice, keep the blender running as you drop the pieces, one at a time, through the lid's fill hole.

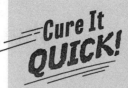

Cure It QUICK!

TRIUMPHANT TRIAD TONIC Worldwide studies show that a mixture made of apple cider vinegar, garlic, and honey can help alleviate the symptoms of almost every ailment under the sun, including high blood pressure, asthma, joint pain, obesity, muscle aches, infections—and the common cold. To make your own supply, simply combine 1 cup each of apple cider vinegar and raw honey and eight peeled garlic cloves in a blender. Mix on high for 60 seconds. Pour the mixture into a glass jar that has a tight-fitting lid, and let it sit in the refrigerator for five days. Then every day, ideally before breakfast, take 2 teaspoons of the blend stirred into a glass of water or fruit juice. Researchers especially recommend using 100 percent grape juice or freshly squeezed orange juice.

Chapter Ten

Delectable
Desserts

Vinegar for *dessert*?! Yes indeed! As unlikely as it may sound, vinegar adds not only renowned health benefits but also delicious flavor to cakes, pies, cookies—even ice cream! What's more, it can stand in for ingredients you may be out of and help you solve or prevent culinary dilemmas ranging from dry cakes to weepy frosting. So don't just stand there! Haul out your baking gear—and your vinegar stash—and whip up one of these sweet treats.

DARK CHOCOLATE PEANUT BUTTER FUDGE

The fudge fans in your crowd will love this easier-than-pie treat. But it's not just delicious—thanks to the healthy helpings of peanut butter and dark chocolate, it also delivers plenty of protein and antioxidants to boot.

YIELD: 9–12 squares	PREP: 5 minutes	COOK: 10 minutes

3 ½ cups of sugar

1 ½ cups of evaporated milk

½ cup of unsalted butter

¼ cup of corn syrup

1 tbsp. of white vinegar

3 cups of peanut butter

1 cup of marshmallow cream

1 cup of dark chocolate chips

1. Combine the sugar, milk, butter, corn syrup, and vinegar in a large pan. Cook over medium heat, stirring constantly until the mixture comes to a full boil (about 5 minutes).

2. Add the peanut butter and marshmallow cream, and stir until smooth.

3. Pour half of the hot batter into a bowl, and stir in the chocolate chips. Pour the contents into a pan lined with wax paper, and top it with the remaining mixture. Let it cool, and cut it into squares.

A+ Ingredients

EVAPORATED MILK
Promotes strong bones

PEANUT BUTTER
Supports healthy blood pressure

DARK CHOCOLATE
Enhances heart health

KITCHEN CAPERS

The next time you make fudge, try this neat, clean cutting routine: Once the candy is cooled and firmly set, slice through it with a pizza cutter. The result: nice, tidy squares with no muss and no fuss!

INSTANT GRATIFICATION

A Light and Sweet Holiday Treat

It seems that between Thanksgiving and New Year's Day, the heavy, calorie-laden desserts never stop coming. So, at your next winter holiday gathering, offer your guests a change of pace with a seasonal fruit salad featuring pears, tart apples, and grapes topped with a dressing made from 2 parts honey to 1 part balsamic vinegar. It makes an especially useful addition to a buffet because—thanks to the vinegar—it can sit on the serving table for the duration without the fruit turning brown. Plus, it's absolutely mouth-wateringly delicious.

STRAWBERRY-BALSAMIC PIE

The superstar combo of balsamic vinegar and strawberries turns out a mighty fine performance in this nutritious variation on the classic custard pie.

YIELD: 6–8 servings   **PREP:** 15 minutes   **BAKE:** 1 hour

⅓ cup of unsalted butter

2 eggs

½ cup of water

¼ cup of balsamic vinegar

1 cup of sugar

3 tbsp. of all-purpose flour

10–12 firm, ripe strawberries, sliced

9-inch pie shell

1. Melt the butter over low heat, and set it aside to cool.

2. In a small bowl, beat the eggs until they're frothy. Add the butter, water, and vinegar, and stir until thoroughly blended.

3. Mix the sugar and flour in another bowl, then add the liquid ingredients, and beat. Fold in the strawberries, and pour it all into the pie shell.

4. Bake at 325°F until a toothpick inserted in the center comes out clean (about 1 hour). Serve warm or let cool to room temperature. Refrigerate any leftovers.

A+ Ingredients

EGGS
Support memory and cognition

BALSAMIC VINEGAR
Promotes weight loss

STRAWBERRIES
Boost immunity

KITCHEN CAPERS When you need to roll out some pastry dough, and you don't have a rolling pin, use an empty, straight-sided wine bottle. To keep the pastry cool, fill the wine bottle about halfway with water, close it securely with a bottle stopper, and refrigerate it for 30 minutes or so before you start working.

CULINARY Q & A

? I always seem to find rust spots in my baking pans, no matter how carefully I wash and dry them. Is there any way to prevent this nuisance?

! There is! After you've turned off the oven and removed your baked goods from their pans, wash the pans and dry them with a dish towel. Then put the pans in the still-warm oven. The residual heat will be just enough to completely dry all the surfaces—including those nooks and crannies that are impossible to reach with a dish towel. No more worrying about pesky rust spots!

ROSE PETAL ZUCCHINI CAKE

This unique dessert is tailor-made for serving on a summer's day, when the enticing scents of flowers are filling the air—and zucchini is bursting out of every garden in town. Plus, it's packed with nutrients and good flavor, too!

YIELD: 10–12 servings	PREP: 20 minutes	BAKE: 1 hour

1 cup of unsalted butter
at room temperature

2 cups of sugar

4 large eggs

1 ½ cups of shredded zucchini

2 tbsp. of minced fresh
rose petals

2 tbsp. of minced fresh rose-
scented geranium leaves*

3 cups of unbleached
all-purpose flour

1 ½ tsp. of baking soda

1 ½ tsp. of ground cardamom

1 tsp. of salt

⅓ cup of rose petal
vinegar**

¼ cup of buttermilk

1 cup of chopped pecans,
lightly dusted with flour

Not all types are edible, so don't make substitutions.

**See the Q & A box on page 21 for a recipe.*

1. Grease and flour a 10-inch tube or Bundt pan, and set aside.

2. Cream the butter and sugar in a bowl until light and fluffy. Add the eggs one at a time, beating thoroughly after each addition. Mix in the zucchini, rose petals, and geranium leaves.

3. In another bowl, combine the flour, baking soda, cardamom, and salt. Add the mixture to the creamed ingredients, and beat well. Then add the vinegar and buttermilk, again beating thoroughly. Stir in the nuts.

4. Pour the mix into the prepared pan, and bake at 350°F until a toothpick inserted in the center comes out clean (about 1 hour). Cool for 10 minutes in the pan, then invert onto a cooling rack.

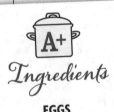

A+

Ingredients

EGGS
Promote memory

ZUCCHINI
Aids weight loss

ROSE PETALS
Promote healthy skin

The pretty pink flowers of rose-scented geraniums are also edible. Use them to decorate cakes, or freeze them in ice cubes and add them to iced tea, fruit juices, or sparkling water. Just make sure that these and any other flowers you consume have not been treated with chemicals of any kind.

KITCHEN CAPERS

SENSATIONAL SPICE STAND-INS

It's frustrating, all right: You're getting set to make a special dessert and discover that you're lacking one, or maybe more, of the spices called for in the recipe. Well, don't get all hot and bothered. Just consult this handy table. Chances are you have something on hand that'll work just as well as your AWOL ingredient. **Note:** *All spices listed are ground versions. Unless otherwise specified, use an equal amount of the substitute in place of the ingredient you're missing.*

If You Don't Have ...	Substitute ...
Allspice	Cinnamon or a dash of either cloves or nutmeg
Apple pie spice	For each teaspoon, substitute ½ teaspoon of cinnamon, ¼ teaspoon of nutmeg, ⅛ teaspoon of allspice, and a dash of either cloves or ginger.
Cardamom	Ginger
Cinnamon	For each teaspoon, substitute ¼ teaspoon of either allspice or nutmeg.
Cloves	Allspice
Cream of tartar	For each teaspoon, substitute 2 teaspoons of white vinegar
Ginger	Allspice, cinnamon, mace, or nutmeg
Mace	Allspice, cinnamon, ginger, or nutmeg
Nutmeg	Cinnamon, ginger, or mace
Pumpkin pie spice	For each teaspoon, substitute ½ teaspoon of cinnamon, ¼ teaspoon of allspice, ¼ teaspoon of ginger, and ⅛ teaspoon of nutmeg.

BALSAMIC ROASTED PLUMS

Plums don't get much "airplay" in dessert circles, but they shine like stars when you give them a venue like this. Plus, they are full of healthy vitamin C and are low in calories, too!

YIELD: 4 servings	**PREP:** 10 minutes	**COOK:** 25 minutes

12 plums, unpeeled, halved, and pitted (about 3 ½ lbs.)

½ cup of balsamic vinegar

½ cup of water

6 tbsp. of sugar, divided

10 whole black peppercorns

¼ tsp. of pure vanilla extract

8 fresh rosemary sprigs, divided

1. Arrange the plums in a 13- by 9-inch baking dish. Combine the vinegar, water, 4 tablespoons of sugar, peppercorns, and vanilla in a bowl. Whisk until the sugar is dissolved, and pour over the plums. Tuck 2 rosemary sprigs into the liquid. Sprinkle the remaining 2 tablespoons of sugar over the top.

2. Bake at 400°F until the plums are tender and the skin on some of them begins to split (about 20 minutes). Using a slotted spoon, transfer the plums to a serving platter.

3. Strain the vinegar mixture into a pan, discarding the solids. Bring to a boil and cook on medium-high heat until the liquid is reduced to roughly ¾ cup (about 5 minutes). Pour the syrup evenly over the plums, garnish with rosemary sprigs, and serve.

A+ Ingredients

PLUMS
Support weight loss

BALSAMIC VINEGAR
Promotes skin health

ROSEMARY
Helps relieve stress

KITCHEN CAPERS

If you cut into a melon only to find that its flavor was not quite up to snuff, don't toss it! Put some life into it by pouring honey-sweetened thyme vinegar on each slice. Your taste buds will love it!

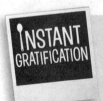

INSTANT GRATIFICATION

Herbal Tea & Vinegar Sorbet

Choose your favorite herbal tea mixture and team it up with a compatible herb- or fruit-infused vinegar in this tasty sorbet. Steep four herbal tea bags with 1 quart of boiling water for 15 minutes. Remove the tea bags and add ½ cup of sugar and ¼ cup of flavored vinegar. Stir until the sugar is dissolved, and refrigerate the mixture until it's thoroughly chilled (30 minutes or so). Then transfer it to an ice cream machine and freeze according to the manufacturer's instructions. The result: a refreshing and healthy treat!

CRANBERRY-APPLE CRISP

The crunchy pecan topping in this dish adds vitamins and minerals that boost your brain, heart, and bone health. Use a mixture of apple varieties to deliver a range of flavors.

YIELD: 6–8 servings   **PREP:** 15 minutes   **COOK:** 40 minutes

1 cup of all-purpose flour

⅓ cup of light brown sugar

⅓ cup plus 1 tbsp. of granulated sugar

¼ tsp. of grated orange zest

⅓ cup of unsalted butter, softened

½ cup of chopped pecans

6 apples, peeled, cored, and sliced

1 tbsp. of cranberry-orange vinegar

½ cup of dried cranberries

1. Combine the flour, brown sugar, ⅓ cup of granulated sugar, and orange zest. Use your fingers to work in the butter. Then mix in the pecans and set aside.

2. Sprinkle the apples with vinegar and the remaining 1 tablespoon of sugar. Mix in the cranberries. Transfer the filling to a 9-inch-square baking dish, and spoon on the pecan topping evenly.

3. Cover with foil, and bake at 375°F for 20 minutes. Remove the foil, and continue baking until the top is crisp and brown and the apples are tender (about 20 more minutes).

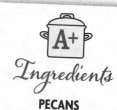

Ingredients

PECANS
Help build strong bones

APPLES
Help ease joint pain

CRANBERRIES
Maintain oral health

KITCHEN CAPERS Whenever you finish the last of a stick of butter, save the wrapper and use it to grease baking pans. (A ziplock bag in the freezer makes a perfect holding "tank.") The residue on the wrapper supplies just the right amount of product, and also makes it a snap to apply.

CULINARY Q & A

? Is there a quick way to soften butter when it's straight from the fridge? I tend to wait too long to take it out of the fridge and end up heating—and mistakenly melting—it.

! There are a couple of tricks for speeding up the process. Simply grating the cold butter into a bowl will bring it down to room temp faster. You can also cut the stick into squares, put them into a bowl, and set it in a pan of warm—not hot!—water.

STRAWBERRY GRANITA

Granitas are closely related to sorbets and sherbets, but they have one advantage over other frozen desserts: You don't need an ice cream machine to make them! This teams up the favorite—and highly healthy—Italian duo of balsamic vinegar and strawberries.

YIELD: 1 quart	PREP: 20 minutes	CHILL: 3 hours

2 pints of fresh strawberries, hulled and sliced

1 cup of sugar

2 tbsp. of freshly squeezed lemon juice

Balsamic vinegar

1. Put a 9- by 13-inch nonreactive metal pan and a large metal spoon in the freezer to chill for 15 minutes.

2. Puree the strawberries, sugar, and lemon juice in a blender for 15 seconds. Pour it into the chilled pan, and freeze until it's semi-solid and icy around the edges (about 1 hour). Stir using the cold spoon. Freeze for another hour, and then mix again.

3. Return it to the freezer until it's completely frozen but still soft enough to scoop (about 1 hour).* Serve immediately in chilled dessert bowls with a cruet of balsamic vinegar so that each diner can drizzle it onto the granita to taste.

   If the mixture freezes solid, break it into large pieces, put them in a food processor, and pulse until they're coarsely chopped.

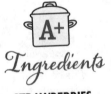

Ingredients

STRAWBERRIES
Promote healthy vision

LEMON JUICE
Helps maintain liver health

BALSAMIC VINEGAR
Supports healthy blood pressure

Here's a no-fuss, no-muss way to hull strawberries: After you've washed the fruit, hold a wide plastic soda straw up to the bottom of the berry and push. The hull will glide right out, taking the stem with it.

KITCHEN CAPERS

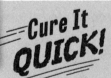

Cure It QUICK!

MITIGATE THE MEAT EFFECT No matter how much you enjoy a T-bone steak, it can leave you feeling like you've swallowed a pillow. Fortunately, there's a simple, scrumptious antidote: mangoes. These tropical fruits contain enzymes that help break down protein and can put your system back in shape fast. The next time you're serving a meat-centered meal, offer mango granita for dessert. To make 6 servings, mix 4 cups of mango puree (made from very ripe fresh mangoes) with ¾ cup of Marvelous Mango Vinegar (see page 20) and a pinch of salt. Pour it into a shallow pan and freeze until hard (at least three hours). Shave it into chilled glass dishes and serve.

PERSIMMON-APPLE CAKE

If you've never eaten a persimmon, imagine the taste of an apricot dusted with cinnamon. These often-overlooked fruits make a perfect pair with apples in this dessert!

YIELD: 6 servings | **PREP:** 20 minutes | **BAKE:** 30–40 minutes

1 large apple, peeled and chopped into ½-inch cubes

⅛ cup plus ½ cup of raw honey

⅛ cup plus ½ cup of water

1 tsp. of ground cinnamon, divided

¼ tsp. of ground ginger

2 or 3 ripe persimmons, skinned and seeded

1 ½ cups of unbleached all-purpose flour

1 ½ tsp. of baking soda

½ tsp. of salt

¼ cup of applesauce

¼ cup of orange juice

1 tbsp. of apple cider vinegar

½ tsp. of pure vanilla extract

1. Grease and lightly flour a 9-inch baking dish.

2. Combine the apple, ⅛ cup of honey, ⅛ cup of water, ½ teaspoon of cinnamon, and ginger in a pan. Cook over medium-low heat, stirring frequently, until the apple softens (about 10 minutes). Stir in the persimmons, and set aside.

3. In a bowl, combine the flour, baking soda, and salt with the remaining ½ teaspoon of cinnamon. In another bowl, mix the applesauce, orange juice, vinegar, and vanilla with ½ cup of honey and ½ cup of water. Make a well in the center of the dry ingredients, and add the applesauce mixture. Stir, then fold in the apples and persimmons.

4. Pour into the pan, and bake at 350°F until a toothpick inserted in the center comes out clean (30 to 40 minutes). Cool in the pan for about 15 minutes. Remove and serve.

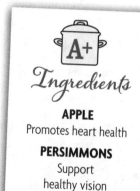

A+

Ingredients

APPLE
Promotes heart health

PERSIMMONS
Support healthy vision

ORANGE JUICE
Fights inflammation

KITCHEN CAPERS

Although they are delicious and nutritious, persimmons that grow native to the United States are smaller, less juicy, and have more seeds than Japanese varieties. Because of this, cultivated Japanese varieties are the kinds you will typically find in U.S. supermarkets.

SUPER SPICE CAKE

A handful of spices gives this cake a nutritious kick. And the aroma it gives off while it's baking is heavenly. Serve plain or topped with vanilla ice cream.

YIELD: 8 servings	**PREP:** 20 minutes	**BAKE:** 1 hour

1 ½ cups of sugar

½ cup of canola oil

2 large eggs

¾ cup of milk

¼ cup of Mighty Spicy Vinegar*

2 cups of unbleached flour

1 tsp. of baking soda

1 tsp. of ground allspice

1 tsp. of ground cinnamon

1 tsp. of ground cloves

1 tsp. of ground coriander

1 tsp. of ground nutmeg

½ tsp. of salt

½ cup of chopped walnuts

½ cup of dried fruit

* Recipe on page 14. Or substitute balsamic vinegar.

1. Grease and flour a 9-inch-square baking pan, and set aside. Beat the sugar and oil in a bowl until light and creamy. Mix in the eggs, milk, and vinegar.

2. In another bowl, combine the flour, baking soda, spices, and salt. Then toss ¼ cup of the spice mixture with the nuts and fruit. Stir the remaining dry ingredients into the sugar-oil mixture, then fold in the nuts and fruit.

3. Pour into the pan and bake at 350°F until a toothpick inserted in the center comes out clean (about 1 hour). Serve warm.

KITCHEN CAPERS

If you're short on eggs in a recipe, substitute 1 tablespoon of vinegar for each missing egg. **Note:** *This will work only if there is another leavening agent, like baking powder, baking soda, flour, or yeast in the recipe.*

A+

Ingredients

CANOLA OIL
Promotes brain function

WALNUTS
Help alleviate symptoms of SAD

DRIED FRUIT
Boosts immunity

INSTANT GRATIFICATION

Champagne Vinegar Dessert Syrup

This sweet, tangy blend makes a perfect topping for vanilla ice cream, pound cake, or any kind of berries. To make ⅔ cup of syrup (6 to 8 servings), mix ¾ cup of packed brown sugar, ⅔ cup of champagne vinegar, and ¼ cup of water in a 2-quart nonreactive pan. Simmer over medium heat, and cook for 15 minutes, or until reduced to ⅔ cup (check by pouring the syrup into a heat-proof measuring cup). Cool to room temp before serving, or refrigerate, covered, until ready to use.

FESTIVE FRUIT & CHEESE PIE

Guests are coming over and you want to serve them a tasty treat? This no-bake pie is as delectable as a dessert can get—and full of heart-healthy apricots and peaches, too.

YIELD: 6–8 serving   **PREP:** 25 minutes   **CHILL:** 30 minutes

3 oz. of cream cheese at room temperature

¼ cup of sugar

1 tbsp. of milk

1 tbsp. of grated orange zest

⅔ cup of heavy cream

9-inch graham-cracker piecrust

6 apricots, pitted and thinly sliced

2 large peaches, peeled, pitted, and thinly sliced

½ pint of blueberries

½ cup of red currant jelly

1 tbsp. of balsamic vinegar

1. Stir the cream cheese in a bowl until smooth. Then mix in the sugar, milk, and orange zest until combined. Add the cream, and beat until smooth and thick. Pour it into the pie shell.

2. Arrange the apricots, peaches, and berries in a pattern on top of the filling.

3. Melt the jelly in a small pan over very low heat. Then stir in the vinegar. Using a pastry brush, spread the glaze over the fruit. Refrigerate until ready to serve, but no longer than 30 minutes.

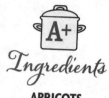

Ingredients

APRICOTS
Enhance digestive health

PEACHES
Help calm anxiety

BLUEBERRIES
Boost liver function

KITCHEN CAPERS To make a 9-inch graham cracker crust, mix 1 ½ cups of graham cracker crumbs, ⅓ cup of sugar, and 6 tablespoons of melted unsalted butter in a bowl. Press the mixture tightly onto the bottom and sides of the pan. Then chill or bake the crust according to the directions in your recipe.

CULINARY Q & A

? It never fails that when I'm making pies or pastries, the phone rings at the very time my hands are covered with sticky dough. Is there a quick way to remove it?

! Yes! Whenever you're working with dough, keep a small bowl of cornmeal close by. Then, when you're interrupted, grab a handful of the stuff and rub it into your skin. It'll remove the dough much more quickly than washing your hands in soap and water.

BALSAMIC PEACH BUNDT CAKE

Creamy vanilla yogurt, balsamic peaches, and a cool burst of mint make this cake a splendid summertime dessert. And those same ingredients give your health a welcome boost with loads of calcium, iron, fiber, and antioxidants.

YIELD: 10–12 servings	PREP: 20 minutes	BAKE: 1 hour

- 3 tbsp. of balsamic vinegar
- 3 tbsp. of brown sugar
- 1 tbsp. of chopped fresh mint
- 4 large ripe peaches, peeled and diced
- 3 cups of all-purpose flour
- 1 tsp. of baking soda
- 1 tsp. of salt
- ½ tsp. of ground cinnamon
- 2 sticks of unsalted butter at room temperature
- 1 ½ cups of granulated sugar
- 6 large eggs at room temperature
- 1 cup of vanilla Greek yogurt
- 1 tsp. of pure vanilla extract

1. Grease and flour a 10-inch Bundt pan and set aside. Whisk the vinegar, brown sugar, and mint in a bowl. Then lightly bruise the mint with a wooden spoon. Add the peaches, toss gently, and set aside.

2. In a large bowl, mix the flour, baking soda, salt, and cinnamon until well combined.

3. In another bowl, beat the butter and granulated sugar until light and fluffy. Add the eggs, one at a time, beating each until thoroughly blended. Fold in half of the flour mixture, followed by the yogurt and the rest of the flour mixture. Add vanilla, and beat a final time.

4. Spoon ⅓ of the batter into the pan. Drain the peaches, and top the batter with ⅓ of the fruit. Repeat the process twice, ending with a top layer of peaches. Bake at 350°F for about 1 hour. Cool 15 minutes in the pan, then remove and cool completely. Serve it plain or with whipped cream or vanilla ice cream.

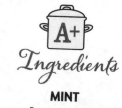

A+

Ingredients

MINT
Promotes good digestion

PEACHES
Maintain skin health

GREEK YOGURT
Boosts immunity

KITCHEN CAPERS

It's not easy to evenly grease all the curves and grooves in a Bundt pan—unless you know this simple trick: Do the job using very soft or melted butter and a pastry brush. You'll get perfect results every time!

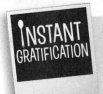

Vinegar Sugar Cookies All the cookie monsters in your family will love tucking into these colorful confections. To make 3 ½ dozen cookies, cream 1 cup of softened unsalted butter with ¾ cup of sugar until light and fluffy. Beat in 1 tablespoon of white vinegar and ½ teaspoon of pure vanilla extract. In a separate bowl, combine 2 cups of all-purpose flour and 1 teaspoon of baking soda. Gradually mix the dry ingredients thoroughly into the butter-sugar mixture. Roll the dough into 1-inch balls and arrange them 2 inches apart on greased baking sheets. Flatten to ¼-inch-thick rounds, and sprinkle with colored sugar. Bake at 350°F until the edges are lightly browned (8 to 10 minutes). Remove from the oven and cool for 1 minute before transferring the cookies to wire racks. Store in an airtight container.

FRESHEN UP FAST!

Whether you find yourself with leftover baked goods, or you want to make a stash to keep in the freezer, these guidelines will help you keep those treats safe, sound—and as tasty as they were fresh from your oven. Freeze freshly baked goods as soon as possible after they've cooled to room temperature. Use sturdy, airtight, moisture-proof freezer bags or rigid containers. Refrigerate leftovers wrapped in plastic wrap, aluminum foil, or plastic bags.

Tasty Treat	Refrigerator Storage Life	Freezer Storage Life
Cakes (with or without frosting)	4–5 days	3 months
Pies, custard	2–3 days	Do not freeze
Pies, fruit	3–4 days	6–8 months
Cookie dough	4–5 days	2–3 months
Cookies, baked	1 week (keep at room temperature)	3 months
Cookies containing cream cheese or cream frosting	3–5 days	3 months

GREEN-TOMATO MINCEMEAT PIE

The spicy filling in this pie originated during World War II, when nothing went to waste. As a bonus, it can be made ahead of time and frozen—just as big a convenience today!

YIELD: 4 servings   **PREP:** 1 hour   **BAKE:** 45 minutes

2 lbs. of green tomatoes, coarsely chopped

1 lb. of apples, peeled and chopped

1 cup of packed light brown sugar

1 cup of raisins

½ cup of apple cider vinegar

½ cup of cold water

1 tbsp. of grated lemon zest

2 tsp. of cinnamon

¼ tsp. of allspice

¼ tsp. of cloves

¼ tsp. of salt

2 piecrusts

1. Combine all the ingredients, except for the piecrusts, in a large pan. Boil over high heat, stirring constantly. Reduce the heat to low, and simmer, uncovered, stirring frequently until the tomatoes and apples are tender, and the mixture has thickened (about 45 minutes).

2. Press one piecrust into a 9-inch pie pan and fill it with the mincemeat. Cut a 2-inch hole in the center of the second crust, and lay the crust over the filling. Turn the excess pastry under, and flute the edges.

3. Bake the pie on a rimmed baking sheet at 375°F for 45 minutes, or until the crust is golden. Cool 30 minutes before cutting, and serve warm.

 KITCHEN CAPERS Boost the nutrients in a homemade piecrust by using a blend of 1 part all-purpose flour and 1 part whole-wheat pastry flour. Or replace up to 25 percent of the flour with cornmeal or wheat germ.

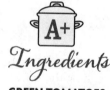

A+

Ingredients

GREEN TOMATOES
Support healthy eyes

RAISINS
Relieve congestion

LEMON ZEST
Supports bone health

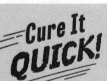 **Cure It QUICK!**

FEED YOUR BRAIN DESSERT Studies have found that eating berries regularly can improve your memory, reduce the risk of developing diseases, delay cognitive aging, and more. Up your intake of these anti-aging miracle workers with this recipe: Combine 1 cup each of strawberries (hulled and quartered), raspberries, and blueberries, ½ cup each of balsamic vinegar and sugar, and 2 tablespoons of water. Simmer over low heat and cook, stirring frequently, until the berries are slightly soft (three to five minutes). Serve warm over pound cake, vanilla ice cream, or cheesecake.

OIL & VINEGAR CAKE

This recipe combines the health-giving goodness of extra virgin olive oil and balsamic vinegar in a confection that's worthy of a dessert menu in a five-star fine-dining restaurant.

YIELD: 8 servings	**PREP:** 10 minutes	**BAKE:** 1 hour

1 ½ cups of all-purpose flour

1 cup of sugar

½ tsp. of baking powder

½ tsp. of baking soda

¼ tsp. of kosher salt

2 large eggs

¾ cup of milk

½ cup of extra virgin olive oil

2 tsp. of lemon zest

4 tbsp. of balsamic vinegar

1. Grease and lightly flour a standard-size loaf pan. Mix the flour, sugar, baking powder, baking soda, and salt in a large bowl. In another bowl, beat the eggs and whisk in the milk, olive oil, and lemon zest. Gradually fold the egg mixture into the dry ingredients.

2. Pour the mix into the pan, and bake at 350°F until a toothpick comes out clean (about 1 hour). Cool the cake in the pan for 5 minutes, then turn it out onto a rack to cool completely.

3. In a nonreactive pan, heat the vinegar until it's reduced to about 2 tablespoons. Pour the reduction over the cake, and serve.

A+ Ingredients

EGGS
Promote skin health

MILK
Helps build healthy teeth

OLIVE OIL
Promotes weight loss

KITCHEN CAPERS When a cooled cake refuses to budge from its pan, lay a thick, clean towel in the kitchen sink, without plugging the drain. Pour a kettle of boiling water over the towel, and set the pan on top of it. Leave it for a minute or two, and the cake should slide right out.

CULINARY Q & A

? My family loves angel food cakes, but every time I make one, it falls as it's cooling. Is there a secret to making the cake hold its shape?

! There is, and it couldn't be simpler. When the cake is done, take it from the oven and immediately set it upside down on the neck of a wine bottle. Wait 30 minutes, then turn the cake over and remove it from the pan. It'll come out perfectly!

CHOCOLATE-CHILI BUNDT CAKE

Chili powder in a chocolate cake? It sounds crazy, but the heat in this recipe enhances the flavor of the chocolate in a way you won't believe!

YIELD: 10 servings	PREP: 15 minutes	BAKE: 35–40 minutes

2 cups of all-purpose flour, plus more for dusting

¾ cup of dark cocoa powder

1 tsp. of baking soda

½ tsp. of chili powder

1 cup of sugar

¼ tsp. of salt

1 cup of whole milk

½ cup of melted coconut oil

2 eggs

2 tbsp. of apple cider vinegar

1 tsp. of pure vanilla extract

1. Lightly grease and flour a 10-inch Bundt pan. Sift the flour, cocoa, baking soda, and chili powder three times into a bowl. Mix in the sugar and salt. In another bowl, whisk the last five ingredients.

2. Combine the two mixtures, and whisk until the batter is smooth. Pour it into the prepared pan.

3. Bake at 350°F until a toothpick inserted in the center comes out clean (35 to 40 minutes). Cool for 10 minutes in the pan, remove, and dust with flour.

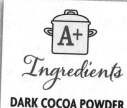

A+
Ingredients

DARK COCOA POWDER
Helps relieve stress

MILK
Helps build strong bones

COCONUT OIL
Promotes youthful skin

KITCHEN CAPERS To keep the cut sides of cake fresh and moist, put it into an airtight container with some sugar cubes, a few apple slices, or a slice of fresh bread. Or put the cake on a plate, along with the moistening agents, and wrap it tightly in plastic wrap.

INSTANT GRATIFICATION

Old-Time Vinegar & Molasses Taffy

Taffy pulls were popular forms of entertainment back in the Roaring Twenties, when this recipe originated. Here's all there is to it: Mix 2 cups of molasses, 1 cup of white sugar, 1 tablespoon of unsalted butter, and 1 teaspoon of white or apple cider vinegar. Boil for 20 minutes, stirring constantly. Then beat the mix by hand until it's smooth and creamy, and pour it into a buttered 8- by 8-inch pan. When the batter is cool enough to handle, pull it into long strips until the candy is satiny and light-colored. Cut the strips into desired lengths, and wrap in wax paper.

RICOTTA-ORANGE CHEESECAKE

This dessert packs a potent protein punch, a major dose of antioxidants, and more! But that's not all. This out-of-the-ordinary cheesecake is also full of fantastic flavor.

YIELD: 10 servings	PREP: 10 minutes	BAKE: 1 ¼ hours

⅔ cup of sugar

⅓ cup of all-purpose flour

2 cartons (15 oz. each) of whole-milk ricotta cheese

5 egg yolks, beaten

1 tbsp. of orange flower water

2 tsp. of grated orange zest

1 ½ tsp. of pure vanilla extract

¼ tsp. of ground nutmeg

Pinch of salt

1 cup of orange juice

2 tbsp. of balsamic vinegar

1. Combine the sugar and flour in a bowl. Add the next seven ingredients. Pour the mixture into a greased and lightly floured 9-inch springform pan.

2. Bake at 300°F until the top is golden brown (about 75 minutes). Transfer to a rack and cool. Cover and refrigerate for 2 to 3 hours.

3. Cook the orange juice over high heat until it's reduced by half. Stir in the vinegar, and set aside to cool.

4. Remove the cake from the pan, and cut. Serve each slice with a spoonful of orange sauce.

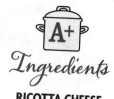

A+ Ingredients

RICOTTA CHEESE
Enhances bone strength

EGG YOLKS
Support heart health

ORANGE JUICE
Promotes skin health

KITCHEN CAPERS When you need just egg yolks or whites for a recipe, and you don't have an egg separator, set a funnel on top of a glass. Crack each egg gently, then break it open over the funnel. The white will flow into the glass, leaving the yolk behind.

CULINARY Q & A

? When I'm only using egg yolks in a recipe, can I store the whites?

! Absolutely! In a tightly covered container, they'll be fine in the refrigerator for up to four days. In the freezer, they'll last for up to six months. The most convenient way to freeze egg whites is to put one in each section of an ice cube tray, then pop the frozen cubes out and store them in a freezer bag or rigid container. Remove as many as you need at a time and thaw them overnight in the refrigerator.

PINEAPPLE-COCONUT CRUNCH

In this winner, two tropical all-stars deliver a healthy burst of flavor that'll tickle every sweet tooth around. And it's one of the simplest desserts you can make!

YIELD: 6–8 servings	**PREP:** 20 minutes	**BAKE:** 20–25 minutes

6 cups of diced pineapple

¼ cup of granulated sugar

3 tbsp. of Fruity Vinegar*

2 tbsp. of raw honey

1 cup plus 1 tbsp. of flour

1 tsp. of cinnamon, divided

½ tsp. of nutmeg

2 cups of shredded coconut

1 cup of packed brown sugar

1 cup of uncooked oatmeal

1 cup of unsalted butter

* Recipe on page 16.

1. Combine the pineapple, granulated sugar, vinegar, honey, flour, ½ teaspoon of cinnamon, and nutmeg in a bowl. Mix well, and pour into a lightly greased 2 ½-quart casserole.

2. In another bowl, combine the coconut, brown sugar, oatmeal, and remaining ½ teaspoon of cinnamon. Cut the butter into the mixture until it resembles a coarse meal. Sprinkle it evenly over the pineapple mixture.

3. Bake at 350°F until the pineapple is slightly tender and the top is golden brown (20 to 25 minutes). Serve warm or cold with fresh whipped cream or ice cream.

KITCHEN CAPERS

When you're baking, always make sure you are using the center rack, unless the directions say otherwise. If you've got more than one pan going at a time, keep them at least 2 inches away from the oven walls and from each other.

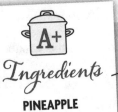

A⁺ Ingredients

PINEAPPLE
Boosts immunity

COCONUT
Supports brain function

OATMEAL
Promotes healthy blood sugar

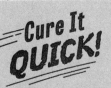

Cure It QUICK!

CAST YOUR EYES ON STRAWBERRIES They're dynamite at fighting off the free radicals that cause damage to your eyes as you age. And this classic Italian favorite is a wonderful way to enjoy them: First, halve 1 quart of fresh, ripe strawberries. Place them in a shallow dish in a single layer, and sprinkle with 4 teaspoons of sugar. Cover tightly with plastic wrap, and let sit at room temperature for at least two hours, shaking the contents occasionally. Thirty minutes before serving, drizzle 1 tablespoon of balsamic vinegar over the berries.

PEACH-RASPBERRY COBBLER

Peaches and raspberries are the leads in this colorful production. They are known to help fight free radicals that can cause premature aging, cognitive decline, and some diseases.

YIELD: 6–8 servings   **PREP:** 30 minutes   **BAKE:** 40 minutes

5 cups of ripe peaches, peeled, pitted, and cut into ¼-inch slices

5 tbsp. plus ¼ cup of granulated sugar

3 tbsp. of instant tapioca

Pinch plus ½ tsp. of salt

1 ½ cups of raspberries

2 tbsp. of Marvelous Mango Vinegar*

2 cups of all-purpose flour, plus more for dusting

4 tbsp. of packed brown sugar, divided

2 tsp. of baking powder

6 tbsp. of unsalted butter, cut into small pieces

1 ¾ cups plus 1 tbsp. of heavy cream

½ tsp. of vanilla extract

* Recipe on page 20.

1. Combine the peaches, 5 tablespoons of sugar, tapioca, and the pinch of salt in a bowl. Gently mix in the raspberries and vinegar. Spoon the mixture into an 8- by 8-inch baking dish.

2. In another bowl, combine the flour, ½ teaspoon of salt, 3 tablespoons of brown sugar, and baking powder. Cut in the butter until small clumps form. Slowly mix in ¾ cup of the cream until just combined.

3. Knead the dough until it holds together. Roll it out into a ½-inch-thick sheet. Cut the dough with your choice of cookie cutters, and lay on top of the peach mixture. Brush with 1 tablespoon of cream, and sprinkle with the remaining 1 tablespoon of brown sugar. Bake at 350°F until the pastry is golden brown (about 40 minutes).

4. Beat the remaining cream in a bowl until it begins to foam. Add the remaining ¼ cup of granulated sugar, one small spoonful at a time. Beat until the mixture holds soft peaks, then mix in the vanilla extract. Spread the whipped cream onto the warm cobbler, or serve it on the side.

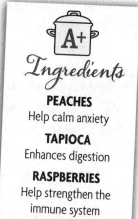

A+

Ingredients

PEACHES
Help calm anxiety

TAPIOCA
Enhances digestion

RASPBERRIES
Help strengthen the immune system

KITCHEN CAPERS

If a recipe calls for brown sugar and you're out, make your own. If you need light brown sugar, mix 1 cup of granulated sugar with 1 tablespoon of molasses. For the dark version, use 2 tablespoons of molasses per cup of white sugar. Store any leftovers in an airtight container.

BERRY-BALSAMIC CHOCOLATE MILKSHAKE

The classic chocolate milkshake gets a flavor and health "makeover" with the addition of berries, banana, soy sauce, and a honey-enriched balsamic topping. Once you've tried this nutrient-rich version, traditional milkshakes may never cut the mustard again.

YIELD: 2–3 servings	PREP: 25 minutes

1 cup of balsamic vinegar

2 tbsp. of raw honey

1 tbsp. of cornstarch

1 tbsp. of soy sauce

2 cups of frozen mixed berries

1 cup of chocolate ice cream

1 cup of milk

1 frozen banana

Whipped cream

1. Combine the vinegar, honey, cornstarch, and soy sauce in a nonreactive pan. Bring the mixture to a boil, whisking constantly. Reduce the heat to medium-low and simmer, stirring frequently, until thick (about 15 minutes). Set aside.

2. Put the berries, ice cream, milk, and banana in a blender. Process on low until thick and creamy.

3. Serve each shake with whipped cream and a few teaspoons of the balsamic glaze. Refrigerate the remaining glaze for up to 3 weeks.

If your whipping cream is just beginning to sour, simply whisk in ⅛ teaspoon of baking soda. It will counteract the lactic acid in the cream. Taste the cream before using it to make sure the flavor is A-OK.

KITCHEN CAPERS

A+

Ingredients

BERRIES
Promote brain health

MILK
Supports oral health

BANANA
Boosts skin health

INSTANT GRATIFICATION

Old-Time Hard Candy

If you've never tried homemade hard candy, whip up this classic treat. Combine 2 cups of sugar, ½ cup of white vinegar, and 2 tablespoons of unsalted butter in a nonreactive pan. If you like, add a few drops of flavored extract and a few drops of food coloring. Boil over medium-high heat, stirring frequently, until the liquid reaches 270°F, or until a few drops dropped into very cold water separate into hard threads. Pour onto a large greased cookie sheet and cut the still-warm candy into 1-inch squares. When they're cool enough to handle, roll each square into a ball with your hands. Let them cool completely, and store them in an airtight container at room temperature.

CRAZY CAKE

Also known as Wacky Cake, this simple dessert rose to fame in the 1940s, when wartime rationing often left bakers without standard ingredients like eggs and butter.

YIELD: 15 servings   **PREP:** 15 minutes   **BAKE:** 35–40 minutes

3 cups of unbleached all-purpose flour

2 cups of granulated sugar

⅓ cup of dark cocoa powder

2 tsp. of baking powder

1 tsp. of salt

1 tsp. of pure vanilla extract

2 tbsp. of white vinegar

¾ cup of vegetable oil

2 cups of cold water

Powdered sugar or frosting

1. Combine the dry ingredients in an ungreased 9- by 13-inch baking pan. Make three holes in the mixture, each one an inch or so in diameter.

2. Pour the vanilla into the first hole, the vinegar into the second, and the vegetable oil into the third. Pour the water evenly over the surface. Then mix with a wire whisk until blended. It's fine if it contains some small lumps.

3. Bake at 350°F for 40 minutes. Cool, then top with powdered sugar or any frosting.

Ingredients

UNBLEACHED FLOUR
Boosts metabolism

DARK COCOA POWDER
Helps relieve stress

VEGETABLE OIL
Promotes cellular health

KITCHEN CAPERS Since Crazy Cake contains no eggs, it relies on flour alone for its form and texture, so it's crucial to use a high-protein, all-purpose, unbleached flour that has more holding power than regular flour can deliver—and offers up more nutrition to boot!

CULINARY Q & A

? I have some infused balsamic vinegars, but I don't know how to use them! I have both dark and white versions, infused with chocolate, vanilla, cherry, and other fruits.

! Try using them as a flavorful, healthy boost to homemade desserts! Here are a few ideas: Add a few drops of a dark balsamic to any chocolate-based dessert, including cakes, brownies, fudge, or fondue. Use vanilla or any fruit-infused white version in lighter desserts or atop poached peaches. **Note:** *Use a light hand, especially when adding to baked goods so you don't affect the texture of the finished product.*

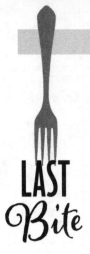

SECRETS TO SWEET SUCCESS

PERFECTIONISM PAYS OFF

When you're whipping up cakes, pies, cookies, or any other oven-generated sweet treats, success lies in the details. Here are five tips for top results:

1. Read the recipe in full before you start. Knowing ahead of time what you have to do and when you have to do it can help you avoid a culinary disaster.

2. Have all of your ingredients prepared, measured, and set out on the counter before you start working. You'll greatly reduce your risk of making a blunder.

3. Always use butter at the temperature and consistency called for in the recipe. If not, it can dramatically affect the texture of your baked goods.

4. When a recipe specifies room-temperature eggs or dairy products, obey that instruction, or the end product may not come out correctly.

5. Get—and use—an oven thermometer. Unless you have a brand-new or regularly calibrated oven, it's all but guaranteed that its temperature is somewhat inaccurate. Even if it's only a little bit off, it could ruin the dessert you've just spent a lot of time preparing—not to mention waste the ingredients.

BREAD TO THE RESCUE

What happens when cookies come out of the oven exactly the way you like them, but after you've stored them in your cookie jar for a day, they've turned dry, hard, and stale? You'll likely end up dumping them right in the trash—what a waste! But here's an easy solution: The next time you place freshly baked cookies into your cookie jar, just grab a slice of bread (any kind will do), a hoagie roll, or a hot dog bun. Tuck it in with the cookies, and close the lid. The bread will dry up any moisture, while the cookies stay moist, soft, and tender. Then you can continue to enjoy them for as long as they hold out—yum!

Baking a fruit pie can make a major mess of your oven. The simple solution: Cut four small slits into the top crust and shove a short piece of tube-shaped pasta (like ziti) into each one. The juices will bubble up the "tube" and back into the pie—instead of running into the oven. When the pie has finished baking, just pull the pasta out and toss it in the trash.

SWEET WORK FROM SOUR STUFF

In addition to being a key ingredient in some mighty tasty desserts, white vinegar can also take care of trouble with your favorite homemade treats. Here are six ways to put it to work in your kitchen:

Tone down the sweetness. Have you ever whipped up a special dessert only to have it turn out so sweet that it almost tasted like pure sugar? Well, next time, just add a teaspoon of vinegar to the recipe. It'll reduce the sweetness without changing the overall flavor or overpowering the other ingredients.

Fluff up meringue. If you beat in 1 teaspoon of vinegar for every three egg whites, then that tasty topping will be fluffier and more stable to boot!

Make flakier piecrust. Simply add 1 tablespoon of vinegar to the recipe. You'll have the best pies in town!

Bake moister cakes. One teaspoon of vinegar mixed into the other ingredients will improve the moistness and flavor of any cake—whether it's made from scratch or a boxed mix.

Make finer frosting. Mix in several drops of vinegar as you beat the icing. It'll turn out smooth, shiny, and creamy—with no sugaring. To keep boiled icing from hardening, stir in ⅓ teaspoon of vinegar as the frosting is cooking.

Firm up Jell-O®. Add in 1 teaspoon of vinegar per box of gelatin. It'll help the gelatin hold its shape even in hot weather. And it'll be easier to cut.

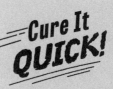

Cure It QUICK!

MAKE A MIGHTY MIX
How can a cake from a boxed mix possibly improve your health? When you beef it up with pumpkin—that's how! This famous pie ingredient also happens to score high marks in health-care circles for its ability to help keep your vision sharp, your ticker in tip-top shape, and your immune system running on all cylinders. Here's the drill: Empty a box of yellow cake mix and one 13-ounce can of pumpkin puree (not pie filling) into a bowl. With a mixer, beat the duo to get a thick batter. Pour it into a lightly greased 7- by 11- by 2-inch baking pan. Bake at 350°F until a toothpick inserted into the center comes out clean (about 28 minutes). While the cake is cooling, mix 1 ½ cups of powdered sugar, 3 tablespoons of apple cider vinegar, and ¾ teaspoon of pumpkin pie spice to form a thick but pourable glaze (add more sugar or vinegar if needed). Pour it over the still-warm cake, keeping some to serve on the side. Then dig in!

INDEX

honey mustard, 132
Honey-Vinegar Beets with
    Mushrooms, 196
measuring, 104
raw, 281
in remedy recipes, 24, 41, 337
shelf life of, 271
Summer Switchel, 324
Honeydew melon, 95, 280
Horseradish, 38, 39, 188, 290
Hot dogs, 129, 131, 238
Hot peppers. *See also* Cayenne
pepper; Jalapeño peppers
    benefits of, 49, 52, 128, 286, 301
    handling tips, 128
    Pickled Grapes with
        Rosemary & Red Pepper, 126
    Scoville scale, 181
    Ultra-Easy Hot-Pepper
        Vinegar, 22
Hot-pepper sauce, 37, 39, 114
Hot-pepper vinegar, 236
Houston, Sam, 52, 316
Hummus, 259

I

Ice cream and ices, 344, 346, 358
Ice substitutes, 303, 312
Immune boosters, 50, 119, 120,
    186, 300
Indigestion, 312
Indoles, 189
Inflammation, 256, 288
Infused vinegar
    commercial vinegar for, 11
    described, ix
    egg, 11
    flower, 24
    vs. fortified, 25
    fruit, 8, 16, 17, 328
    herbal, 12, 15
    hot-pepper, 22
    spice, 14
    tips for making, 28

tips for using, 322, 359
vegetable, 23

J

Jalapeño peppers, 142, 154, 177,
    202, 277
Jars and containers
    filling, 127
    metal lids on, 13
    number needed, 117
    sterilizing, 4, 115
    washing, 7
    wide-mouth, 9
Jell-O®, 361
Joint pain, 328, 332. *See also*
    Arthritis
Juniper berries, 292

K

Kale
    benefits of, 70, 185
    Black-Eyed Peas with Garlic
        & Kale, 185
    Kale & Kielbasa Soup, 151
    Kale & Yukon Gold Potato
        Salad, 70
    in remedy recipes, 56, 296
    salad with peaches, 71
    softening, 185
Ketchup
    benefits of, 52, 251
    Cranberry Ketchup, 130
    Healthy Homemade Ketchup, 127
    Mushroom Ketchup, 128
    tomato, 129, 130
Kidney health, 160
Kielbasa, 151
Kitchen equipment,
    deodorizing, 53, 62, 65
Kiwifruit, 288, 316

L

Leeks, 157, 302

Leftovers, freezing, 97. *See also*
    specific foods
Legumes. *See* Beans, dried;
    Black-eyed peas; Lentils
Lemons, lemon juice
    benefits of, 42, 44, 142, 156, 278
    juicing, 295, 313
    Lemon-Ginger Tonic, 322
    Lemon Roasted Chicken, 224
    substitute for, 16
    Wake-Up Call Lemon
        Marinade, 47
Lemon thyme, 51
Lentils, 73, 153
Lettuce, storing, 109, 219, 305
Libido, 258
Light cream, 162
Lime juice, 54, 95, 158, 252
Liquor, shelf life of, 271
Liver function, 74, 296, 325
Lung disease, 88
Lutein, 56, 189
Lycopene, 127, 189, 217, 280

M

Macaroni, 91
Macular degeneration (ARMD), 56
Madeira wine, 46
Malt vinegar
    benefits of, 73, 132
    described, ix
    malt vinegar–tarragon dip, 282
    Malty Mustardy Coleslaw, 73
    Merry Malt Vinegar, 7
    substitute for, 63
Malt vinegar salt, 8
Mangoes
    benefits of, 56, 136, 177
    Gingery Mango Barbecue
        Sauce, 56
    Mango Chicken Chili, 177
    Mango Chutney, 136
    Marvelous Mango Vinegar, 20
    in remedy recipe, 346